ealth

Care

y Years

Series editor: Angela Fisher

OCR
National Level 3

www.heinemann.co.uk
✓ Free online support
✓ Useful weblinks
✓ 24 hour online ordering

01865 888058

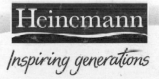
Heinemann
Inspiring generations

Heinemann is an imprint of Pearson Education Limited, a company incorporated in England and Wales, having its registered office at Edinburgh Gate, Harlow, Essex, CM20 2JE. Registered company number: 872828

www.heinemann.co.uk

Heinemann is a registered trademark of Pearson Education Limited

Text © Angela Fisher, Mary Riley, Hilary Talman, Marion Tyler

First published 2006

10 09
10 9 8 7 6 5 4 3 2

British Library Cataloguing in Publication Data is available from the British Library on request.

ISBN: 978 0 435 44977 3

Acknowledgements

Every effort has been made to contact copyright holders of material reproduced in this book. Any omissions will be rectified in subsequent printings if notice is given to the publishers.

Photo acknowledgements

Page 1: Getty Images/PhotoDisc; **page 51**: Alamy Images/Stock Connection Distribution; **page 52**: Corbis; **page 55**: Getty Images/PhotoDisc; **page 68**: Brand X Pictures; **page 77**: Corbis; **page 90**: Harcourt Education Ltd/Gareth Boden; **page 101**: Getty Images/PhotoDisc; **page 104**: Corbis; **page 113**: iStockPhoto/Silvia Cook; **page 118**: Corbis; **page 126**: Getty Images/PhotoDisc; **page 128**: Photos.com; **page 151**: Richard Smith; **page 155**: Corbis; **page 182**: Getty Images/PhotoDisc; **page 187**: Getty Images/PhotoDisc; **page 199**: Photos.com; **page 205**: Getty Images/PhotoDisc; **page 216**: iStockPhoto/Joshua Sowin; **page 242**: Corbis; **page 249**: Everyday Sport; **page 259**: Getty Images/PhotoDisc; **page 268**: Photos.com

Photo research by Susi Paz

Edited by Stephanie Richards
Index compiled by Catherine Harkness
Typeset and illustrated by Saxon Graphics Ltd, Derby
Original illustrations © Harcourt Education Limited 2006

Printed by Scotprint
Cover photo: Alamy

Websites

Please note that the examples of websites suggested in this book were up to date at the time of writing. It is essential for tutors to preview each site before using it to ensure that the URL is still accurate and the content is appropriate. We suggest that tutors bookmark useful sites and consider enabling students to access them through the school or college intranet.

Contents

Introduction

This book is designed to give support for students wishing to gain the *Level 3 OCR Nationals in Health and Social Care.* It aims to provide a guide for the teaching of the knowledge, understanding and skills that you will need to complete a course of study.

At *Level 3 OCR Nationals in Health and Social Care*, there are **four** mandatory units:

1 Working to quality practice in care settings

2 Working with service users in care settings

3 Behavioural awareness in care

4 Applied practical care in settings

These are units which **must** be covered in order to achieve the certificate award. You also need to consider which **optional** units will best help you to work towards a career of your choice. What you must remember is that you have to complete **two** optional units in order to gain the full **Certificate in Health, Social Care and Early Years at L3.** The **optional units** included in this book are:

16 Anatomy and physiology for health care

17 Health education and promotion

There are other optional units available for you to choose but they are not contained within this book. These two have been chosen as they appear to be very popular for the six-unit award.

It is very important that you complete **six** units in order to achieve the full Certificate in Health, Social Care and Early Years. For the Diploma and Extended Diploma, additional optional units will be needed, for example:

- Diploma 4 mandatory units and 8 optional units
- Extended Diploma 4 mandatory units and 14 optional units

Features of the book

Throughout the book there are a number of features that relate theory to practice in a health, social care and early years context. These are:

In this unit you will learn
A list of the knowledge that you will need to have covered.

Consider this
Points for discussion, in the form of questions that will help you to understand to apply the knowledge.

Key points
Explanations of important items of vocabulary, or concepts.

Theory into practice
Activities you can do to help practise the skills that you learn in the classroom.

Activities
Examples of questions that can be used to check that you have learned and understood the topics included in a particular section.

Case studies

Examples of 'live' situations that have been found in the world of health, social care and early years which will enable you to see how some theories are applied and, in other cases, how they are not applied.

Assessment activities

These are activities that need to be completed in order to produce the relevant material for the portfolio evidence required for assessment.

Assessment

The assessment for all portfolio units will be made by your tutor. Portfolio evidence will be graded by using the AO (Assessment objectives) and the **grading criteria**. Whether you achieve a **Pass**, **Merit** or **Distinction** will depend on how well your work matches the grading criteria. An External Visiting Moderator will visit your Centre to check that correct grades have been awarded for the work you have completed.

A range of experienced professionals have contributed their experience to this book in order to provide you with knowledge from the occupational sector that will equip you to develop your particular interest in the units.

We hope you will enjoy your *OCR Nationals in Health and Social Care* and wish you good luck and every success in achieving your qualification and in your future work or study.

Angela Fisher

Unit 1 Working to quality practice in care settings

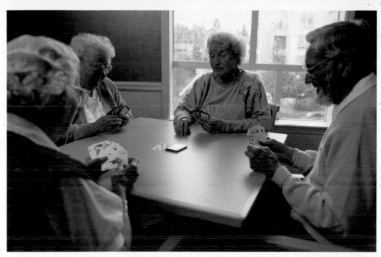

Quality practice means happy and contented service users

Introduction

What is quality practice?

The term 'quality practice' is one that is frequently used in all care settings, but you may find it difficult to break the term down into meaningful parts. What do you understand by the term 'quality practice'?

Quality practice in a care setting means upholding service users' human rights, such as the right to marry and the right to freedom from torture.

A care setting will want to make sure that all of its workers follow guidelines that maintain effective quality practice. In their day-to-day tasks, care workers will be required to show that they are able to:

- demonstrate in their behaviour that they are treating individuals as equal by using body language and oral communication to show respect and maintain dignity
- record information that is accurate and which clearly differentiates between fact and opinion. This information will be securely stored

- make sure that service users' choices are listened to and their views and beliefs are valued
- use a non-judgemental approach when working with and speaking to service users
- use systems that provide support and confidentiality and that demonstrate a willingness to help to promote service users' rights
- help service users with the complaints procedures and advocacy services if they have a need to do so.

Remember: the management and staff are responsible for setting the tone and atmosphere in a setting, and for having systems in place that provide efficient service. Good relationships with service users, relatives, other professionals and the outside world are formed when guidelines are set and followed, and quality service is maintained.

In this unit you will learn

Learning outcomes

You will learn to:

- promote service users' rights and responsibilities
- promote equality and value the diversity of service users in care settings
- maintain service users' confidentiality
- find out how a care setting is affected by legislation, codes of practice and policies and how these help to promote equal opportunities
- consider the routes of redress available to service users
- conduct a survey to find out how a care setting promotes quality practice.

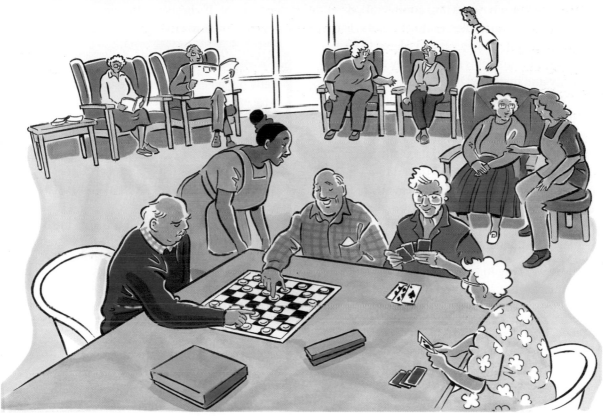

High quality services maintain service users' rights

Service users' rights

Service users' rights are no different from the rights that all human beings have. Just because a person decides to live in a residential home or goes into hospital for treatment does not mean that they have fewer rights than anyone else. Rights are broadly divided into:

- human rights
- rights that are provided by legislation.

Human rights are a set of values. They reflect the way that individuals should act towards one another. Examples of human rights include:

- the right to life
- the right to freedom from slavery
- the right to hold free elections
- the right to marry
- the right to freedom from torture
- the right to a fair and public trial
- the right to freedom of expression.

Human rights are an entitlement that everyone has, regardless of ethnic origin, gender, age or class. They promote and encourage acceptance of others. The Human Rights Act of 1998, implemented in October 2001, allows people in the United Kingdom to seek **redress** if they believe their human rights have been infringed by any public organisation.

Organisations in health, social care and early years that are affected by the Human Rights Act are:

- residential and nursing homes
- public services
- voluntary organisations
- charities.

Anyone working in a health, social care or early years setting is affected by the Human Rights Act. Any organisation that carries out a public function or carries out work in a public area will have to take human rights into consideration when planning and implementing its work. For example, a private nursery is considered to be a public area, because it is registered by the local authority and inspected by Ofsted, and it must therefore ensure that services are provided within the Human Rights Act. Similarly, any community services that are provided to allow people to remain in their own homes by providing support have to make sure they are, in their day-to-day tasks, operating within the requirements of the Act. In other words, they must ensure they do not prevent anyone from receiving what is rightfully their legal entitlement.

For those working in health, social care and early years, questions arise as a result of the Human Rights Act. Examples are given below:

- Protecting life
  - Is it right to switch off life support machines?
  - Is it right to close residential and nursing homes, resulting in reduced life expectancy?
- Degrading treatment
  - Is it right not to protect children from abuse?
  - Is it right to neglect service users in residential homes?
- Rights to liberty
  - Is it right to make a compulsory admissions order for a person to be admitted to hospital under the Mental Health Act?

Human rights prevent **social exclusion**. Factors that contribute to social exclusion are given in the table below.

All individuals have moral rights. Sometimes, maintaining human rights means imposing obligations on others. We all have to accept this in order to live alongside one another in peaceful co-existence. If rights are not accepted, people can go to court to enforce their rights.

Theory into practice

Carry out an interview to find out what factors have influenced one person's development.

Without naming the person, discuss your findings with others.

Activity

Maxine

Maxine is 76. She has lived alone since the death of her husband 20 years ago. She has become very forgetful and often wanders around the streets in the middle of the night. She sometimes lights the gas ring on her cooker and then puts an empty pan on top. It is only neighbours who smell burning who prevent a fire from breaking out.

Maxine's house is full of rubbish as she never throws anything out. The smell is quite awful. Maxine has been assessed by a psychiatrist and has not been found to be mentally ill. The neighbours are so worried that they would like Maxine to be removed from her home.

1 What rights does Maxine have?

2 What rights do Maxine's neighbours have?

3 How could the situation be best resolved?

4 With another person, write a case study showing a difficult situation relating to rights that has arisen in an early years setting.

5 Produce your questions and answers.

6 Exchange your case study with another pair and answer the questions. Discuss the answers with the other pair.

Factors contributing to social exclusion	How this will affect the individual concerned
Unemployment	Low self-esteem Only basic needs can be met
Poor housing	Likely to have increased health problems, frustration and anger
Poor education	Lack of knowledge, poor skills, less likely to obtain employment
Family break-up	Increased stress, lack of trust, unable to form good relationships with others
Low income	Lack of access to education, health services, food

Service users' rights to make decisions in consultation with others

Service users have the right to make their own decisions or at least to be involved in any decisions that concern them. All service users should be presented with options, not given solutions. Such options should be explained so that the service user has a wide range of information to consider from which they can make their decision. Whenever there are options, there are also risks. Care workers have a responsibility to present both sides of a situation so that the service user can weigh up the advantages and disadvantages.

Sometimes, it may seem hard for a service user to make a decision, and on other occasions it may seem both quicker and easier for the care worker to make the decisions for the service user, particularly if the service user has difficulty in communicating. However difficult the situation, the care worker should not make the decisions for the service user. Everything necessary must be done to ensure that the service user has their right to choose and to be consulted about the decisions that will affect them.

Service users may wish to make decisions, for example, about:

- the treatment they are hoping to have
- the activities they may wish to join
- the food they wish to eat

- the clothes they wish to wear.

Participating in decision-making can help a service user to:

- feel in control of their lives
- feel valued
- be independent
- maintain their chosen lifestyle.

Some service users may be restricted or limited in some way about the type of lifestyle they are able to have. This could be because they have chosen to live in residential care or because they have limited mobility or because they have a disability. Others may need the help of an **advocate** to help explain to them the options that are available, particularly if they have a mental disability or if they have a learning disability.

If a service user is not involved or consulted about their personal choices, their individual rights under the Human Rights Act are being **violated** under Article 3, which relates to 'the right to freedom from inhuman and degrading treatment'. By not acknowledging human rights, care workers would be denying individual rights and treating service users with a complete lack of respect.

When care workers in a setting are busy or short staffed, it is very easy to bypass the service user and not allow them their rights.

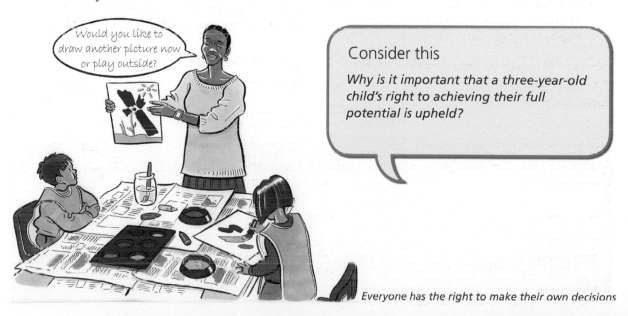

Would you like to draw another picture now or play outside?

Everyone has the right to make their own decisions

Consider this

Why is it important that a three-year-old child's right to achieving their full potential is upheld?

The table below lists other service users' rights that must be upheld.

Right to confidentiality

Confidentiality means keeping the information given to oneself, that is, not sharing it with anyone who does not 'need to know'. It means making sure personal and private information cannot be accessed by others. Any information given by the service user should not be **disclosed** without the service user's permission. Providing quality care involves keeping personal information safe. Personal information can include:

- information being discussed, e.g. care workers discussing proposed treatment with the service user
- written information, e.g. a care plan being stored safely
- electronic records, e.g. a person's medical history being stored securely, with only authorised personnel having access.

Service users' rights	How rights could be applied
To express preferences	Service users may wish to express preferences including: - the GP they will have - which services they may want - the preference for a female care worker when bathing rather than a male if they are female - what time they will go to bed.
To make choices	When options are possible, service users may wish to make choices. They can do this if they are given information about the advantages and disadvantages of each option. They may wish to make choices about: - the time they get up or go to bed - when and at what time they have a bath - what they would like to eat.
To develop their full potential	A service user can be of any age. They may be a 3-year-old attending a playgroup, an adult visiting a GP surgery or an older adult in a residential home. Whatever their ability or age, the service user should always be encouraged to meet their full potential. This can be achieved by: - having individualised action/learning plans - providing activities that are both challenging and stimulating - assisting the service user to reflect and analyse the experience.
To make complex decisions	Making difficult decisions requires: - information about what is available - discussing the options and looking at each from different perspectives - decision-making about the best solution for the situation the service user finds themselves in. Care workers must take the time to have discussions with the service user and to make sure service users have understood the information presented.
To understand, regardless of age and ability	Effective communication is essential when considering choice, consultation, difficult decisions and expressing preferences. The care worker will need to use language the service user can understand, speak at a pace that is appropriate, and use skills of clarifying and summarising to ensure all that has been said has been understood.

> **Disclosure** means passing on personal information, given by a service user in confidence and considered to be a secret between the service user and the care worker.

- intends to harm themselves
- intends to harm others
- is involved in a criminal activity.

Care workers should never make a promise not to pass on personal information. They should explain to the service user that they will not pass on personal information unless there is a very good reason to do so.

Disclosure of information can be necessary in special circumstances, for example, if a service user:

> **Consider this**
>
> *A friend of a patient demands to know what is wrong with her friend. What should the response be? Why?*

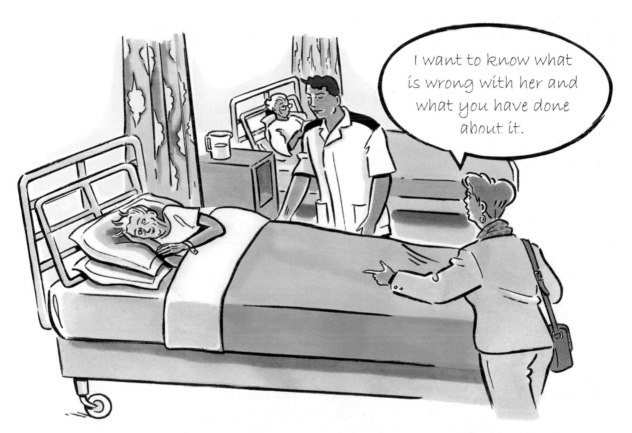

What should be the response?

Roy

Roy is 20 years of age and has learning difficulties. His parents found they could not look after him any longer and arranged for him to live at Barchester Court Residential Home. The residential home looks after people who have learning difficulties, from the age of 17 upwards.

Roy tells his mother, when she visits, that he is unhappy and that the staff are talking to others about him. They also barge into his room and tell him what he is to wear.

When he was in the kitchen on the previous day Roy found his notes lying on the side. He knew one of the other residents had read them, as he made comments about them to Roy.

1 Explain the rights Roy has while staying at Barchester Court Residential Home.

2 Explain how the staff at Barchester Court could put the situation right.

3 What does 'to keep things confidential' mean?

4 Describe the different ways that the staff at Barchester Court could keep information confidential.

Ways of supporting service users to exercise their rights

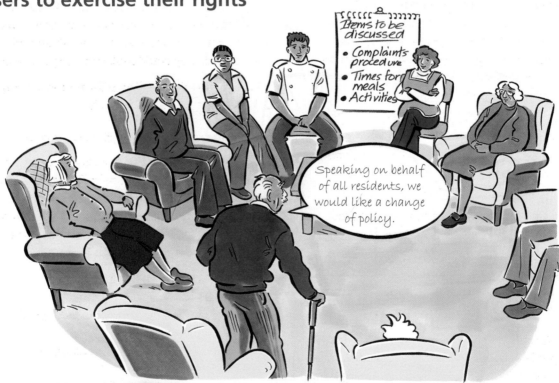

Service users should be encouraged to put forward ideas

People's voices need to be heard

Staff at any care setting should be supportive of service users. There are a number of ways in which this can be achieved, including:

- listening to service users
- giving accurate information
- giving up-to-date information
- finding out facts
- giving encouragement

- maintaining confidentiality
- providing an advocacy service.

Care workers should encourage service users to speak and to express their opinions. This can be done through:

- careful listening
- encouraging the service user to put forward opinions and ideas
- making notes to make sure ideas are not forgotten and to show the service user their thoughts are valued.

Many settings have regular committee meetings with service users, allowing a discussion of ideas and to raise matters of concern. In some settings, one or two people are voted to be on a management committee and are able to put forward the ideas and opinions of the whole group.

Even at a very young age, children are encouraged to contribute to the way a setting is run. At schools, even at primary level, school councils are formed. Representatives from each class meet to discuss ideas and to put forward the opinions of their own group.

> ### Theory into practice
>
> Try to visit a care setting to find out about how the voices of their residents are heard. Make notes to help you with building your portfolio.
>
> Discuss your findings with others in the group to see how methods at different care settings vary.
>
> You could do this while on work placement if this is part of your course.

Such meetings are not 'one-way events'. Ideas and guidance are sent back to the classroom or to the residents of residential and nursing homes as a result of the discussion. This enables everyone to have their voices heard and not to feel left out.

Up-to-date information

Providing information that is out of date will not help a service user. For example, if a service user is enquiring about the different types of treatments available, it is no use telling him or her what was available three years ago. One or more of the services could no longer be in existence! Similarly, if a service user is enquiring about early years services, information from a previous year may no longer show all that is available. Being up-to-date with information is very important.

There may also be situations where a service user may need to try out a service to see if it meets their need. They may not fully understand what is involved and observation or participation may help them to determine their choice.

Many decisions service users have to make can be quite complex. Large amounts of information should be broken down into manageable-sized portions so that a service user can understand and make decisions most appropriate to their circumstances. Not to do so means service users could feel overwhelmed. This shows a lack of respect on the part of care workers. As a result, service users are not likely to feel valued and, even worse, they could make a wrong decision.

At the centre of providing information is being able to communicate effectively.

Appropriate help and advocacy

There will be occasions when service users need someone to speak on their behalf. Care workers will need to be aware of such situations, They should be prepared and, if required, ready to act on behalf of the service user. Such occasions include when:

- a service user has a disagreement
- a problem has to be resolved
- a service user is too young to understand
- information is needed
- a service user has learning difficulties
- a service user is ill
- a legal matter has to be dealt with
- a service user is upset.

If a care worker thinks that an advocate is required, they should discuss this with their line manager and with the service user, clearly explaining why an advocate may be necessary.

Advocacy can be used to enable a service user who cannot speak out for themselves to communicate their needs and wishes to others. It is not accepted practice for care managers to act as advocates and to make decisions on behalf of service users, as they may be too close to the situation, and the service users' needs may be in conflict with the needs of the organisation.

An advocate may be a member of the service user's family, a close friend of the service user or a trained volunteer who works alongside the service user. Working alongside the service user enables the advocate to get to know the service user well and enables them to represent the service user's interests.

There are two main forms of advocacy used in care settings:

- citizen advocacy
- self-advocacy.

Citizen advocacy usually offers support to the service user so that they can communicate their wishes. The advocate can then speak on behalf of the service user.

Self-advocacy is a process where service users are trained and supported to speak out for themselves. They develop the skills necessary to speak on their own behalf and, by doing so, are involved in decisions about their own lives and also become independent.

Consider this

Why is it important that a service user who cannot speak for themselves has a person to speak on their behalf?

Tensions between rights and responsibilities

Balancing rights against responsibilities

Balancing services users' rights against their responsibilities can cause **tensions** and disagreements. Service users have a responsibility towards those who are offering the service. They also have rights. Balancing these two perspectives could at times be very difficult. For example, if a service user with a mobility problem wants to walk around the gardens of the residential home after they have eaten breakfast, but no one is available to accompany the person because the home is short-staffed, tensions could arise. The service user has the right to go for a walk around the gardens, but the care workers have a responsibility to ensure the service user is safe.

Similarly, tensions could arise if a service user wanted a late breakfast, when breakfast is only served between 8.00 and 9.00 a.m. The service user has the right to choose to have their breakfast later, but the responsibility of care workers, because of their routines, is to finish serving breakfast at 9.00 a.m. and to move on to other responsibilities.

> ## Consider this
>
> *Sonia is watching a programme on TV. Four other residents want to watch a film on another channel. How can care workers balance service users' rights against their responsibilities?*

Balancing needs against resources

Service users have a right to have their needs met. Each service user will have specific needs. Although these may appear to be the same as other people's needs, they may require different applications. Settings, such as a hospital, often have to make very serious decisions. A child may need major surgery that involves a great many specialists and support staff, the cost of which could be £1,000,000 or more. For the same money, they could do 250 hip replacement operations. Which should they do? Needs and resources have to be balanced.

On a smaller scale, a child in a reception class may have very challenging behaviour. If the teacher spends nearly all of her or his time with the child, the behaviour of this child becomes acceptable. However, the other members of the class are not having the attention they need to help them with their work. The teacher has to balance needs against the resources available. In this case the resources are human resources, i.e. herself or himself.

Sometimes, the unavailability of resources can create tensions in care settings. For example, some older people with disabilities may benefit from time in the hydro-pool. There may only be one pool, but a number of service users who would benefit from using it. Because the pool has only single occupancy and there is only one teacher, some service users may not have their needs met. Similarly, a residential home may only have one or two wheelchairs but five or six would be needed if a number of older people were taken out on a day's visit. The residential home may not be able to afford to hire additional wheelchairs, so some residents may have to be left behind. Such difficulties related to resources have to be balanced, one against the other.

> ## Consider this
>
> *A hospital has one older, seriously ill adult, who may die if they do not have a heart bypass operation which will cost £3,000. The hospital has ten service users waiting for essential lung operations caused by smoking. Without the operations, the service users' condition will deteriorate rapidly and they will be able to do very little. The hospital has to choose between doing the heart bypass operation or the lung operations. Which would you choose? Why?*

Role boundaries

Care workers are encouraged to be as **objective** as possible when working with service users and not to become emotionally attached. If working with a service user for a long period of time, an emotional attachment may form. Such a situation could be very difficult and could have the effect of 'clouding the judgement' of the care worker, so that they become **subjective** rather than objective. They may wish to care for the service user entirely on their own, being very critical of any other care worker who is trying to carry out their role. For example, a care worker responsible for distributing medication and overseeing service users taking their medication maybe very firmly carrying out their responsibilities with a reluctant service user. The care worker who has formed an emotional attachment may try to interfere or criticise the way in which the care worker who is responsible for medication is working. Such attitudes can cause tension.

> ## Consider this
>
> *Why is it important for care workers to be objective rather than subjective?*

Legal requirements and organisational needs

Legislation is intended to set standards and to help maintain the rights of service users. All health, social care and early years settings have to work within the boundaries of legislation, both in relation to staff and to service users. Some examples of legislation that apply to care settings are listed in the table below.

All settings are required under the Care Standards Act 2000 to have a complaints procedure in place. This is usually accomplished through printing a mission statement or information pack which is handed to service users. It is essential that a service user fully understands how the complaints procedure is carried out by the setting. If a service user does not know how to complain, they have no way of standing up for themselves.

Tensions between an organisation and a service user can arise because the setting has to work within the boundaries of the law, but the service user may be seeking a solution which is outside the boundaries of the law. An example is given in the following case study.

Case study

Fion

A report is received by social services from a neighbour who has stated that Fion, a 5-year-old child who lives next door, is frequently appearing with bruises and can be heard crying at night because she is apparently being left alone.

After some immediate research, the social worker pays a visit to Fion's home. During their discussions, the parents admit to hitting Fion and locking her up in her room while they go out to the pub.

They say they will not let this situation happen again.

Legislation that supports rights	Purpose
Access to Health Records	Allows service users to see medical history that relates solely to themselves
Care Standards Act	Sets standards, e.g. having a complaints procedure in place
Children Act	The **paramountcy** of the child
Data Protection Act	Relates to access and storage of records
Disability Discrimination Act	Prevents discrimination towards people with disabilities
Human Rights Act	Protection of life, freedom from torture and inhumane behaviour
NHS and Community Care Act	Allows choice about where to receive care and sets standards within settings
Mental Health Act	Provides for the rights of individuals who have mental health needs
Race Relation Act	Prevents discrimination

In the case study opposite, the social worker must act within the law. The parents are virtually requesting that the social worker ignores the law, forgets what he or she has heard and does nothing about it.

While on the one hand the parents may be willing to reform their ways, on the other hand the social worker must follow legislation as set out in the Children Act. Tensions between the service user and the social worker are apparent. The requirements of the law must be followed.

> ### Consider this
>
> *Madeline, who has severe arthritis and difficulty with mobility, wants to remain in her own home and have support to help her live as normally as possible. The occupational therapist assesses Madeline and states that she should go into a nursing home.*
>
> *What are the tensions between Madeline and the social worker? How are these best resolved?*

Tensions within individuals

Sometimes individual service users may be 'at odds with themselves'. They may be suffering from a mental illness or be confused. They may have taken offence at something that has been said or may have misunderstood a point that has been made.

Whatever the reason, the person could be:

- aggressive
- withdrawn
- isolated
- angry
- upset.

Their behaviour will mirror their feelings. Care workers need to be able to successfully calm a person. They need to establish some common interests or a mutual respect between the two parties. The care worker will need to understand the service user's point of view and to create an atmosphere of trust. This will help to meet the individual's self-esteem needs and will help to build links between the service user and the care worker.

The care worker will need to negotiate with the service user, which may take time, and give the service user the necessary facts. The service user's expectations will need to be structured by gently introducing ideas. The care worker will need to be careful not to argue, as this approach could cause the service user to become aggressive or withdrawn. A positive outcome is important when concluding negotiations. If a solution can be found, then the situation will be resolved and the service user will feel valued and have improved self-esteem.

> ### Consider this
>
> *Why might a child in a nursery school be at odds with themselves?*

Tensions between service users

There are occasions when tensions erupt between service users. This could be for a variety of reasons, for example:

- emotional distress
- using swear words
- difficulties over choosing TV programmes
- irritating behaviour
- poor personal hygiene
- aggressive behaviour.

In most cases, tensions can be resolved by care workers adopting a calm, **non-confrontational** manner. Talking calmly to a service user and listening to their side of the situation can help them to think things through and come to an amicable solution. The service user needs time to think quietly. They also need to feel that they have not been undermined and that they are valued. They should not be made to feel foolish or be ridiculed by others.

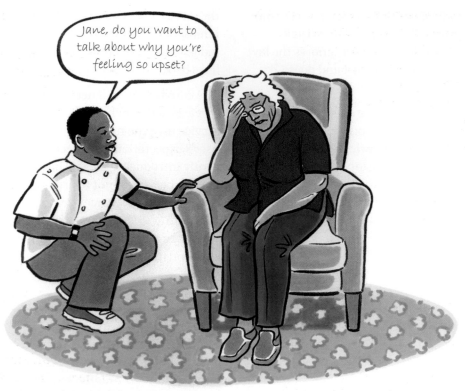

Jane, do you want to talk about why you're feeling so upset?

A care worker may need to negotiate with the service user

Case study

Joan, May and Maria

Joan was wrapping up her Christmas presents. She was being helped by May and Maria who also lived at the residential home. Several presents had been successfully wrapped by the three residents. May and Maria were talking and laughing about an incident they had seen when out on a visit. Joan was not included in their conversation.

Suddenly, Joan threw the scissors and the tape she had been using across the room and started swearing and shouting at May and Maria. Joan didn't want their help, she didn't like them and she didn't want to be anywhere near them.

Maria and May shouted back. They told Joan she was 'a stupid old fool' and that they didn't want to help her any more or even speak to her. In fact they didn't want to be in the same room as her.

May and Maria picked up their walking aids and bustled out of the room. Joan began to cry.

A care assistant hurried in to see what the fuss was about.

In this case study opposite, disagreement arose because Joan had been left out of the conversation between May and Maria. She had mistakenly thought that both were laughing at her and this made her feel foolish and unwanted. Two care workers were required to supply tea, listen and to talk to both sets of residents. Fortunately, by tea-time, friendship had been re-established! A confrontational manner would not have resolved the problem.

Sometimes, a **compromise** has to be made. It is not always possible to satisfy the rights of a service user. Listening and using effective communication skills are essential if solutions are to found. Through discussion, it may be possible to meet half way in order to resolve the issues that arise.

Consider this

How would you deal with the situation described in the case study below?

Case study

Howden Playgroup

Two parents arrived at Howden Playgroup, both seeking to see the play leader urgently. Both were very angry. One of the children had spoilt the painting of the other by knocking the painting out of the child's hand and treading all over it. The nursery nurse in charge of the painting group knew what had happened and had just told the children to 'stop being silly and not to do it again'.

The child whose picture was ruined had hit the other child. Both were crying by the time the parents met them from playgroup, and were inconsolable.

Both parents wanted the other child punished. One wanted the other child to be banned from attending the playgroup again.

Tensions between service user and the organisation

We have already discussed the service users' needs, and tensions that can arise between these and the organisation. It must be remembered that all service users have the right to:

- confidentiality
- choice
- not to be discriminated against
- practise their cultural and religious beliefs
- make a complaint
- have access to their health records
- equal and fair treatment
- protection
- safety and security
- be given clear and accurate information.

Organisations must comply with these rights. To do so, they will have in place policies and guidelines to provide a safe and secure environment for all who use their facilities. Policies for individual settings could be those that are specific to that setting or they could **originate** from a parent organisation. For example, the NHS has policies which settings such as hospitals, GP practices, health centres and clinics use as a basis for their own individual policies.

The role of any policy is to ensure that service users' rights are upheld, and staff are provided with guidelines so that the best possible care is available.

Quality practice requires not denying one service user or one service user group the same quality of opportunity or service that a different group receives. It means having in place procedures to prevent the abuse of service users and which promotes **empowerment**. In this way, service users will be as independent as possible and feel in control of their own lives.

Assessment activity 1.1 Promoting service users' rights and responsibilities

Case study A: Ida

Ida is living at Brecon Nursing Home for adults with learning difficulties. Although the ownership of Brecon has recently changed, most of the staff have remained, but two new workers are being introduced, one to the day shift and the other to the night shift.

When Ida's parents placed her in the residential home they had asked to see the policies and checked the systems that were in place to maintain quality practice. However, Ida tells her parents that she is very unhappy and wants to move out.

She says she is unhappy because:

- she has to wear other people's clothes, not her own
- she is not asked what she would like to eat; food is just put in front of her
- a strange person visited her and said he was her GP and wanted to examine her
- she is bored as she is not given anything to do all day
- when she asked about complementary approaches to health she was given a list published three years previously
- she heard some service users talking about her and other service users
- she found her notes and those of the service user whose bedroom was next door, on her chair.

Case study B: Ian

Ian is a 5-year-old boy who attends Fairway Primary School. He is in the reception class with a group of twenty-three other children of similar age. He enjoyed school when he first started but now, during his second term, he dislikes going to school. His parents have tried to find out why he feels this way. Ian tells them:

- he is bored because when he finishes his work he is given nothing to do
- he is told what he must eat for dinner and has to eat it even if he does not like it
- other children are asked which task they would prefer to do, but he is told that he has to paint
- he is told that he will have to wear a jumper from lost property as he does not have a school uniform jumper to wear

- he heard the teacher talking about him to other staff and to other parents, in front of the children in his class.

Ian's parents are quite worried about what they hear and make an appointment to speak to the teacher. At the meeting, they ask if there are any other primary schools in the area. They are given a list that was printed eight years earlier.

Activity

Choose either case study A **or** case study B. Answer the questions that follow for your chosen case study.

You have been asked to prepare a guide that will be useful to anyone wishing to use the setting you have chosen. Within the guide, you will include information about quality practice, illustrating how to promote service users' rights and responsibilities.

1. In the guide, explain in detail **three** rights that service users have. Try to give examples to illustrate the points you make.

2. In the guide, explain, giving a comprehensive account, how service users at the chosen care setting could be supported to exercise those rights.

3. What tensions might arise between service users and care workers in the case study chosen?

4. Arrange (with your tutor's permission) to visit a care setting similar to the setting in your chosen case study.

5. Prepare some questions to take with you to find out how quality care is provided and how a correct balance can be maintained when tensions do arise.

6. Trial the questions on other people to see if any adjustments are required. Make any adjustments that are necessary.

7. Visit the setting to find out about quality care and how a correct balance can be maintained when tensions do arise.

8. Write up your findings from the visit for the guide that you are producing. Make sure you give examples to illustrate the points made and explain them, making reference to theory.

Origins of discrimination

> ### Key point
>
> **Discrimination** is considering a **race**, culture or type of person to be of less value than one's own. To discriminate is to deliberately act against a group of people or to favour one group above another.

Society is made up of different types of people, each having their own traditions, beliefs and culture. Some people consider their own race or culture to be **superior** or better than others. They have a narrow view and think the beliefs and values they hold are the only correct ones to have. They are not prepared to be open to the values and beliefs of people from other cultures. Unfortunately, such people try to influence others to their way of thinking.

Historical perspective and oppression

From before the times of the slave trade, **oppression** has existed throughout the world. Oppression means committing acts which cause misery to others. History shows how the slave trade caused misery to others, with white men physically taking black people from their homes and making them work in a strange land for no reward, and not being concerned whether they were ill or died.

The importance of human life has now been accepted in the majority of countries in the world. In some countries, however, there is still an unacceptable level of aggression, where military might is used to oppress and exploit people both within their own country and outside their own country.

Most western countries have adopted **democracy**, which means they are governed,

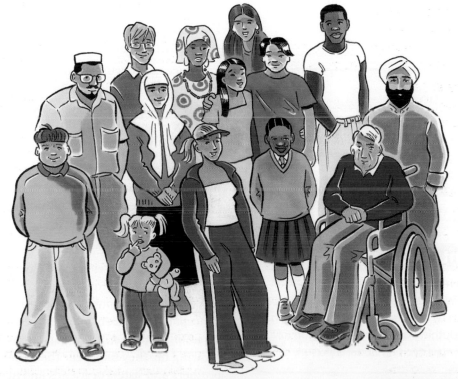

The UK is a multicultural society

both politically and economically, through the wishes of the majority of those living in their country. Democracy depends on the principle of individuals voicing their opinions, even if they are different from those who are in government.

A democratic society allows individual rights, choice and freedom. This is in line with human rights and promotes racial equality, anti-discrimination and sexual equality. Discrimination can take many forms, including:

- *racism* – being discriminated against because of the colour of your skin or your culture
- *sexism* – being discriminated against because of your gender
- *homophobia* – being discriminated against for being gay or lesbian
- *disablism* – being discriminated against because of a physical, mental or sensory impairment.

The way people are brought up and the experiences they have can influence the way they react to others. People can be discriminated against because of their class, education, the location in which they live or the income they have. Discrimination means non-acceptance of others. Care workers need to be sure that this type of behaviour is not displayed in their work.

Consider this

Why is it important for care workers to have some historical perspective of how oppression has contributed to discrimination?

Key point

Prejudice is making a decision about a person without knowing anything about them. It is judging them by a particular characteristic, e.g. their looks, clothing or accent. It usually involves making an unfair decision about a person.

Case study

Trudi

Trudi, aged 55, was working as a nurse in the accident and emergency department of a hospital. She was having a busy evening and was feeling quite tired when a service user was brought in with cuts all over his face, arms, hands and legs.

Trudi noticed the service user had ear-rings in both ears, another in his nose and another in one eyebrow. His clothes were made of leather that was well-worn and smelt badly.

Trudi's attitude was unsympathetic as she assumed he had been in a fight and had brought disaster upon himself. She made these judgements on his appearance. She was very surprised when the young man spoke. 'I can see what you're thinking, but you're wrong,' he said. 'I am not a street lout. I'm an undercover police officer and was beaten up while on duty.'

Trudi realised that she had displayed prejudice. She had allowed her own views to be clouded by the appearance of the person in front of her. This type of attitude can lead to discrimination.

Development of prejudice and discrimination

Prejudice may occur because it is an easy way to group people together and to give them a label. This form of grouping people together could have developed from a variety of sources, as shown in the illustration opposite.

Not being prejudiced means not viewing a group of people as being 'less worthy than ourselves'. Prejudice can lead to discrimination. It can cause a person to treat another with less respect and to think of them as inferior.

Assumptions and prejudicial views are learned and do not come naturally. For example, children will notice skin colour, but they will not have a concept that one skin colour is 'better' and superior to another. They learn this view. When growing up, they may hear their parents, brothers and sisters or friends and neighbours

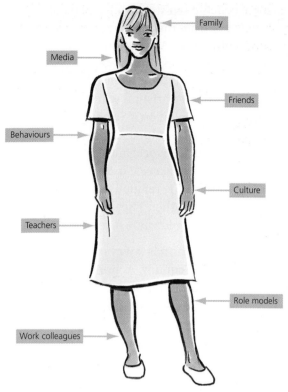

Family
Media
Friends
Behaviours
Culture
Teachers
Role models
Work colleagues

Sources of prejudice

- *gender* – e.g. subjecting women to harassment
- *age* – e.g. thinking of older people as being a burden
- *disability* – e.g. not placing any value on people who are not able-bodied.
- *sexuality* – e.g. not tolerating people with different sexual preferences.

Attitudes such as those given above demonstrate prejudice and affect working practice. For example, black and Asian people are often the target of discrimination. They are shouted at in the street, verbally threatened and sometimes prevented from being employed or from gaining deserved promotion at work.

While attitudes to women have changed since women obtained the right to vote in 1918, there are many men who still consider that a woman's place is in the home carrying out domestic and child-rearing responsibilities. It is only recently that women have begun to be promoted within large organisations, even though they have demonstrated the ability take control and be strategic planners and organisers. The 'glass ceiling' effect still exists to a certain degree.

express jokes or opinions about others that are detrimental. They may then grow up to express them as their own point of view.

Care workers need to examine carefully their attitudes, views and opinions to make sure these are not being reflected in the day-to-day tasks they perform.

> **Consider this**
>
> *How could prejudice affect the work of a teacher in a reception class?*

> **Consider this**
>
> *What do you think is meant by the term 'glass ceiling'?*

Basis of discrimination

Discrimination is centred on people's attitudes and beliefs. These attitudes and beliefs can influence their behaviour. Factors that can influence individuals to discriminate against others include:

- *race* – e.g. not tolerating people whose skin colour is different

Vulnerable people, such as those with disabilities, are often looked down upon, patronised or ignored. How often is a person in a wheelchair ignored when being taken out? A conversation is often held about them as though they were not present! Some people in society consider that because a person in a wheelchair has a bodily dysfunction, they are mentally affected as well! This is a form of discrimination.

Sexual orientation can also be the focus of discrimination. While people who are **bisexual** or **homosexual** are tolerated more sensitively in today's society, there are still those who are verbally and physically abusive towards them.

A care worker must not allow themselves to be influenced by the sexual preferences of the people they care for. Service users must be able to make their own choices about sexual orientation, whether they are able-bodied, young or disabled. Quality practice means not ignoring, neglecting or verbally harassing those whose sexual orientation is different from the care worker's own. They must be given equality of access to the care they need.

Discrimination according to age can operate at both ends of the age spectrum. There can be discrimination against children, where children have their rights withheld, because it is considered that they are not old enough to make their own decisions. At the other end of the age range, older people are often thought of as being 'past it' and have very little to contribute. It is often forgotten that older people have a great deal of experience to offer and that many are members of committees or voluntary organisations, still contributing a great deal to society.

> ### Consider this
>
> *Name three ways in which older people are discriminated against. Why do you think this happens?*

Links between prejudice and discrimination

Beliefs and actions

Values are things that people count as important. Service users from different cultures have different values. They may also have different beliefs, which could vary from the care worker's own. For example, a service user may believe in Islam, Judaism or Christianity. Being aware of the differences and day-to-day requirements of service users who have different beliefs is an important part of a care worker's role.

Personal beliefs often stem from a person's upbringing or from their experiences, although this is not always so. A person who is a follower of Judiaism will, for example, want to celebrate their holy day on a Friday, while a Muslim will not eat pork, and a Christian will want to celebrate their religion on a Sunday. A service user's belief must be valued. Care workers must ensure they value all world faiths by arranging specific activities for service users. They must not behave as though one religious belief is more important than another. They must avoid being prejudiced and should value diversity.

Anti-discrimination is a way of making sure people are treated equally. Actions that can support anti-discrimination are those that promote procedures and systems to ensure that discrimination does not, as far as is possible, occur.

Treating people equally does not mean treating everybody the same. It means treating service users in a way that ensures they have equal access to all services they need. It also means making sure service users get equal benefits from services. The aim of an anti-discrimination policy is to make sure all the population feels they are valued, regardless of their colour, belief, sexual orientation, age or disability.

Discrimination needs to be challenged. This can be done in a variety of ways, as shown in the table on the next page.

The best interests of service users must be upheld if quality practice is to be meaningful. In care settings, a number of approaches can be used to prevent discrimination, including:

- recording information
- having a complaints procedure
- providing an advocacy service
- using language that can be understood
- having recruitment policies in place
- ensuring staff development
- maintaining staff development.

How to challenge discriminatory behaviour	Action
Challenge all forms of racism	Be assertive. Ask the person what they mean by the remark(s) they have made
Speak out when unacceptable behaviour is seen	Report the discrimination to a line manager or talk to the person yourself to point out how their behaviour is discriminatory
Encourage service users to report incidence of discrimination	Make sure service users know how and to whom they should speak if they are discriminated against in any way
Keep calm	Do not shout or argue. Speak quietly and let the person know that you are not happy with what has happened

Types of discrimination

There are two main forms of discrimination. These are:

- **indirect** discrimination, e.g. only printing information in one language which could exclude a number of people from accessing it
- **direct** discrimination, e.g. talking to someone disrespectfully.

Indirect discrimination is subtle and not obvious. Sometimes it is unintentional and arises because a person has not given sufficient thought to a situation. Service users are undermined by indirect discrimination and often experience inequality even when individuals are apparently being treated the same. Indirect discrimination occurs when a condition is made for one group which is harder than for another to meet. For example, a primary school makes a rule that no

> **Consider this**
>
> *In small groups, think of three ways that indirect discrimination could be shown in a care setting.*
>
> *Share your findings with the whole group.*

Activity

Sertina

Sertina attends Dukes Nursery School. Various activities are provided for her and the other children to do. There is a dressing-up corner where clothing from different cultures is made available for the children to use. They also have a Wendy house with dolls that are Chinese, Asian, Afro-Caribbean and white European. Throughout the year, the nursery school celebrates events from different world faiths.

One morning Sertina wants to play with the cars and the train, but two of the boys also want to play with these toys. A nursery nurse tells Sertina to let the boys play with the cars and the train and she can have the doll.

1 Explain how the nursery school values the beliefs of individual service users.

2 How is the nursery school not paying attention to issues relating to gender?

3 How could the nursery school make sure that all its staff are aware of anti-discrimination issues?

4 Explain how language could be used in an anti-discriminatory way at the nursery school.

5 Explain the term 'basis of discrimination'.

headwear is to be worn inside the building. For western Europeans this would not be a problem, but for a child who is a Muslim and whose family follow the tradition of their faith, this could be difficult to accept.

Direct discrimination is where individuals are openly treated differently because of their race, colour, gender, sexual orientation, age, class or disability. Obvious unfair treatment shows prejudice and is intentional. An example of direct discrimination is excluding someone who has a different colour from joining a group. Or it could take the form of parents lobbying a nursery school trying to prevent a child who is known to have HIV from being admitted.

Effects of discrimination

Whether discrimination is direct or indirect, it can have a serious physical, emotional, intellectual and social effect on an individual, particularly if the discrimination is regular and systematic. It can lead to depression and low self-esteem, and can completely destroy a person's belief in themselves.

Abraham Maslow developed the idea of a 'hierarchy of need'. He considered that as people go through life they develop or **self-actualise**. In order to fully reach self-actualisation, the more basic needs at the bottom of the hierarchy have to be met. The diagram below shows how discrimination can affect an individual at each stage.

Repeated episodes of discrimination are likely to have an impact on an individual's physical, intellectual, emotional and social development as one can affect another. For example, if a person becomes depressed they may fail to socialise. This could negatively affect them because they will not be receiving any intellectual stimulation through conversation. Increased isolation could cause them to be 'vegetative', which means they could be sitting around a lot and could therefore put on weight. The combined effect could result in:

● tendency to illness
● mental ill health
● insecurity
● an inability to build relationships
● poor performance.

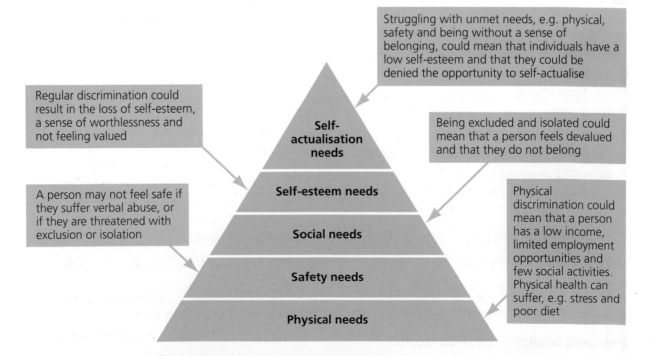

Maslow's hierarchy of need showing how discrimination can affect each stage of our development

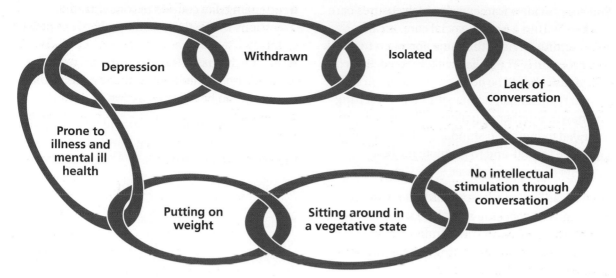

A perpetual cycle of decline

Ways of promoting equality and diversity

Care workers' own practice

Care workers need to be very much aware of their own values, but must allow service users the right to have their own values too. They must ensure they do not undermine others when their views and opinions differ from their own. This is part of empowering the service user, helping them to make their own choices and decisions. A care worker should make sure they are well informed and knowledgeable in order to avoid being prejudiced. They should have examined their own attitudes and values to make sure they know themselves well and are not unjustly judging others.

Service users who do not experience equality in the service they receive are **marginalised**, that is, they are pushed to the edge of the group or to the fringes of society. This means they are cut off from cultural, social and economic activities and do not exercise their rights. Disempowerment means they could be deprived of choice, are not consulted and lose control over the decision-making process. In practice, this could mean they fit in with the service, rather than the service fitting in with them.

Promoting equality and diversity means:
- understanding and not showing prejudice
- understanding and valuing the benefits of diversity
- understanding the basis of discrimination
- understanding one's own beliefs and not making assumptions.

> **Consider this**
>
> *How would a care worker in a residential home understand the benefits of diversity?*

Organisational practice

Good work practice promotes service users' rights. The organisation will have a set of goals or standards which all care workers should follow to provide quality care. For example, many organisations will have in place standards of behaviour relating to care workers' day-to-day relationships with service users. Such standards will provide guidance about:

- what to do when dealing with vulnerable people
- what to do if a service user wishes to make a complaint
- what to do if offered a gift by a service user
- how to record information.

Policies provide a framework which ensures care workers within a health, social care or early years setting all have the same approach to a task or a procedure. The policy will give guidelines on how a task should be done or to whom the staff should report in particular situations. A setting will have a number of policies, all of which are intended to maintain standards of care, to give guidance to staff and to promote the best interests of the service user.

If an organisation sets standards, it must have the means of checking that these standards are met. Staff development and training is one way this can be achieved. Training can take many forms. For example, it can mean:

- being supervised and receiving training while carrying out a task

- attending day courses or longer training sessions where there is input about specific topics
- having discussions with managers or supervisors to find out how the goals of the setting can be reflected in day-to-day tasks.

Policies arise from legislation and help to ensure quality practice by showing how to implement theory in day-to-day tasks.

Quality practice means making sure the setting is meeting the standards that have been set and finding out how well the setting is meeting legislation and codes of practice. It means checking that policies and procedures, staff development and recording systems are all being maintained so that service users' rights are maintained.

System or procedure monitored	What is being checked?
Complaints procedures	Is there an easy-to-use complaints procedure in place? Do staff and service users know how to follow the complaints procedure?
Recording procedure	Are records relevant, up-to-date and legible? Who has access? How are they stored? What systems are in place for updating and deleting records?
Staff appointment procedures	Is there a range of ages and people from different cultures on the appointments panel? Are questions asked without discrimination/without bias?
Health and safety procedures	Are there named staff for first aid and health and safety? Is there guidance about the frequency of safety surveys/audits? Are policies in place for dealing with emergencies?
Staff development and training	How frequently is formal training carried out? What individual needs do staff have? What are the needs for group training? How are staff being assessed? What needs are being noted from the results of assessment?
Communication procedures	Is communication with service users appropriate? Are there clear lines of communication between management and staff, and between management and service users?
Supervision of staff	Is there a policy in place relating to staff supervision? Is the policy being implemented? Are any changes needed to the policy?
Equality and diversity policies	Is there a policy in place to ensure that equality and diversity exist? How is it being implemented? Have any complaints been registered? Have they been dealt with? How?

To carry out such checking, settings need to **monitor** their systems. For quality practice, the table opposite shows examples of some of the monitoring that takes place within an organisation.

The performance of a setting is also monitored by an independent person. Inspections can be carried out by:

- the National Care Standards Commission, who inspect nursing and residential homes
- the Social Services Inspectorate, who inspect the services provided by social services
- Ofsted, who inspect early years establishments.

Such external audits are compulsory.

Formal and informal structures

Formal structures are those that arise as a result of legislation. These include:

- policies
- codes of practice
- regulations.

These will be examined later in the unit.

Informal structures could include:

- meetings with residents
- chats with small groups and individuals
- representatives collecting the views of others to put forward at a formal meeting, e.g. school council meetings or formal committee meetings.

These have been discussed earlier in this unit.

Assessment activity 1.2

Promoting equality and valuing diversity

Case study A: Ida

Ida is living at Brecon Nursing Home for adults with learning difficulties. She is very unhappy because she feels she is being discriminated against.

Case study B: Ian

Ian is a 5-year-old boy who attends Fairway Primary School. He and his parents feel that they have been discriminated against.

Activity

Choose case study A **or** B (see Assessment activity 1.1):

1 Produce a handout, leaflet or other material that could be used by staff at your chosen setting to explain the origins of discrimination. Remember to include the historical perspective, the results of oppression and the development of discrimination and prejudice.

2 Produce materials that could be used in a training session to explain to staff at the setting:
   - the types of discrimination
   - the effects of discrimination
   - how a care worker's own prejudice and beliefs could influence their work.

3 Produce information for the guide you started in Assessment activity 1.1 to explain in detail to the staff at the setting how to promote equality and diversity of service users. Try to include reasoned judgements in your explanation.

4 Show how your chosen care setting could, through organisational practice, have formal and informal structures in place to promote equality and diversity. Give examples to illustrate the points you make and try to make connections between theory and practice.

Key point

Confidentiality comes from the word 'confide' which means to tell someone you trust, secret information they will not pass on.

Confidentiality is keeping personal information to oneself and not sharing it with others unless it is on a 'need to know' basis. Confidentiality is based on trust between the care worker and the service user. The service user must feel confident they are able to talk to the care worker without the information being passed on. A care worker will have access to information which is both sensitive and personal.

There may be times when care workers face **dilemmas** about respecting confidentiality. For example, if a care worker is told that the service user is thinking of harming themselves, this must be shared with the appropriate named person in case the service user does inflict harm on themselves. Any information held about the service user is, however, protected by law.

Legislation

Data Protection Act

There are eight main principles to the Data Protection Act which apply to paper and computer records. These principles guide the way health, social care and early years services deal

Principle of Data Protection Act	How legislation is applied in care settings
Personal data must be obtained and processed fairly and lawfully	Service users should know about all records kept and be told why they are being kept.. Service users must be told with whom information will be shared and why, and asked to give their permission. The service user must be told of their rights to access the information.
Personal data must be held only for one specified and lawful purpose	There must be a lawful purpose to hold the data on individuals, for example, to provide, monitor and review services.
Personal data must be relevant, adequate and not excessive	Organisations should only keep information they need to provide services, nothing more, nothing less.
Personal data shall be accurate and kept up-to-date	Before recording the facts, they should be checked. Service users' records should be reviewed regularly to make sure all the information is correct. Changes to service users' circumstances must be recorded.
Personal data must not be kept for longer than is necessary	There must be a disposal date for records. The setting must destroy the records when that date is due. Adoption records and records of those who have committed offences may be kept for 100 years.
Personal data must be processed in accordance with rights of data subjects	All individuals have the right to access their data and rights as to when data can be passed on and to whom. They have control over their data.
Personal data must be kept secure from unauthorised access, alteration or disclosure, loss or destruction	Paper records must be stored safely. A system for the removal and return of files must be in place. Records kept on a computer must only be accessed by those authorised to do so, using a password. Computerised records should be backed up regularly.
Personal data should not be transferred to a country outside the European Economic Area	Only if the country agrees to an adequate protection system can records be transferred. This could apply when the NHS arranges with another country, e.g. France, to provide operations for UK residents.

with information they hold about service users. Staff in all care settings therefore need to be aware of the responsibilities that the Act places on them.

The legislation makes it necessary for every care setting to have a nominated member of staff who will act as 'controller of data'. All care staff must follow the principles of the Data Protection Act.

Activity

Data Protection

1 Carry out secondary research (see Qualitative data, p 272) and explain when a person would not have control of their data.

2 Invite a care manager or supervisor of a care setting to your centre (with your tutor's permission) to find out how confidential information is managed at their setting.

3 For each of the eight main principles of the Data Protection Act, describe what would happen in the care setting.

Access to Personal Files Act

The Access to Personal Files Act 1987 and the Access to Personal Files (Social Services) Regulations 1989 give people the right to access material held by authorities, recorded about themselves, after 1 April 1989.

The Access to Personal Files Act states that social services should let service users see information about themselves unless there is good reason for not doing so. This is similar to the Data Protection Act, which allows service users to have access to any personal details. However, information about other people must be removed before a service user has access to the records.

Access to Medical Records Act

This Act gives service users the right to have access to health information written about them after November 1991. This covers all written records and not computer records, which are already accessible as a result of the modifications made under Section 21 of the Data Protection Act.

The service user must make a direct request to the service provider, for example, at an outpatient consultation, otherwise requests should be made in writing. Written requests are usually dealt with by an administrator who will have to get permission from the service provider before any information can be released. A charge can be made for giving this information to the service user.

Information held in medical records will only be available to other people if the service user gives their consent. This is usually a signed consent form.

Case study

Harry

Harry, who is 55 years of age, has moderate learning difficulties and lives in a small residential home in the community.

While being helped to get ready for bed, Harry tells a care worker that some of his medals have been stolen. Harry appears to be very concerned about this and repeats his concerns several times. The care worker tells him, 'Not to worry, I expect you are mistaken. Just settle down and forget all about it.'

Harry then hands a file over to the care worker. The file contains all the personal records for Bobby Cairnes, whose room is next door. Harry tells the care worker that the file had been left on his bed.

1 Name a piece of legislation that requires the care worker to take action about the complaint Harry has made.

2 Explain what the care worker should have done when Harry told him about his missing medals.

3 Explain which pieces of legislation apply to the security of paper-based personal records.

4 Explain what should happen to maintain the security of paper-based records at the care setting.

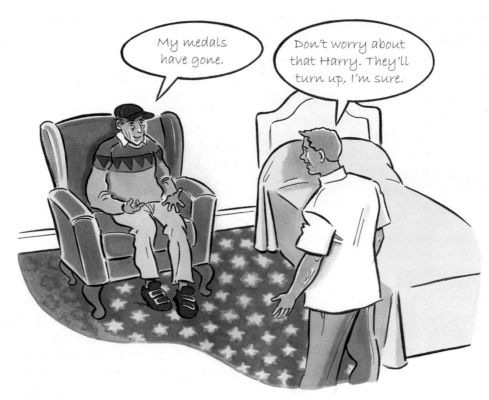

Speech bubbles: "My medals have gone." / "Don't worry about that Harry. They'll turn up, I'm sure."

Ignoring Harry's complaint is not acceptable behaviour

Organisational requirements

Policies

Policies arise out of legislation. They provide a framework which ensures that care workers within a health, social care or early years setting, or across a number of settings, all have the same approach to a task or procedure. The content of a policy will give guidelines on how a task should be done or to whom staff should report in the case of a particular occurrence. An organisation could have a number of policies, all of which are intended to maintain standards of care, to give guidance to staff and promote the best interests of the service user. Examples of policies include those covering:

- confidentiality
- moving and handling
- access to records
- health and safety
- complaints
- recruitment
- equal opportunities
- communication.

Policies are usually kept in a folder and placed in the staff rest area or lounge. A copy will be kept in the manager's office. Service users will probably be given a copy in the form of a Mission Statement when they use or are admitted to a setting.

> **Confidentiality policy**
>
> The controller of all confidential information is Mrs F ...
>
> Two care workers, AB and CH, will hold the password to computer data ...

Procedures in organisations

A procedure sets out exactly what a care worker must do in a particular situation or in relation to particular task. For example, if a person makes a complaint, what must a care worker do? The procedure gives instructions as to exactly what steps to take.

Recording information

Information should only be recorded when it is necessary for the organisation to carry out its duties and responsibilities. A care worker must decide which information is fact and which is opinion, and only the facts should be recorded about service users. The Data Protection Act gives very clear instructions about what can be recorded, how it should be recorded, and what should be recorded relating to a particular individual. All information must be:

- **legible**
- accurate
- up-to-date.

It is important to make sure that information is correct, as incorrect information could lead to a person receiving the wrong treatment. Also, records can be used as evidence in a court of law, a **tribunal** or a formal enquiry. Being able to communicate effectively, through accurate record-keeping, is a basic part of good practice that all care workers should maintain. Records can include those listed in the table below.

Records	Examples
Written	Letters, memos, assessments, reports, messages, policies, procedures, review documents
Electronic	e-mails, internet information, networking information

Care workers need to be clear about the purpose of records. That is, they need to think about:

- who will be reading the records
- what they are to be used for
- what the care worker hopes they will achieve.

Care must be taken not to include:

- too much information, e.g. do not include padding
- too little information, e.g. do not be too brief.

When completing records, it should always be remembered that service users can access it and ill-feeling can arise if there are inaccuracies or if points have been made that are insensitive or judgemental.

Storage and security

Storage of information can be:

- **manual**, e.g. using a filing system/cabinet
- electronic, e.g. using a computer.

All records of service users must be protected. Access to information must be controlled to prevent unauthorised people from seeing it. Records kept manually should be placed in a locked room, with access limited to certain nominated people. The records themselves should be stored in locked filing cabinets within the room, to make doubly sure that they are protected. Many large organisations set a time when records can be accessed, after which the protected area is locked and access is only available if an emergency arises. Most care settings will have a clear policy relating to the storage of records. Part of a Control of Records Policy for a residential home is given on the next page.

Records held on a computer are likely to require each person who wishes to access information to have an identity number to enable them to do so. Each person is given a password and this prevents unauthorised people from gaining entry to personal information. It is possible that some care workers will be **restricted** or limited to particular information on the computer. For example, care workers involved in providing personal care would not need to have access to financial aspects of the care setting.

A large organisation, such as a Trust hospital, may have a system known as 'ownership' of information or data. All information coming into the organisation is given an 'owner' or person who is responsible for the storage and security of

Control of records

1 Each set of records will be maintained in a secure location within the home's administration offices, and in such a manner as to prevent deterioration or spoilage. Records will be collated and filed in an orderly fashion and indexed so as to be easily retrievable.

2 A Quality Records Log will be maintained which will identify the following for each set of records, taking into account statutory requirements as applicable:
   2.1 Location of storage
   2.2 Disk references, where records are stored on computer
   2.3 Length of time records are kept
   2.4 Responsibilities for maintenance and control
   2.5 Staff who are authorised to have access to individual sets of records.

3 Records will be kept in accordance with Data Protection legislation.

the information they hold. People who have such responsibility have to:

- keep a record of all the information they hold
- explain to others how the information can be used
- agree, with the person responsible, who can access the information
- agree what type of access is permitted for each user.

Activity

Organisational requirements

1 Explain how a policy helps to maintain quality practice. Use examples to illustrate the points made.

2 What is meant by the term 'control of records'? Explain how this would be applied in a care setting of your choice.

3 Explain how data kept electronically on a computer can be protected in a day care centre.

4 Why must service users' personal information be kept confidential?

5 Design a leaflet or handout or other material to explain to staff at a day care centre how records should be stored.

Care workers' responsibilities when handling confidential information

Who might see or hear the information?

Disclosing personal information in a situation where others can see or hear it is not acceptable. Care workers should not speak about service users where others can hear and they should not leave notes where others can read them. Care workers have the responsibility to ensure that information is not disclosed, unless on a 'need to know' basis, and should remember:

- not to talk about people by name in public places, so that they cannot be identified
- to move to a room where a door can be closed if they wish to share information
- not to discuss the care of others with service users
- to use initials in written reports
- not to leave written records where other people can read them.

A service user's file should be returned immediately to the secure area as soon as it has been finished with.

Who might have access to the information?

Even though every service user's information has to be kept confidential, there is no such thing as 'complete' confidentiality. This is because information about service users has to be shared among other care workers within a setting or with care workers in other settings, if the service user is using more than one service. Service users' relatives must not be given information unless the service user has given permission.

Care workers must follow the policy and procedures of the care setting to ensure service users' information is kept confidential. Care workers can also provide support by:

- ensuring service users know and understand how confidentiality will be maintained
- ensuring service users know that their permission will be required before information can be passed on

- making sure they follow all policies and procedures relating to confidentiality
- being aware of the requirements of legislation, e.g. the Data Protection Act.

Disclosure of information

Care workers should never make a promise not to pass on personal information. They should explain to the service user that they will not pass on personal information unless there is a very good reason for doing so.

Proof of identity

Before exchanging information with another worker, it may be necessary to have proof of the identity of the other person. Many care workers have official badges which are easily recognisable, so identification is not a problem. If you are at all unsure, information should not be exchanged.

Support available

Support from colleagues

It often helps to talk things over with colleagues when in doubt about the best course of action to take. This does not mean talking about the actual problem or issue, if it is confidential, but to explore all the possibilities available. Talking and sharing often helps to find a solution. A colleague may have had experience of a similar problem or issue and would be able to explain what happened as a result.

Support from line managers

A line manager will be familiar with legislation, policies and procedures within the care setting. If a care worker has a concern, they should share that concern with the line manager as soon as possible. The line manager will provide advice and guidance, but if the issue is major the line manager may prefer to deal with it themselves.

> ## Consider this
>
> *Think of a situation in a hospital when disclosure may be necessary.*

Assessment activity 1.3

Service users' rights to confidentiality

Case study A: Ida

Ida is living in Brecon Nursing Home. Ida feels that confidentially has not been maintained in the home as notes have been left lying around and care workers have been heard talking about service users to other service users and to staff.

Case study B: Ian

Ian is a 5-year-old boy who attends Fairway Primary School. He and his parents feel that confidentiality has not been maintained at the school because notes about Ian's history have been left lying about where other children and parents could read them, and teachers and children have talked about Ian in front of other parents and the children in the class.

Activity

Choose case study A **or** case study B.

1 Produce a leaflet or a handout to give a detailed and accurate definition of confidentiality.

2 Explain how legislation and policies relating to confidentiality will affect the care setting chosen.

3 Arrange to visit a care setting (with your tutor's permission) or arrange for a representative from a care setting to visit your centre, to find out how good practice relating to confidentiality is maintained in care settings. Prepare some questions in preparation for this visit.

4 Using different sources of information, explain how the care setting could maintain good practice when dealing with confidentiality.

5 Produce a handout or a leaflet or other material to explain to the staff what is meant by 'disclosure'. Give examples to illustrate the points made.

6 Give a presentation, including presenter's notes, or use other methods, to explain to the staff how colleagues and line managers can provide support. Use different sources of information, making your presentation as detailed as possible.

Laws are made by those in government. They must be understood and implemented by care settings, care workers and service users within the settings. The purpose of laws is to:

- promote standards and quality
- inform individuals and organisations about standards that must be in place
- inform individuals on rights and freedoms.

Key features of legislation
Key features relating to race

The Race Relations Act 1976 makes discrimination on the grounds of race, either direct or indirect, illegal.

> **Key point**
>
> **Race** relates to colour of skin, place of origin, nationality, or ethnicity.

The Act includes discrimination that occurs in:

- housing
- education
- employment
- public and private clubs
- entertainment
- the provision of goods and services.

Care settings are affected by this legislation as they fall within the boundaries of 'goods and services'.

Victimisation is also illegal under this Act as it is unlawful to treat someone differently because they have made a complaint about discrimination.

The Race Relations Amendment Act 2000 (which does not replace the Race Relations Act) extends the legislation previously passed and requires public authorities to provide 'fair and accessible services and to improve opportunities in employment'.

All those who provide health, social care and early years services are affected by the Act. The NHS, for example, is affected as it has a general, statutory duty to eliminate unlawful racial discrimination and to promote equality of opportunity and good relations between individuals from different racial groups. To treat a service user or a member of staff less favourably than another is unlawful. The NHS has produced a good practice guide called *Improving Working Lives* which focuses on the actions required to tackle racial harassment at work. Within the document, under 'A Case for Action', guidance and help is given on topics such as:

- recruitment and retention of black and minority ethnic staff
- clinical governance
- using people's talents to the full
- avoiding litigation costs.

Examples of how the Act would be applied in settings are given in the table below.

Discrimination in a setting	Action in a setting
Language	Not allowing a service user to speak their first or preferred language when they receive visitors from the same race
Naming a person	Calling a service user by a name that is not their own because it is easier to pronounce
Employment	Not employing a person because of the colour of their skin
Harassment	Not recording incidents of harassment between: • service users and staff • service users • members of staff

Consider this

What is harassment? Give examples.

Consider this

How could racial discrimination manifest itself in the reception class of a primary school?

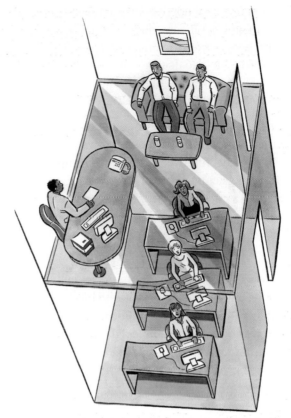

The glass ceiling effect

Key features relating to gender

The Sex Discrimination Act 1975, revised in 1996, applies equally to men and women. It makes it illegal to discriminate according to gender in areas of recruitment, selection, promotion and training. It is also unlawful to discriminate because a person is married. The Act covers:

- direct discrimination – where one person is treated differently because of their sex
- indirect discrimination – where conditions are applied to a situation which favours one sex over the other
- victimisation – where a person is treated less favourably because they have complained about sex discrimination in the past.

Many women work in low-paid jobs such as care assistants, domestic workers or kitchen assistants. Barriers such as prejudice, attitudes and lack of rights often prevent women from gaining promotion to senior positions. This is known as 'the glass ceiling effect'. Women can see the top jobs, are often qualified and have the skills to do the top jobs, but can be prevented from accessing them because of outdated attitudes relating to child-rearing and domestic chores.

The Sex Discrimination Act does not change these attitudes, but it does provide rights for women. It also prevents women from being the subject of jokes that are biased against them, and from sexual harassment.

Consider this

What do you think is the effect of the 'glass ceiling' on women?

The Sex Discrimination Act set up the Equal Opportunities Commission to promote equal opportunities for men and women.

Key features relating to disability

The Disability Discrimination Acts (1976, 1995, 1998) are concerned with preventing discrimination against people with disabilities. They cover housing, transport, employment, access to education, and obtaining goods and services. The original Act is constantly in the process of being reviewed and improved, especially in the area of public transportation. Many of the provisions relating to employment of disabled persons came into force on 1 December 1998.

The Act does not apply to prison officers, fire fighters, police officers, members of the armed forces, people working on ships, aircraft and hovercrafts. It also does not apply to employees working wholly or mainly abroad or to organisations who employ fewer than 15 people.

The Act does apply to permanent, temporary and contract workers, as well as full-time employees. It covers any employees or potential employees with a 'physical or mental impairment', which has long-term effects on their ability to carry out day-to-day tasks. It also covers people who have had a disability in the past. The 'long-term effect' is taken to be at least 12 months.

Employers must not discriminate against an employee with a disability or who has had a disability in the past (whether they are actually employed or could be employed in the future). This includes ensuring that the interview and selection process, the practices and rules of the company and the premises of the employer do not put a disabled person at a disadvantage compared with a person without a disability. This also includes promotion opportunities, training, pensions and other benefits.

The 1975 Disability Act made it unlawful to discriminate between men and women. In other words, women must not be treated less favourably than men. The Act makes it unlawful to discriminate on the grounds of marital status for either sex.

> ## Consider this
> *Why should it be unlawful to discriminate between men and women?*

Other responsibilities an employer has to a disabled employee include:

- providing supervision
- modifying instructions or reference manuals so that they are, for example, in large print or Braille

- allowing absences from work/rehabilitation related to an employee's disability
- modifying or purchasing new equipment to meet a disabled employee's needs.

Any adjustments must be reasonable, bearing in mind the cost to the employer, the disruption it will cause and the effectiveness it will have in removing or preventing any disadvantage to the disabled employee.

Any employees who believe that they have been the subject of discrimination can apply to an Employment Tribunal within three months of the date of the discrimination. The Employment Tribunal can:

- make a declaration about the rights of the disabled employee
- order the employer to pay compensation to the disabled employee
- recommend that the employer take reasonable action within a certain period of time to prevent or reduce any disadvantage to the disabled person or to make reasonable adjustments.

As from 1 October 1999, Part 3 of the Discrimination Act came into force. Amongst other things, this part of the Act relates to adjustments service providers have to make to ensure access by disabled people to their services. This includes, for example, providing poor-sighted people with information in large print, Braille or tape, providing hard-of-hearing people with written information or providing wheelchair access and allowing guide dogs onto premises.

Key features relating to equal pay

The Equal Pay Act of 1970 works with the Sex Discrimination Act in that it states that all people who carry out equal work should receive the same pay. For example, a care assistant in a residential home who is doing exactly the same job as another should not receive different pay.

In 1983 the Equal Pay Amendment Act was brought into being to ensure that the Equal Pay Act met European Community law.

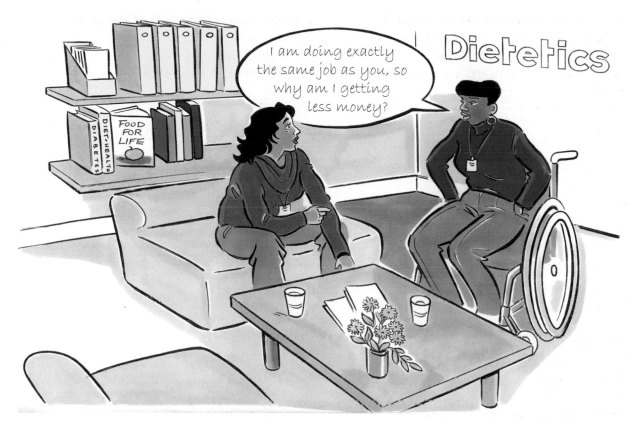

The Equal Pay Act states that all people who carry out equal work should receive the same pay

Activity

Thembelihe

Thembelihe is African-Caribbean. She works in a hospital as a nurse. She enjoys her job but recently she has been upset as one of the male nurses keeps following her about, making jokes about women. On several occasions, he has touched her in inappropriate places, but afterwards he says it was an accident as he was not looking where he was going.

1 Explain which Act could help Thembelihe in this situation.

2 What actions should Thembelihe take? Why?

3 Thembelihe's friend, Patience, also works in the hospital. She has a disability but is a dietician. When talking to another dietician who is doing the same work, Patience discovers that she is earning less. Explain which Act would help Patience. How would it help?

4 Prepare a presentation (with presenter's notes) to explain to care workers in a residential home:
   ● the Sex Discrimination Act
   ● the Disability Discrimination Act.

Key features relating to children

The Children Act 1989 requires local authority social services departments to provide services and support for children and young people and their families, including disabled children. The Act covers children and young people under 18. Key features of the legislation are:

● it aims to protect children who are at risk – the paramountcy principal
● children have the right to be heard

- children's wishes have to be taken into consideration
- support should be provided to keep families together, where this is possible.

The services provided under the Children Act 1989 can include:

- social work
- help with housing and support
- equipment and adaptations
- occupational therapists or other specialists
- short-term breaks
- counselling
- interpreters
- an advocate or representative for individuals or families
- benefits advice.

Under the Act, the County Court has the ability to protect a child by making him or her a ward of court and placing him or her under the protection of the court and the Official Solicitor. The Court also has the ability to make orders that can remove a child from a home, or other protective action.

The Children (Scotland) Act 1995 and the Children (Northern Ireland) Order 1995 have similar provisions for children's services in Scotland and Northern Ireland.

Key features relating to human rights

The subject of human rights has been dealt with early on in this unit. Below is a summary of the Human Rights Act 2000.

Countries who have signed up to the UN Convention on Human Rights must secure the above rights for everyone in their jurisdiction, and individuals must also have an effective remedy to protect those rights in the country's courts without the need to go to the European Court of Human Rights. The role of the European Court of Human Rights is to determine whether the domestic courts have been true to the Convention.

All national courts and tribunals must take into account the case law of the European Court of Human Rights. The Human Rights Act covers England, Wales, Scotland and Northern Ireland.

Key point

Summary of rights under the Human Rights Act 2000

The right to:

- life (Article 2)
- protection from torture and inhuman or degrading treatment or punishment (Article 3)
- protection from slavery and forced or compulsory labour (Article 4)
- liberty and security of person (Article 5)
- a fair trial (Article 6)
- protection from retrospective criminal offences (Article 7)
- protection of private and family life (Article 8)
- freedom of thought, conscience and religion (Article 9)
- freedom of expression (Article 10)
- freedom of association and assembly (Article 11)
- marry and found a family (Article 12)
- freedom from discrimination (Article 13)
- property (Article 1 of the First Protocol)
- education (Article 2 of the First Protocol)
- free and fair elections (Article 3 of the First Protocol)
- the abolition of the death penalty in peacetime (Sixth Protocol)

Codes of practice

Codes of practice set out the standards of professional practice required from care workers. Codes of practice contribute to the standard of care provided because they can be monitored, by observation, to check whether they are being implemented. Codes of practice set out procedures that are to be followed by professional care workers when carrying out their day-to-day tasks. Some apply to specific settings, while others affect how individuals work when working across a number of settings. The table below shows how the Nursing and Midwifery Council code of practice is applicable to health care, and its main function.

Home Life: a Code of Practice for Residential Care was first published in 1984. Some of its recommendations include the quality care checked by inspectors, such as:

- staff qualities should include responsiveness to, and respect for, the needs of individuals
- staff should have the ability to give competent and tactful care, while enabling residents to retain dignity and self-determination
- when selecting staff, at least two references should be taken up
- an applicant's curriculum vitae should be checked and all convictions should be disclosed
- changes in duties should be made clear
- minimum staff cover should be designed to cope with residents' needs at any time
- in small homes where staff carry out a range of responsibilities, these must be understood by staff.

Code of practice	Main function
Nursing and Midwifery Council	Recently formed, the code of practice states that registered nurses and midwives should: • respect all service users as individuals • obtain consent before giving treatment • protect confidential information • co-operate with others in a team • maintain professional knowledge and competence • be trustworthy • act to identify and minimise risks to service users.

Code of practice	Main function
Equal Opportunities Commission (EOC)	The EOC has published a code of practice which removes all instances of sexual discrimination. An equal opportunities policy can be developed by an organisation or setting and should include: • the statement • the implementation plan • the monitoring policy • the evaluation of the policy • targets.
Special Educational Needs (SEN)	Primary and secondary schools follow the guidelines given within this code of practice. It is also recommended for use in health, social service or any other service concerned with the education of children with SEN. Actual policies and procedures recommend: • early identification • mainstream provision, if possible • LEAs to make multi-disciplinary assessment • annual review of the child's assessment • the child's view to be considered

The table above gives two examples of other codes of practice that exist in health, social care and early years settings.

The Mental Health for Social Workers code of practice, published in March 1999 by the Department of Health, gives guidance to registered practitioners, managers and staff at hospitals and mental nursing homes, and to approved social workers, on how they should proceed when carrying out duties under the Act. The guidance includes giving service users:

● recognition of their basic human rights
● respect for their qualities, abilities and diverse backgrounds
● assurance that account will be taken of their age, gender, sexual orientation, social, ethnic, cultural and religious background, and that general assumptions will not be made on the basis of any one of these characteristics
● any necessary treatment and care in the least controlled and segregated facilities compatible with ensuring their own health and safety or the safety of others.

Organisational policies

Policies exist in all settings. Their purpose is to provide a detailed account of the approach the

Activity

Codes of practice

1 Work in pairs to carry out some research about one of the following:
   ● Equal Opportunities Commission code of practice
   ● Special Educational Needs code of practice
   ● Mental Health for Social Workers code of practice.

2 Arrange to visit a setting (with your tutor's permission) to find out how the code of practice you have investigated is applied in the care setting. Alternatively, a care worker could be invited to your centre.

3 On your own, prepare a presentation (with presenter's notes) to show others:
   ● the content of the code of practice
   ● how it is applied in the setting.

setting will take towards a particular procedure or issue. Policies are specific to each care setting. Policies that may exist in a setting include those relating to:

● complaints
● health and safety

- first aid
- recruitment
- equal opportunities
- staff training
- assessment.

Policies are developed to make sure that standards are maintained and that service users' rights are upheld.

Complaints policy

A complaints policy gives details of the procedures that should be followed if a complaint is made. The policy will show:

- who has responsibility to deal with the complaint
- how a complaint should be made
- how an outcome is to be achieved.

Health and safety policy

Employers who have more than five employees must have a health and safety policy. In a care setting, health and safety policies should cover:

- infection control
- correct lifting techniques
- standards of hygiene
- cleanliness in food preparation areas
- safe disposal of clinical waste
- heating, lighting and ventilation
- cleaning processes
- observations and measurements.

Equal opportunities policy

Equal opportunities policies have been discussed earlier but, to remind you, such a policy should include:

- the service provider's position relating to equal opportunities
- clear definitions of unfair discrimination, victimisation and harassment
- details of the procedures to be followed when service providers have been subjected to discrimination
- who is responsible for implementing the policy.

Mission statements

Mission statements are used by service providers and organisations to highlight their aims. A mission statement can be used:

- as a starting point for expressing the vision, beliefs, intentions and practices to which the service provider is committed
- to articulate the values which the organisation seeks to uphold
- as a reminder to all who work in the setting of their ultimate goals
- as a way in which the organisation can be judged in meeting quality practice.

Mission statements are usually included as an introduction in promotional documentation for the setting and are often displayed in the foyer so that they are immediately visible. Part of a mission statement for a residential home is given below.

> ### Policy 10: Mission Statement
>
> It is the objective of Barchester Court to provide care to all service users to a standard of excellence which embraces fundamental principles of good care practice, and this may be witnessed and evaluated through the practice, conduct and control of quality care in the home. It is a fundamental ethos that those service users who live in the home should be able to do so in accordance with the home's 'Statement of Values', reference Policy 12.
>
> It is the objective of the home that service users should live in a clean, comfortable and safe environment, and be treated with respect and sensitivity to their individual needs and abilities. Staff will be responsive to the individual needs of service users and will provide the appropriate degree of care to assure the highest possible equality of life within the home.
>
> To meet these clients' needs, the care home ...

How legislation and policies are applied to care settings

Legislation relating to equality of opportunity and equal rights has to be applied in all care settings. The regulations are incorporated into various types of documents which are used by care settings to make sure the care provided meets the required standards. Service users, care workers and care managers all need to know about documents such as:

- codes of practice
- policies
- citizen's charter
- government charters
- codes of conduct.

Each of the documents imposes responsibilities on service providers and care workers. If anyone fails to implement the requirements, they can face prosecution or sanctions may be imposed, such as fines or even being closed down, if it is the setting that is at fault.

Care workers should ensure that they know, for example, what legislation, policies and charters are applicable to their setting by examining, reading and seeking advice from care managers or supervisors at the beginning of their employment. They should also ensure that they keep their knowledge up-to-date throughout their employment, particularly when changes occur.

Care managers have a responsibility to ensure that care workers and service users know about the information and are aware of what actions to take if a situation or infringement should arise.

Assessment activity 1.4

Legislation, codes of practice and policies

Case study A: Ida

Ida is living in Brecon Nursing Home. The training officer has decided that care workers need updating on legislation, codes of practice and policies that relate to the home. He is organising a training day for the staff. He also wants the staff to be aware of how these apply to the setting and how they contribute to service users' rights.

Case study B: Ian

Ian is a 5-year-old boy who attends Fairway Primary School. The training officer has decided that staff need updating on legislation, codes of practice and policies that relate to the school. She is organising a training day for them. She also wants the staff to be aware of how these apply to the setting and how they contribute to service users' rights.

Activity

Choose case study A **or** case study B.

1 Arrange to visit a setting (with your tutor's permission) to find out about:
   - **two** pieces of legislation and how they are applied
   - **one** code of practice and how it is applied
   - **two** policies and how they are applied.

Alternatively, you could arrange for a care worker or manager to visit your centre to give the information required.

2 Prepare questions to help you find out the information required.

3 Trial the questions and make any adjustments necessary.

4 Use the questions to collect the information needed.

5 Research **two** pieces of legislation that relate to the chosen setting. Give a comprehensive account of how the legislation should be used by the setting to promote equal opportunities.

6 Choose **one** code of practice that relates to the setting chosen. Provide detailed information, using different sources, about its content, giving examples, to show how it should be applied in the setting to promote equal opportunities.

7 Choose **two** policies that apply to the setting chosen. Give detailed information, using different sources, about their content. Show, by giving examples, how they should be applied by the setting.

Complaints procedures in settings

Complaints procedures should be made available to all service users in any health, social care or early years setting. If a service user feels that they have not received the care they expected, or that their rights have not been met, they have the right to complain.

For example, the NHS has a national complaints procedure – see opposite.

NHS staff will do whatever they can to make sure you are treated properly. But sometimes things go wrong.

You have every right to complain if the services you receive fall short of what you expect.

Here is what you do if you are not happy with any aspect of the NHS.

The first step is to contact the local organisation with which you are unhappy to seek local resolution of your complaint.

If you are still unhappy, you can ask for an independent review to take place.

Finally, if your complaint is still not resolved to your satisfaction, you should contact the health service commissioner.

Source: www.nhs.uk

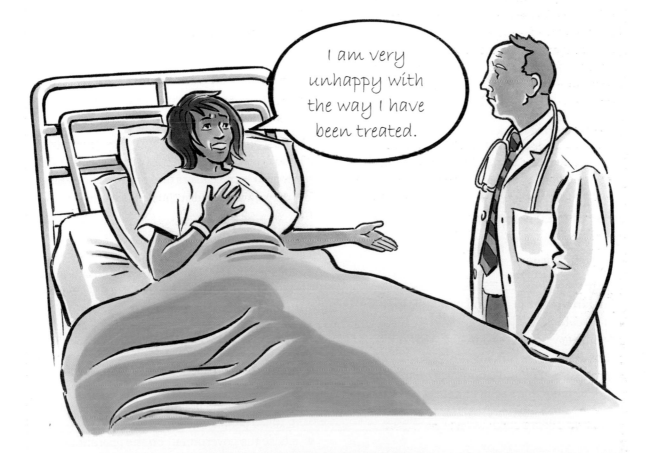

You have a right to complain if the services you receive fall short of what you expect

Workers' roles and responsibilities

All care workers have a responsibility to the service users they are caring for to make sure that they have no cause for complaint. Any complaint which arises must be dealt with promptly to prevent the situation becoming worse. Details of the complaints procedure are usually provided to the service user on or before their arrival at a setting.

When a service user makes a complaint, the care worker must inform their supervisor/manager. This is to ensure that the complaint is dealt with effectively.

Service users' access to complaints procedures

If a service user has a complaint to make, the process should be straightforward. They should complain to the manager or person in charge of the care setting. If the service user feels the complaint has not been dealt with in a suitable manner, then they should complain to the registration authority, for example, social services for residential care homes. If the complaint is not sorted out, the service user should seek support from organisations who have experience in dealing with such issues. Addresses of such organisations are usually included in the package of information provided for the service user on admission. Alternatively, the Citizens Advice Bureau (CAB) will provide the information required.

Support for service users

When making a complaint, service users can seek support from:

- care workers
- an advocate, e.g. a friend or a professional advocate
- voluntary organisations, e.g. Age Concern, Citizens Advice Bureau
- professional organisations, e.g. solicitors, Commission for Racial Equality.

Organisations that offer support and redress

Commission for Racial Equality

The Commission for Racial Equality (CRE) was set up by the Race Relations Act 1975. The CRE is responsible to the Home Office and has a duty to:

- work towards the removal of all discrimination
- promote equality of opportunity and good relations between persons of different racial groups
- review the workings of the Act and draw up proposals for improving and amending it
- give advice to people with complaints of discrimination and, in some cases, represent people in court.

The CRE provides information and advice to people who feel they have suffered racial harassment or discrimination. Its aim is to make sure that policies and procedures are implemented to provide equal treatment for all.

Equal Opportunities Commission

The Equal Opportunities Commission (EOC) was set up by the Sex Discrimination Act 1975. It has a legal duty to enforce both this Act and the Equal Pay Act 1970.

The EOC publishes leaflets and gives guidance on all issues linked to equal opportunities and offers support to service users and organisations who feel they have been discriminated against.

Disability Rights Commission

The Disability Rights Commission (DRC) was established by the Disability Discrimination Act 1995 and started work in April 2000. The main duties of the commission are to:

- work towards removing all discrimination against disabled people
- promote equal opportunities for disabled people
- encourage good practice in the treatment of disabled people
- advise the government on the operation of the Disability Discrimination Act 1995.

The DRC provides help for disabled people by providing information and advice, preparing and reviewing statutory codes of practice and making sure there are arrangements to access goods, facilities, services and premises.

Survey of care settings

Organisations that provide health, social care and early years services are known as **providers**. Services can be broadly divided according to the care they provide, for example:

- *health care* – e.g. hospitals, dentists, GPs
- *personal care and support* – e.g. day care centres, home care assistants, independent living centres
- *early years care and education* – e.g. childminders, playgroups, nurseries
- *voluntary care* – e.g. hospices
- *private care* – e.g. nursing homes, residential homes, private hospitals.

Health care is usually in the statutory care sector and includes services that are provided by the NHS and local authorities (i.e. services that have to be provided by law). Social service provision is also statutory and includes the provision of social workers.

Care services in the private sector are provided by profit-making organisations which make a charge for their services. Such services are not provided by law. The private sector can include such services as hospitals, dentistry, complementary therapies, residential homes, nursing homes, playgroups, childminding and nurseries.

The voluntary care sector provides services and advice. Voluntary organisations often 'plug the gap' where statutory services are not providing any services. Sometimes they work with statutory providers. For example, the Women's Royal Voluntary Service (WRVS) works with local authorities to provide meals for older people who live in their own homes, but who find it difficult to cook for themselves. Voluntary organisations include, for example, charities, day care centres, support groups, hospices, parent and toddler groups. Voluntary groups are not-for-profit making organisations. Sometimes, a voluntary service will charge a small fee for the service they are providing, but this money is often used to pay the cost of their overheads, for example, petrol if delivering meals-on-wheels.

All service providers must provide quality care for those who are using the services. To make sure that the services are doing this, regular inspections are made by people who are trained to check that standards are being maintained. For example, for early years settings, Ofsted check that standards meet the quality that is required.

Quality practice

Service users' rights and equality of opportunity have already been discussed in this chapter.

What are the care values?

Providing quality care means applying the care values when working with service users. The care values are based on ideas about human rights. These are the rights to which all people are entitled. A care worker will want to 'act in the best interests of the service user'. This means valuing them as an individual and treating them in a way that we would want to be treated ourselves. A care worker will, therefore, show that they value each individual by applying the care values in the day-to-day tasks that they do.

In health and social care organisations, there are three main components of the care values. These are:

- fostering service users' rights
- fostering equality and diversity
- maintaining confidentiality.

Each of these care values can be broken down, as follows.

Service users' rights
Rights include:

- the right to be different, e.g. sexual orientation, beliefs

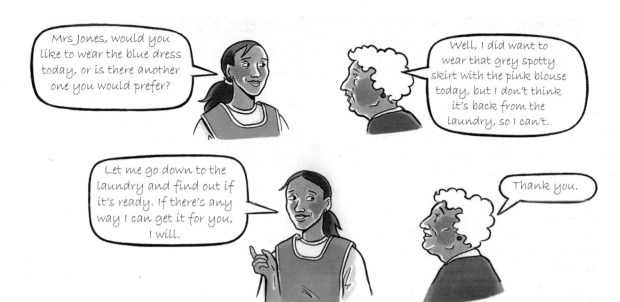

Service users' rights include the right to make their own choices

- freedom from discrimination, e.g. not to be singled out and treated differently
- confidentiality, e.g. to have all personal information kept private
- choice, e.g. to be able to make their own decisions and to be consulted
- dignity, e.g. to be treated with respect
- effective communication, e.g. to have things explained and to be listened to
- safety and security, e.g. to be protected from harm
- privacy, e.g. to have their own space which is not invaded by others without consent.

Equality and diversity

Fostering equality and diversity means:

- understanding and not showing prejudice, stereotyping and labelling
- understanding and valuing the benefits of diversity
- understanding the basis of discrimination, such as gender, race, age, sexuality, disability or social class.

Activity

Applying the care values to achieve quality care

Ahmed works as a nursery nurse in a local nursery school. Bart is working as care assistant in a residential home.

1 Compare how Ahmed and Bart will apply the care values in the workplace. You should consider similarities and differences.

2 Bart is going to take an older person to the toilet. How will he:
- maintain dignity
- use effective communication
- provide choice?

3 Ahmed is responsible for providing a healthy and safe working environment for the children who attend the nursery. What will this involve? Think about organisational policies and legislation when answering this question.

4 Explain how the care values and principles of care contribute to quality practice.

Confidentiality

Maintaining confidentiality means:

- keeping personal information from unauthorised people
- not leaving files containing personal information where others can access them
- having passwords that must be used for accessing electronic records
- not gossiping about service users.

Remember: care values are a statement of the values which underpin practical caring.

Early years care values

Care workers who work in early years care and education settings will need to be aware that there are other values or principles that will need to be applied in their day-to-day tasks. These are summarised in the table below.

Plan the survey

Method

Conducting a survey is a way of gathering information about a subject, in this case to find out how quality practice is achieved and maintained in care settings. Before starting to collect information, you will have to decide which data collecting tool or method(s) will be best to get the information you needed. There are advantages and disadvantages to all data collection tools.

There is a range of methods for collecting information, for example:

- interviewing people
- using questionnaires
- observation of people or situations
- carrying out experiments.

Aspect of early years care	Care value
The welfare of the child	The welfare of the child is the most important core value. Children should be listened to and their views taken into account.
Safety of children	Quality work practice should keep children safe.
Providing a healthy and safe working environment	Safe working practices must exist.
Working in partnership with parents and families	Information about children's development and progress should be shown. Respect must be shown for family traditions.
Children's learning and development	Children should be offered a range of experiences and activities that support all aspects of development: physical, intellectual, emotional and social.
Valuing diversity	Information relating to traditions should be presented in a positive manner.
Equal opportunity	Each child should be offered equality of access to opportunities to learn and develop, and so work towards their potential.
Anti-discrimination	Expressions of prejudice by children or adults should be challenged.
Confidentiality	Information about children and adults should never be shared with others without consent. Secure storage of records is legally required.
Working with other professionals	Liaison with other care professionals should only take place with prior permission.
The reflective practitioner	Early years workers need to reflect on their practices and plan for developing and extending practice.

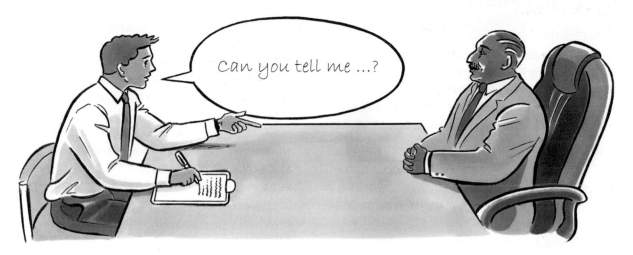

An interview involves asking a person questions face-to-face

Sometimes, more than one method is used to gather information for a survey, depending on the subject matter. For this survey, which is about how quality practice is achieved in care settings, the focus of information-gathering is to be:

- interviews

and/or

- questionnaires.

Such methods will produce both **quantitative** data and **qualitative** data.

Quantitative data is numerical and can be analysed using statistical methods. An example of a question that produces quantitative data would be, 'How many complaints are received in a six month period?' Quantitative data can be displayed using graphs, charts and tables. If a questionnaire were used only to gather information about quality practice, the results could be very limited.

Qualitative data concerns attitudes and opinions and often cannot be produced in numerical form. The participants might talk about their feelings, for example, a service user may say, 'I feel I can complain as it has been clearly explained to me what to do if I need to.' Qualitative data is expressed in words and not in numbers.

Both qualitative and quantitative data can produce useful and meaningful results.

Interviews

An interview involves asking a person questions face-to-face. The person being interviewed has probably consented to take part beforehand. The interviewer will have prepared questions for the interview that will produce the information they need.

When planning your interviews you should:

- ask permission to carry out the interview
- arrange a mutually convenient date and time
- prepare questions to make sure you gather the information you need – you may want to trial questions beforehand to make sure they produce the sort of answers you need
- avoid bias – do not lead the participant on by the way you ask the questions
- consider recording the interview so that you can concentrate on asking the questions and listening to the responses
- maintain confidentiality – do not use the full name of the participant
- prepare a transcript of the interview so that results can be analysed.

Interviews can be structured or in-depth.

Structured interviews

A structured interview is one in which the person gathering the information, the researcher, meets the participant(s) and asks a prepared list of questions, with little **intervention**. The data (information) collected from this type of interview is likely to be quantitative, but some qualitative data will also be gained.

The advantage of using a structured interview is that response rates are usually quite good. The researcher knows who is answering the questions and prompts and probes can be used to encourage responses. The disadvantage of using the structured interview is that it is time-consuming, so that only a small sample can be used.

In-depth interviews

This is where the person collecting the information meets the participant, and the researcher allows the participant to talk freely about a particular topic, in this case quality practice. As the aim is to encourage the participant to get their true feelings across, only qualitative data is collected. The advantage of using an in-depth interview is that participants are able to open up on sensitive issues as there is no structure, and the researcher can explore any interesting areas that arise. The disadvantage is that the interviewer can influence the answers given.

Questionnaires

A **self-completed** questionnaire is one where the researcher hands out questionnaire forms to the participants, who then answer the questions by filling in the answers in the spaces provided. The forms are collected by the researcher when they are completed. This is a way of collecting qualitative data.

The advantages of using questionnaires is that they are cheap, quick, anonymous and a way to collect information without interviewer bias. Participants can also take their time to answer the questions. The disadvantage is that there may be a poor response rate. For a survey that is investigating how quality care is maintained in care settings, a questionnaire on its own may not be the best option.

When using a questionnaire:

- begin with easy-to-answer **closed questions** and work towards questions which need more thought at the end
- include a short introduction that explains why the survey is being carried out, and covers the issue of confidentiality
- ask factual response questions linked to **demographic** factors about the respondent, such as age, sex, ethnicity.

Remember:

- make sure the questions are easy to understand
- do not use questions which allow the respondent to repeat a previous answer
- do not assume the respondents have any previous knowledge of the topics you are asking about
- thank the respondents for completing the questionnaire at the end.

Activity

You have been asked to collect information about how a care setting ensures quality practice.

1 Work in pairs to produce five research questions based on quality practice issues that could be used if you were producing a self-completing questionnaire.

2 Share your questions with another pair within the group and ask them to try answering the questions. Did you get the type of answers you were looking for? Rewrite any questions that were ambiguous or were not successful.

3 As a whole group, discuss the issues that arose when producing the questions.

4 Work in a small group to think about qualitative data that you might want to collect about quality practice. Work out the main topics.

5 Write five questions that could be used in an in-depth interview with a care worker or manager to find out about quality practice.

Plan the survey

Methods to be used

Ideas for the method could come from secondary research, i.e. from the work of others who have already completed similar research topics. Secondary sources can provide data that would be difficult to collect yourself. For example, government papers, research papers and statistics completed after inspection reports may all help you to make decisions about the methods that should be used for conducting the survey.

You will need to produce a plan which provides a framework within which to work. Decisions will need to be made about:

- the aim of the survey, e.g. the overall purpose
- the objectives, e.g. the steps within the aim that you need to take to achieve the outcome
- the timescale for the survey, e.g. start and completion times
- which care setting you will choose. Remember to choose a setting where you know you will be able to obtain all the information you need
- who is to be involved in the research, e.g. care worker or manager
- the method(s) to be used, e.g. self-completed questionnaire, structured interview or both

- the type of questions, e.g. **open** and/or closed, follow-on questions
- how the results are to be presented, e.g. graphs, charts, graphs.

Planning will help you to organise your thoughts and put things into the correct order. A plan for research at a primary school, for example, could look like the one at the bottom of the page.

Sequence of questions

If the survey is to be carried out using an interview, the sequence of the questions cannot be decided upon until the questions themselves are written. Even before that is done, the topics to be included in the survey must be established.

For this survey, the main topics are:

- How are the rights of service users maintained?
- How is equality of opportunity given to service users?
- How are the care values applied by staff?
- How is diversity fostered?
- How is confidentiality maintained?
- Which codes of practice are used?
- How do codes of practice and policies contribute to providing quality care?

Date	Action	Reason for action
6 January ½ hour	Research three secondary sources of information about quality practice. Make notes.	To find out what research has been done previously and the methods used.
9 January ½ hour	Decide on aims, objectives, methods to be used, timescales, care setting, who to gather information from.	To help inform the process, e.g. What do I want to find out?
12 January ½ hour	Letter to care setting to explain the research, to whom I wish to speak, with examples of questions.	To get permission to use the setting and talk to a care worker. To give advance notice of the questions that will be asked.
15 January 1 hour	Plan structured interview questions for teacher and service users, and group together in an organised sequence.	To make sure that there is full coverage of all the topics. To make sure the questions are appropriate and not ambiguous. To make sure all the questions on one particular topic are grouped together.
20 January 1 hour	Visit setting. Ask questions.	To obtain the information needed.

Rights	What do we need to find out?	(Draft)
What rights do children have?	How do teachers make sure children's rights are maintained?	
	How can teachers support children to make sure their rights are maintained?	
	Is this dealt with in staff training?	
	How often does staff training take place?	
	Can you talk me through the type of topics that would be covered?	
	How does staff training help to maintain children's rights?	
	Have there been any occasions when children's rights have not been maintained?	
Advice and guidance	From whom can you seek advice if …	

Each of these topics will need to be broken down into smaller parts or components, as shown in the example above for a primary school.

Once all the topics and the component parts have been listed, the questions can be correctly formed. Remember that the focus of the survey is on quality care practice, so questions must be focused on this topic. Make sure you use both open and closed questions.

Collection of information

You will need to prepare a document for recording the questions and a space to be able to write the answers given. An example is given at the bottom of this page.

An example of an open question in this recording document is, 'What systems are in place to maintain the right to choose?' A follow-on question might be, 'How are these effective?' These questions allow the person being interviewed to give their thoughts and feelings on the subject as well as being able to talk about the facts.

Questions	Answers
1 Can you tell me what rights children have?	
2 What systems are in place to maintain the right to choose?	
3 Do you have a policy to help maintain rights?	
4 Can you give me some idea of what is in the policy? or If you had a policy, what would you want to see included?	
5 Is bullying or not being bullied part of a child's right?	
6 How are new staff made aware of the setting's policies on rights?	
7 What monitoring methods do you have in place to ensure that rights are maintained?	
8 What would happen if a child were denied their rights?	

An example of a closed question in this recording document is, 'Do you have a policy to help maintain rights?' The care worker can answer 'yes' or 'no' to this question.

Sometimes, follow-on questions are required after closed questions. For example, in question 3, if the care worker says 'yes', the follow-on question might be, 'Can you tell me what is in the policy?' If the care worker says 'no', the follow-on question might be the second part of question 4 or 'Why do you not have a policy relating to choice?'

When producing questions for the survey, you may need to include some follow-on questions in order to collect all the information needed and to obtain the whole picture of what is happening.

Before visiting the care setting with the questions and recording documents, it is always a good idea to trial the questions. This means trying them on another person to see if they are clear and unambiguous and that they produce the type of answers that are needed. Questions could be tried out by giving them to other people in your group, to relatives or to friends. Being able to trial questions provides the opportunity to amend any questions that are not clear.

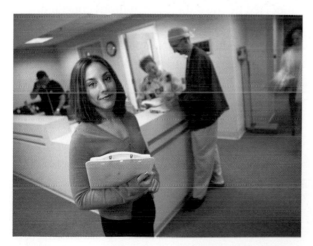

Finding out the answers

Conduct the survey

By this stage, you will have prepared the questions and recording documents and will have arranged a date and time for the visit.

Present and analyse the results of the survey

When all the data has been collected the person who has conducted the survey will need to examine it. As the survey will probably have been conducted through an interview, it is more than likely that the data will be qualitative and will need to be considered question by question. Examining the responses will help you to analyse and interpret the information collected. A questionnaire may also have been used.

Quantitative information can be collated into a table of responses. A frequency table can be used, like the one below.

Information is securely kept in the care setting	Number	Percentage
Strongly agree	10	40
Agree	5	20
Neutral	3	12
Disagree	2	8
Strongly disagree	5	20
Total	25	100

This information can then be presented using a computer spreadsheet. The programme will calculate statistics for you and enable you to create graphs or charts, as in the example on the next page.

Qualitative data is more difficult to present and needs a written description of the findings. This could include flow charts or diagrams to illustrate particular points. Where respondents give similar answers, these can be presented using graphs or charts, as for the quantitative data.

Analysis of qualitative data may seem like writing a report. You will need a summary of comments made – try to give an accurate account of what has been said, but this does not have to be word-for-word. Quotes can be given to clarify and confirm what the care worker or service user has said.

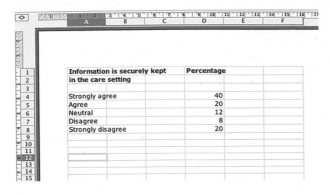

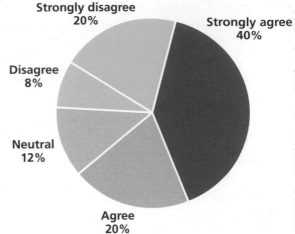

A spreadsheet, and a pie chart created using the spreadsheet

It is important to keep referring back to the questions asked so that a meaningful picture is given, as shown in the example below.

> When asked how the school promotes diversity, the teacher stated that all children had religious education (RE) in which they learned about Christianity, Sikhism, Islam, Judaism, Buddhism and animism. These were the six main religions in the world. Also, when children leave assembly, music from different cultures is played.
>
> All teachers in the school receive training in the use of 'radio aids' so that children with hearing impairment can hear at all times.
>
> Both male and female students are given the same opportunities to take part in all sporting activities. For example, there is a boys' football team, a girls' football team and a mixed football team ...

The analysis makes reference to the question asked and confirms quality practice. Each question asked in the interview should be analysed in this way.

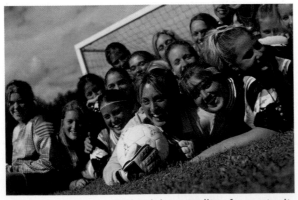

Maintaining equality of opportunity

Drawing conclusions

How are rights maintained? How are diversity and equality fostered? How is confidentiality maintained?

The point of analysing the results of the survey is to draw conclusions about the subject of the survey, in this case how quality care is maintained in the setting. You will need to reflect on the results of the analysis, that is, consider what you have found out and draw conclusions based on your findings.

It is important to make sure the conclusions are supported by the data (information) collected. However, the data may show that some rights are being maintained, for example, confidentiality, but that other rights are not. Whether rights are being partially met or fully met, the conclusions drawn must be supported by evidence from the data collected.

An example of a conclusion supported by evidence from the data is shown at the top of the next page.

From this evidence it is possible to:

- know the question that was asked
- recognise that a conclusion has been drawn
- see that conclusions drawn are supported by evidence, e.g. observation, written policies, answers to questions.

When drawing conclusions, remember they must be directly related to the questions asked.

At Fairway Primary School, I asked how service users' rights were promoted. I was told children were provided with choices about activities, who they would like to sit next to and what they would like to eat. Two examples were given to illustrate the point made. One was giving the children the option of which foods they would like at meal times. I was shown a menu with a range of dishes and was asked to sit and observe how teachers supported the children in choosing their meal. I did note that they gave the children plenty of time to choose their meals and also explained any dishes that they were unfamiliar with.

The teacher also stated that the school supported children's rights by providing safety and security. Doors have electronic locks and only teachers know the code. Fire plans are also located around the building and within the health and safety policy, which I was given. It was clearly stated 'in the event of a fire, teachers on duty will make sure the children are helped from the building to the assembly point. The headteacher in charge will ...'

I was also encouraged to talk to some of the children about rights. I asked, 'What rights do the children have?' Margaret told me that they have the right not to be bullied. She talked about 'bullying' and how the school did lots of things with the children on this subject. Margaret told me how she had entered an anti-bullying story writing competition. She had come second. The aim of the competition was to make people (including the bullies) think about and feel what it was like to be bullied.

Assessment activity 1.6

Conduct a survey

You have been asked to visit a care setting to conduct a survey to find out how they maintain quality practice.

Following the visit, you have been asked to write a report which gives details about how the chosen care setting:

- maintains the rights of service users
- fosters equality and diversity
- maintains confidentiality.

You must plan the survey, conduct the survey and draw conclusions.

1 Decide which care setting you would like to visit (in consultation with your tutor). Draw up a detailed plan for the preparation for the visit, showing the actions you propose to take in order to collect the information, giving reasons for each action.

2 Prepare detailed interview questions that will help you collect the information you need. Trial the questions with others to make sure they are clear and unambiguous.

3 Draw up an appropriate recording document which groups the questions in order within the topic, and which gives a space to record the answers.

4 Write a letter to the care setting asking if it is possible to conduct the survey. Give information about the topics that you need to find out about during the visit and the methods you propose to use for collecting the information. You may wish to enclose a copy of the questions so that the manager can prepare for the visit.

5 Conduct the survey at the care setting.

6 Analyse the results of the survey and present them in the form of a report.

Remember to focus on the questions asked and the responses given. You must also draw conclusions from your findings. The topics on which you must report are:

- how service users' rights are maintained
- how diversity and equality are fostered
- how confidentiality is maintained.

Glossary

Advocate: a person who speaks on behalf of another when the person is unable to represent or speak on their own behalf

Anti-discrimination: making sure everyone is included; being against discrimination

Bisexual: sexually attracted to both sexes

Closed question: a question which requires a specific answer

Compromise: meeting half way by partly giving way on an opinion or view

Confidentiality: keeping information secret

Democracy: allowing everyone the right to express their view

Demographic: relating to the study of the population of an area; population statistics

Dilemma: a difficult situation, involving a choice between two unfavourable options

Direct: to be open; to aim precisely

Discriminate: to favour one group of people above another

Disclose: to make known

Empowerment: enabling a service user to be in control of their lives and to make their own decisions

Homosexual: preferring a same sex partner, e.g. male and male

Indirect: not to be obvious

Intervention: participating and trying to influence the outcome

Legible: able to be read

Manual: done by hand

Marginalised: to be on the edge of; on the outside; not included

Monitor: to check to see how something is going, e.g. quality practice

Non-confrontational: not being aggressive towards others

Objective: a view not distorted by one's personal view or bias (opposite of subjective)

Open question: a question that can have an expanded answer

Oppression: an act of tyranny; an act which causes misery to others

Organisation: a place that provides several services

Originate: to start or begin; to create something; to arise

Paramountcy: of greatest importance

Prejudice: judging a person by a particular characteristic, such as how they look

Providers: people or organisations who give a service or make services available

Qualitative: research that produces data about attitudes and opinions

Quantitative: research that produces data that can be measured

Race: the ethnicity or nationality of a person

Redress: having one's voice heard, e.g. complaint, court hearing

Restricted: kept or confined within limits

Secondary research: existing research that has been completed by others on a similar topic

Self-actualise: to realise fully one's potential

Self-completed: completed by oneself

Social exclusion: to be outside; withdrawn; isolated

Subjective: a view formed from one's personal view or bias

Superior: in a higher position or rank

Tension: difficulties; torn between two things

Tribunal: a group of people appointed to hear disagreements relating to work practices

Victimisation: making a victim of someone; selecting a person or group for unfair treatment or discrimination

Violated: not observed/respected (e.g rights); being the object of violence, e.g. verbal, physical, emotional, sexual

Unit 2 Working with service users in care settings

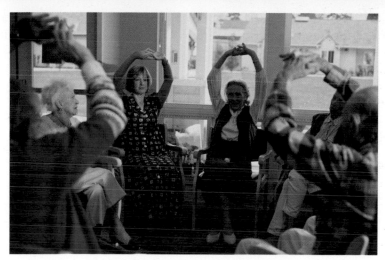

Identifying people can sometimes prove to be difficult

Introduction

How do you identify others? Are you always correct? What signs give you clues about the group they belong to?

Care workers need to understand how to identify service users and how to contribute to trusting relationships with service users if they are to be successful in their work. Knowing our own prejudices, beliefs and opinions and recognising how easy it is be biased and to stereotype people, is of prime importance when caring for others. Behaviour that fails to value service users is easily recognised both by the service user and by other care workers. It disempowers people rather than empowering them.

Effective communication is one way of establishing good relationships and preventing barriers from forming between service users and care workers. Effective communication is about:

- knowing the purposes of communication
- knowing the factors that can contribute to establishing good relationships with service users

- knowing what the barriers are to communication
- knowing the factors that enhance and inhibit communication and their effects
- being able to plan an interaction with a service user or a group of service users
- knowing how to use skills successfully when communicating
- being able to interact with a service user to form an effective relationship
- knowing the different ways in which people communicate in care settings.

Bringing together knowledge and skills to provide a competent approach when working with service users, and having the ability to reflect on the effectiveness of interactions, will give confidence for future work in health, social care or early years settings.

In this unit you will learn

Learning outcomes

You will learn to:

- describe relationships with service users that value them as individuals
- recognise the effects of stereotyping and prejudice on service users
- review the different ways of communicating with service users in care settings, and their purpose
- recognise the effect of barriers on communication
- plan an interaction with a service user to establish and maintain an effective relationship
- interact with a service user to form an effective relationship, evaluating the effectiveness of the interaction.

Different ways people can be identified

Every individual has specific **characteristics** which influence the way they appear to others. It is not just one single characteristic that helps to identify a person, but several, although one characteristic may be stronger than others in some people. People can be identified by their:

- *age* – a person's hair may grow white or become thin
- *gender* – whether they are male or female
- *appearance* – e.g. they look like a child or an older adult
- *place of residence* – e.g. living in a residential home or a nursing home
- *needs* – they may use a mobility aid or have a disability.

Age

As we grow we become aware of the different **life stages** that contribute to our complete life span. For example:

- infancy: 0–3 years
- childhood: 4–10 years
- adolescence: 11–18 years
- adulthood: 19–65 years
- later adulthood: 65+ years.

In each life stage an individual has different characteristics. For example, an infant is young, is cared for and is dependent on its parents or main carer, whereas an adolescent is less dependent on their parents or the main carer and usually wants to 'do their own thing'. An older adult in the final life stage may have lost up to three inches in height, have grey or thinning hair and may have developed wrinkles.

When meeting a service user for the first time, their age may be one of the characteristics that identifies them initially.

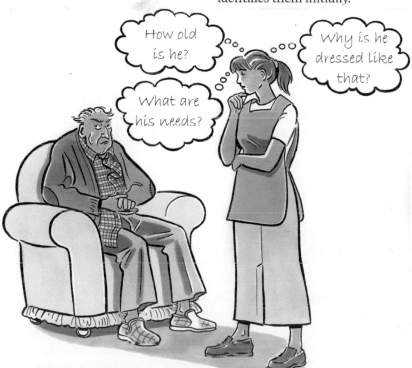

Linking characteristics helps with the identification of service users

Gender

At birth, one of the most frequently asked questions is, 'Is it a boy or a girl?' A baby's sex can have implications for its future life. In western societies it was, until fairly recently, customary for a woman to be the main person responsible for rearing children, while men were the main workers, bringing in wages.

In all countries, infants are born into societies that have well-established norms, values and beliefs. Associated with these norms, values and beliefs are behavioural expectations based on **gender**. The term 'gender' relates to femaleness or maleness. It is a **socially constructed** label that can vary according to the culture into which a child is born. It is putting people into groups according to their male or female characteristics.

In care settings that are particularly involved in the care and education of infants and children, great care must be taken to ensure that specific toys such as buses, trains and cars are not automatically allocated to boys and that dolls and domestic toys are not specifically given to girls.

Similarly, at other life stages, such as adulthood, care workers should not show prejudice about same gender relationships.

> ### Consider this
> *What are the differences between gender and sex?*

Appearance

Judging a person by their appearance can have detrimental results. Such judgements are often based on the norms of the society in which we live. However, some service users may not choose to wear what is expected in that particular society, wishing to appear different from others.

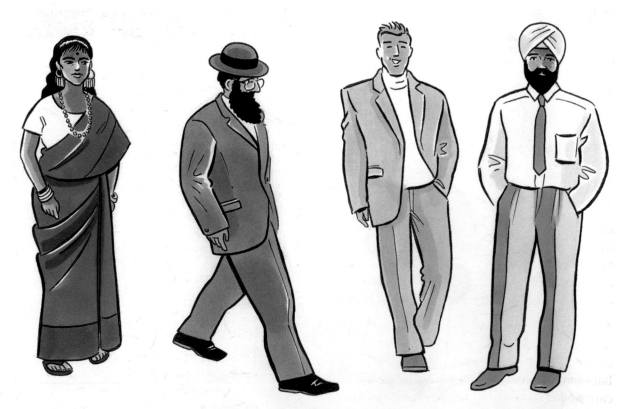

Different cultural codes of dress can assist with identification

Consider this

Look at the group of people at the bottom of the previous page.

What are their cultures? What helps you to identify them?

For example, a wealthy person may wish to dress more as a person who is earning a living rather than as a celebrity. A GP who is faced with a scruffy-looking woman may assume that she has little in the way of financial resources, when in fact she may have more than enough money to meet her required needs and wants.

Appearance can be useful in identifying a service user, when linked with other characteristics.

Place of residence

If a service user visiting an outpatients department gives as their address:

Paddocks Residential Home for Older People, Broadway

it is possible to guess that the service user is in the older adult life stage. This is another characteristic or pointer that helps with identification.

Sometimes, however, the place of residence will not contribute to the identification process. The name of the area in which the person lives may be unknown to the care worker or maybe where people of all ages, backgrounds and cultures live.

A care worker speaking to a child may ask, 'What school do you go to?' The child may give the answer, 'Puddleduck Primary School' or, 'Perry Bar Comprehensive'. From such information, the care worker can determine whether the service user is in the childhood or the adolescent life

stage. Small pieces of information like this contribute to the whole picture.

Needs

Some needs are obvious and will immediately help a care worker to identify the service user. For example, a person who is being pushed by another in a wheelchair, or a service user who is walking by using a zimmer frame, obviously has mobility needs.

Some needs are not so easily identified, however. For example, a person who has a bladder disorder may have to wear a catheter which is hidden beneath their clothing, while a person who is unable to read well or has difficulty with spelling may have dyslexia. It is usually through discussion that such hidden needs emerge.

Theory into practice

Visit a setting and observe how different people are identified. Record your findings.

Activity

Alex

Alex has an appointment at the outpatients department of the local hospital. The medical notes relating to his condition have been mislaid. There is little information about Alex.

1 Make an identification of Alex. Explain how you reached your decisions.

2 Exchange your identification with that made by someone else. What are the differences? Why?

3 Explain why it is important for care workers to identify service users correctly. What characteristics can help them to make their decisions?

4 Prepare four questions to ask a care worker about how they identify different service users.

5 Conduct a short interview with a care worker to find out how they identify service users and how correct identification can contribute to establishing and maintaining effective relationships.

Factors contributing to establishing and maintaining good relationships

Various factors contribute to establishing and maintaining good relationships with service users, including:

- trust
- respect
- confidentiality
- effective communication
- providing choice
- trust.

Many of these factors are part of the **'care values'**. Care values are derived from human rights. They are not laws or related to legislation, but are a form of respect. They are not a *recipe for practice* but a statement showing recognition of worth which indicates quality. The care values focus on treating service users as individuals when providing professional care within day-to-day tasks.

In health and social care settings, there are three main care values that care workers try to apply in all the work that they carry out. These are:

- promoting equality and diversity
- maintaining confidentiality
- promoting individual rights and beliefs.

In early years care and education settings, the care values are known as 'principles of care'. There are ten principles of care, which are:

- understanding the welfare of the child is paramount
- providing for the safety of the child
- providing a healthy and safe working environment
- working in partnership with parents and families
- promoting anti-discriminatory practice
- providing for children's learning and development
- valuing diversity and maintaining confidentiality
- providing equal opportunities
- performing as a reflective practitioner
- working with other professionals.

Consider this

Consider the ten principles of care and compare them with your own working practices. How do think you measure up against them?

Respect

Without respect it is unlikely that a care worker will be able to establish an effective relationship with service users. Respect can be shown in a variety of ways by care workers. For example:

- by calling a service user by their preferred name and not by calling them 'love' or 'dear'
- by allowing them to make choices even if they are different from the choices the care worker would make
- by listening carefully to service users and not holding two conversations at once.

Respect is about treating each service user as an individual, whatever their age or ability. It involves treating them with dignity and valuing them for themselves.

Trust

To trust someone means having complete faith in them. It means believing what a person says and putting yourself in their hands. It takes a great deal of courage for a service user to be able to do this because it means they lose control over their life. This could be through:

- accepting a care worker's advice
- telling a care worker personal information
- asking a care worker to undertake a very important task for them.

Trust is not obtained without first having respect. The two are closely linked. Trust is established by being honest and having reliable, consistent exchanges.

Maintaining confidentiality

Within a care setting, it is not possible to keep all personal information confidential. There may be occasions when other professional care workers, either in the setting or outside, may need to know what has been said.

Occasions when confidential information may have to be disclosed include those in which:

- the service user is intending to harm themselves
- the service user is intending to harm others
- the service user is intending to participate in a crime.

Care workers must ensure that idle gossip does not take place between themselves where others can overhear and are able to identify the person they are talking about. Service users should only be discussed behind closed doors so that information remains confidential.

Service users' notes should be appropriately stored and not left where others can access them. Computers holding personal information should only be accessed by staff who have been given this responsibility as part of their job. The Data Protection Act sets out very clearly which information can be held on computer and for how long. Some of the terms of the Data Protection Act are given below.

If trust is not established, confidentiality is also unlikely to be established and maintained, and therefore good relationships with service users will not exist.

Effective communication

According to Carl Rogers, the way in which communication takes place should be with 'unconditional, positive regard'. This means accepting the service user just as they are without making judgements about them. By expressing approval or disapproval, conditions are imposed on the service user.

Effective communication means sharing information, opinions or ideas in a way that others will understand and will be able to give a response to. A number of factors are involved in the process of communication, as shown in the diagram on the following page.

In a discussion, each person is involved in the process of interpreting and making sense of what is being said and then acting appropriately. In any conversation, a range of **contextualised** clues will be exchanged. This can be through the tone of voice, through the body language used or through the vocabulary and sequence of the words. How these are interpreted will depend very much on our culture. That is, the norms and values we are used to applying.

The relationship between a care worker and a service user is a **partnership**, where the service

Extracts from the Data Protection Act (slightly adapted)

- Service users should be given a copy of any information kept about them which should be clearly explained. This is known as their 'right of access'.
- Service users must be given the right to have any inaccurate information corrected or deleted.
- Service users can complain to the Data Protection Commissioner if they think someone keeping data is not complying with the Act.
- Service users can claim compensation through the courts if they suffer damage through mishandling of information.
- Service users can find out from any person or organisation whether they keep information about

individuals, and if they do, to be told the type of information kept and the purposes for which it is kept.

People keeping personal information **must**:

- obtain personal information fairly and openly
- use it only in ways compatible with the purpose for which it was given in the first place
- secure it against unauthorised access or loss
- ensure that it is kept accurate and up-to-date.

People keeping personal information **must not**:

- disclose it to others in a manner incompatible with the purpose for which it was given
- retain it for longer than is necessary for the purpose for which it was given.

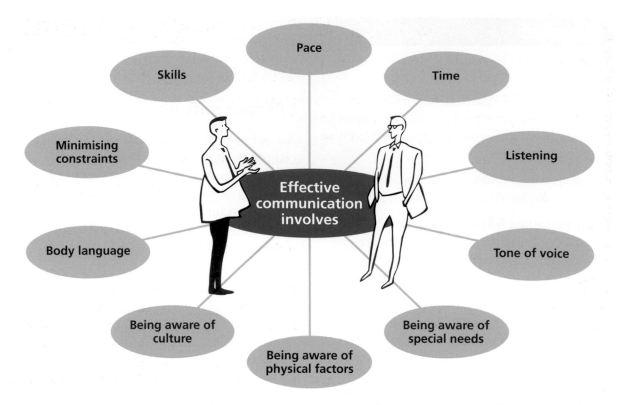

The factors involved in effective communication

user keeps an active role in the decision-making about themselves. Neither the care worker nor the service user is the 'expert'; effective communication means keeping a balance so that an **holistic approach** is applied.

Providing choice

Every service user has the right to make choices, whether the care worker regards them as being acceptable or unacceptable. An **autocratic** approach by the care worker would seek to deprive the service user of power and would lead to domination and the care worker having power over the service user. A **democratic** approach involves the service user and provides them with choice.

Service users will need to have the confidence to make decisions. This means that they must have trust as a central characteristic in their relationship with the care worker. They must also have been given accurate and up-to-date facts and helped to see both the advantages and disadvantages of the topic or information being

provided. When they have this, informed choices can be made.

Anxiety and pressure can cause a service user to make a decision that is not going to be advantageous to their situation. Making hasty decisions, without taking into account all the relevant information, can lead to an inappropriate course of action. Service users must be made aware of the risks when making their choices.

Theory into practice

Try to arrange a visit to a setting to observe the factors that contribute to establishing and maintaining good relationships. Record your observations.

The case study opposite is an example of a care worker not spending sufficient time with the service user to explore the advantages and disadvantages of each type of accommodation. Martha is being hurried into making a decision that could influence the rest of her life. Each aspect of the conversation needs to be explored.

Case study

Martha

Martha is leaving her hostel accommodation, now that she has successfully come off drugs. She has to make a decision about whether to live in shared accommodation with Ricky and Rosalind or whether she wants a bedsit on her own. A care worker is assigned to help Martha make her decision.

Care worker: Well Martha, you know what options you have. Have you made up your mind yet?

Martha: No, it's difficult. I like Ricky and I quite like Rosalind, but I don't really know if I want to share.

Care worker: Well, the alternative is to have a bed-sitting room on your own. You will only have yourself to worry about.

Martha: I might feel very lonely.

Care worker: Make up your mind girl. We haven't got all day!

For example, the care worker could have taken Martha's first answer and helped her to explore her feelings. She could have said, for example:

- What do you think sharing is going to be about?
- What do you think sharing is going to involve, Martha?
- How well do you think you could share in the kitchen?
- What are the advantages of sharing?
- What might you not like about sharing?
- Let's make a list of the advantages and disadvantages of sharing with Ricky and Rosalind.

Having asked these questions and others, the care worker could have given Martha time to think about the answers she has and to meet on another occasion to discuss them. She could also suggest that Martha arranges a visit to talk to Ricky and Rosalind to see if she thinks she would fit into the shared situation.

This is an important decision for Martha. To hurry her was not an acceptable approach. The physical, intellectual, emotional and social aspects had been omitted from the communication process. The focus needed to be much wider and to involve Martha more in the process if it were to be successful.

Assessment activity 2.1

Relationships with service users

Chiedza is an adult and works in a residential home. She fell at work and injured her wrist and is attending Greenacres Day Hospital for minor surgery. She is a Muslim and is anxious that her customs are followed while at the day hospital.

Joy is having day surgery for an ulcer on her leg. She is an older adult and is worried about the procedure.

Mark has opted for day surgery to remove a lump at the base of his neck. He is an adolescent.

Rob's parents have taken him for day surgery as he is unable to pass water without having pain. Rob is 5 years old.

Answer the questions using the information given above and any additional information you may have gathered.

1 Give a comprehensive account of the ways that people can be identified, making connections to show how valuing service users as individuals can contribute to effective relationships.

2 Use evidence from different sources to describe in detail four factors that can contribute to establishing and maintaining good relationships with service users. Give detailed examples to illustrate the points being made.

2.2 Recognise the effects of stereotyping and prejudice on service users

Stereotyping

> **Key point**
>
> **Stereotyping** is making a judgement about a person by their appearance, clothing, accent, etc. It is making an assumption without really knowing anything about them. Inequality arises when negative stereotypes are used. 'Labelling', 'pigeon-holing' or 'categorising' are other names given to stereotyping.

Stereotyping is a **cognitive** activity. That is, it is in the mind and involves the individual's knowledge or belief about something.

Stereotyping is a generalisation about a person or a group of people, often based on views and opinions that are negative and inaccurate. Such views are damaging to others as those who hold them fail to recognise the differences between individuals. Stereotyping means making assumptions that all members of a group are the same, and indeed assuming that a person is a member of a particular group, not an individual. The conversation below illustrates this point.

> *Care worker:* How many children have you got, René?
>
> *René:* I've got three children. No, I haven't, sorry I've got five. I can't always remember so I don't really know.
>
> *Care worker:* Never mind, all older people are forgetful.

The care worker is making a judgement about age. It is untrue that 'all older people are forgetful'. Making such an assumption can hinder effective communication. It is important to remember that some characteristics that generally apply to a particular group do not apply to all individuals within the group.

Another example of stereotyping is the statement, 'All nurses are rude.' It generalises about all nurses, without making any individual distinctions between them.

Stereotyping allows no room for individuality and is usually negative. Its roots come from an individual's deeply embedded way of thinking about others and may be the result of fear or lack of understanding about people who are different from ourselves. These convictions can come from family, friends or from our peer groups. The case study below illustrates this.

> **Case study**
>
> **Amy**
>
> Amy is partially disabled. She is in the reception class of her local primary school. She is a fun-loving child who gets on well with the other children in her class. She has teaching support but is able to join in most of the activities that are organised for her class.
>
> The class has a different teacher for numeracy each day. The teacher gives Amy little attention and often refers to her as 'the child with special needs'. Whenever she talks to Amy she uses very simple 'baby language', rather than using the vocabulary that she uses with the rest of the class.
>
> Amy does not like this attitude and no longer asks any questions. One day the teacher asks the class some questions but first she says to Amy, 'You need not answer, Amy, as you are a wheelchair case and my friends tell me not to expect disabled people and those with special needs to be able answer these harder mathematical questions.'

This is an example of very negative stereotyping which reveals the teacher's lack of knowledge on a particular topic. Her attitude devalues Amy.

Other groups who are frequently stereotyped are ethnic minorities, people who have hearing impairment, people who dress differently and people who are in particular occupations, such as social workers.

Prejudice

Prejudice means having a very judgemental attitude, an attitude which does not take into account the feelings of others. People who are prejudiced do not explore alternative possibilities. Prejudiced attitudes often result in discrimination, which can then lead to negative actions being taken towards individuals and groups. Being prejudiced can take various forms, for example:

- racism – based on a person's race or colour
- sexism – based on a person's biological sex
- ageism – based on a person's age.

To avoid having tendencies towards stereotyping and prejudice, it is important to have a very positive process of **socialisation**. That is, when growing up we need to experience supportive attitudes from our families and friends and have positive environmental experiences.

Prejudice and stereotyping can have a damaging effect on relationships between care workers and service users. Care workers need to ensure that they:

- do not think of themselves as being 'better' or 'above' service users
- do not impose their own values, attitudes and beliefs on service users
- accept service users as they are and not how they would like them to be
- are non-judgemental
- do not take their anger out on service users.

In order to accomplish this, care workers must have respect for service users, value service users' opinions and views, and apply the care values in their work.

There are three main theories relating to the development of prejudice. These are summarised in the table below.

Theory of prejudice	Explanation
Biological theory	Fear of, and hostility to, others; similar to the way animals wish to protect their community
Psychoanalytical theory	The **authoritarian** attitude which suggests prejudice is present in people's personalities
Cultural theory	Negative prejudice which is deeply embedded in a culture

Prejudice can be reduced by encouraging and providing opportunities for contact between social groups or, in other words, by trying to encourage children and adults to meet a wide variety of people from different cultures and races so that there is greater understanding between all.

Activity

Waves Playgroup

Waves is a recently opened playgroup for children aged 1–5 years. It caters for over fifty infants and children from a multi-cultural area of the town.

1 For staff training purposes, using your own words give a definition of:
   - stereotyping
   - prejudice.

2 How do young children acquire stereotyping and prejudice?

3 How could Waves Playgroup make sure stereotyping and prejudice are reduced?

4 In pairs, carry out research on the three theories of prejudice given above. Then, give a presentation to others about one theory you have researched.

To prevent stereotyping and prejudice when communicating with service users in care settings, care workers should:

- examine their ability to see things clearly and objectively, recognising that understanding one's own feelings is the first step to changing biased behaviour
- recognise that individuals deserve to be treated as unique human beings
- treat service users equally, but respond to them as individuals
- extend respect and dignity to all to help build relationships
- condemn stereotyping and prejudice when observed, reporting such instances immediately to line managers.

A care worker who stereotypes and is prejudiced may use **patronising** language which reduces the service user's self-esteem. Such a care worker is likely to use negative body language. This does not show respect to the service user or encourage dignity as set out in the care values.

Misunderstandings can occur between the service user and the care worker as stereotyping and prejudice can distort communication, and the service user may reject the information being given. Speaking harshly to a service user could cause them to withdraw or to respond angrily, which will have a negative affect on relationships.

Factors that can influence self	How we are influenced
Culture	The customs and traditions of the society in which we live will be part of our inner self. Cultures have different customs when communicating. Non-verbal communication may not carry the same message in one culture as it does in another. **Do you consider your culture to be 'better' than another?**
Religion	Not all service users have the same beliefs as our own. What helped us to form our religious beliefs? Most probably family, tradition and friends. **How do your religious views and opinions affect the care you give?**
Education	People follow different routes in education, e.g. the 'traditional' approach of school, college or university, job roles in care, or the less formal approach of leaving school, getting a job and gaining further educational experience 'on the job'. **What is your attitude to education? Do you think the route you followed was better than another?**
Family	Most of our views, opinions and attitudes will have been acquired through socialisation within the immediate family. We will have listened to adults within the family expressing their views and opinions and may have instinctively adopted these as our own. **Do you hold opinions or views that are not truly your own? Are you open to change if you discover that one or some are not factually correct?**
Environment	If we live in a close, rural community, we may look down on those who live in a city. If we have not had the experience of living in a multi-cultural society, our understanding of people with different cultures may be limited. **How has the environment in which you live influenced your opinions?**
Finances	Goals set for some of us in life may have been measured against financial return. For some, lack of money or having just enough money may have been the norm and as a consequence they may have learned to make decisions based on reasoned argument before purchasing goods and services. **How does money influence your decisions and opinions?**
Work	If work has been the norm for your family, do you expect to work? The type of work we do is often influenced by what our fathers and mothers have done before us. If people around us remain unemployed, do we consider them to be of less value? If someone does a different type of job from us, does this mean that they are not equal? **What has influenced your attitude to work? What is your attitude?**

Knowing yourself and your prejudices

The support we give to others will be more reliable if we understand ourselves, for example, what our opinions are on specific topics, what our beliefs are, what values we consider to be important. Having a sound understanding of self helps to prevent prejudice from interfering with the responsibilities we have as professional care workers.

Values, beliefs and opinions are developed through the family, through friends and through those with whom we associate when working or following leisure pursuits. These are learned and not inherited. They are formed through childhood and develop during adolescence and adulthood. A care worker will need to consider, for example, how they are affected by the factors in the table on the opposite page.

> ## Consider this
>
> *Work in small groups to discuss each question in the table opposite.*
>
> *Join together as a whole group to discuss your answers.*

Behaviour that fails to value people

To value a service user means to treat them with respect and dignity and to consider all equal despite their social class, race, nationality or religion. A care worker or anyone who fails to value a service user is not recognising their individual worth. Service users who do not feel valued may feel emotionally threatened and their response could be to become aggressive or distressed. Some service users may find it difficult to manage their own emotions. Care workers should be in full control of their own emotions and should not become angry or threatened but instead should be able to remain calm. Behaviour

that fails to value service users can take a variety of forms:

- threatening behaviour
- sexual harassment
- environmental abuse
- violence
- racial abuse
- verbal abuse and gossip.

Threatening behaviour

One example of threatening behaviour is to shout at a service user. If a service user feels threatened, their immediate reaction may be to retaliate with similar behaviour, even though they may feel frightened.

Threatening behaviour is totally unacceptable on the part of a care worker. This does not mean that the care worker should not have feelings of anger or frustrations, for example, but they should have developed ways to overcome them in order to remain calm and professional. A service user, however, may not be able to disguise their anger or frustration, as they may be very vulnerable and be unable to cope with their circumstances.

Case study

Miles

Miles has been living in a residential home for at least seven years. He is now 78 and has severe dementia. He remembers very little, and constantly repeats himself and asks the same question over and over.

One care worker at the residential home is very impatient with Miles. Miles asks the care worker several times if it is tea time yet. The care worker shouts at Miles and says, 'If you ask me that again, I'll tie you to your bed, you old fool.'

The care worker's response in the case study above is unacceptable. The care worker should have been able to manage the situation better. He or she should have:

- stayed calm
- breathed slowly

- been respectful
- valued the service user as an individual
- given the service user a task to do to divert his attention.

Children can feel very threatened if a teacher or playgroup assistant towers over them. When talking with children, whatever the situation, it is best to be at the same height and to use a firm but sympathetic tone of voice.

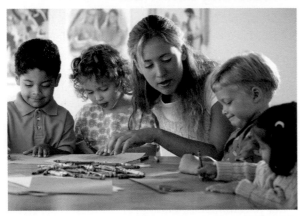

A non-threatening relationship

Violence

If a care worker is violent, for example, hitting, pushing, kicking or assaulting a service user, it is likely that physical, emotional and psychological harm will be caused. The service user will be fearful and intimidated and is likely to be violent in return. If a care worker has committed an act of violence, the service user will not receive the help they need because they will be afraid to ask for it – they may lose their self-confidence. Similarly, if a care worker has been assaulted by a service user, that care worker could become anxious and distressed, resulting in a deterioration in the quality of their work.

Sexual harassment

Sexual harassment involves unwelcome sexual attention or the display of printed material of a sexual nature which gives offence. A service user who is being sexually harassed will be affected emotionally and this could lead to depression and anxiety. They could become withdrawn, keeping information to themselves and be totally lacking in trust.

A female service user who has experienced being touched by a male care worker in personal and private parts of their body, for example, may have a low self-worth and become very angry with others or, in the other extreme, could become very withdrawn, not speaking or sharing anything with others. Any observation of sexual harassment should be reported immediately to a line manager.

Verbal abuse

Saying harsh, hurtful or damaging things is a form of verbal abuse. It also involves falsely accusing someone, shouting and raging at another, constantly criticising, being insulting or patronising. This type of behaviour can leave emotional scars, by lowering self-esteem, as the service user is likely to view themselves in a negative light. A service user who has been verbally abused is unlikely to have confidence in a care worker. It can reduce the trust they have in a care worker, resulting in a break down in the relationship.

Behaviour of this type also shows that the care worker does not value the service user as an individual, is not applying the care values and does not show respect.

Gossip

Gossip is idle chatter about people. It becomes damaging when a person slanders another by divulging confidential information that has been entrusted to them. Such action can cause misery and distress, besides destroying or preventing successful relationships. It can result in hurt feelings and may also harm a service user's reputation, lowering their self-esteem. Gossiping can cause communication to break down between a care worker and service user. For example, if sensitive personal information is revealed, this will affect the service user's ability to trust a care worker.

In the case study opposite, Howard's ability to trust people with personal information will be severely affected. He is less likely to talk about any difficulties or worries he has. Building a good working relationship with Howard will probably be very difficult.

Racial abuse

Racial abuse can include name-calling or racial violence and sends out the message that the person being abused is thought to be inferior. If a service user is being racially abused, they could live in fear of others, worrying about whether they will be safe going out. This could lead to social isolation, depression and anxiety and a low self-esteem. Occasionally, racial abuse could lead a service user to believe that what is being said about them is true, damaging their self-worth.

Environmental abuse

Environmental abuse can include damaging property or leaving a service user in unhealthy or uncomfortable conditions. For example, in a residential home, having the temperature of a bedroom so low that it causes an older person to feel uncomfortable is an environmental abuse. If a room is too cold for comfortable communication, the service user is likely to withdraw from the conversation; if it is too hot, they may fall asleep. If environmental abuse occurs, a service user could be uncomfortable and fearful. Communicating with the service user will be difficult.

Different ways of communicating with service users

Communication in a care setting can take a variety of forms. Whichever method of communication is being used in a care setting, the service user needs to be empowered and should feel that they are valued. Forms of communication include:

- verbal communication, i.e. speaking and listening
- electronic communication, e.g. e-mail
- special methods of communication, e.g. Braille and sign language
- written communication, e.g. care plans
- body language, e.g. smiling.

Communication is an **interaction** between two or more people. It is a two-way process of giving and receiving information.

Verbal communication

In order to have a meaningful conversation with someone, you need to develop the appropriate skills of **social co-ordination**. This means:

- showing an interest
- being interesting
- having the ability to start conversations and end them.

It also means using skills such as listening, clarifying, summarising and knowing how to be **assertive**. Being assertive means not letting the other person take the interaction in a direction that is meaningless, i.e. focusing the interaction on the points that need to be explored.

Professional care workers should know *how* to use these skills when communicating and *when* to use them. The work that is done in care settings depends very much on using effective communication, which requires care workers to:

- **analyse** their own thoughts and think about what they are going to say
- **interpret** the language and non-verbal behaviour of service users
- understand and draw conclusions
- present the next ideas to continue the conversation.

When communicating, messages are sent and information is disclosed. When communicating verbally, messages are encoded by a sender and decoded by a receiver. The diagram below shows this process.

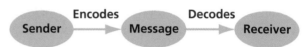

Sending and receiving messages

How would this apply to messages given and received in a care setting? Look at the example below.

> A care worker (**sender**) puts words together (**encodes**) to say, 'Palesha, when do you think we should make your next dental appointment?' (**message**).
>
> The service user (**receiver**) listens, the brain interprets the signal (**decodes**) and then the message is received.

Communication in health, social care and early years settings is likely to be **complex**, because it may have several purposes. Care workers need to be aware that each individual will have their own way of interpreting messages. Effective communication means more than just passing on information. It also means involving the other person.

The process of communicating can be seen as a series of stages in a cycle, as shown in the diagram at the top of the next page.

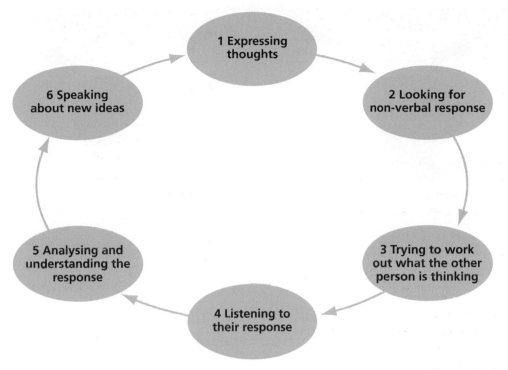

The communication cycle

Here is an example of how the communication cycle works:

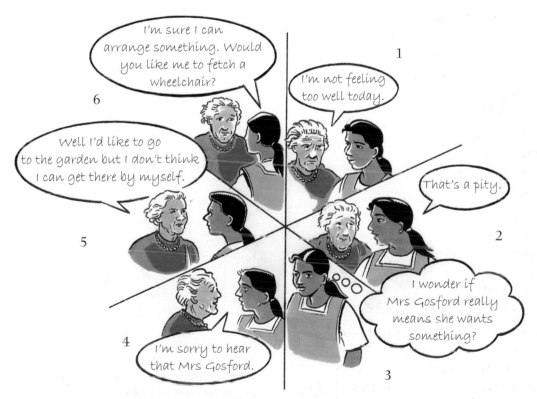

Sending and receiving messages

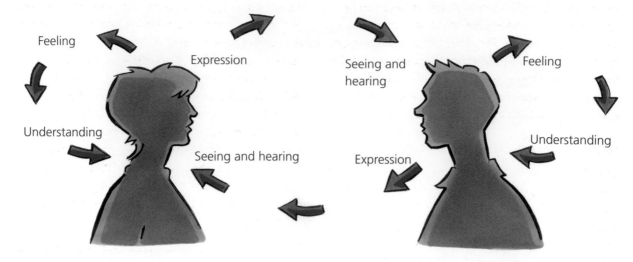

*The communication cycle requires **empathy** and active listening*

Communicating has to be a two-way process where each person tries to understand, interpret or make sense of what the other person is saying. Often it is easier to understand people who are similar to us, for example, a person who has the same accent, or a person who is in a similar situation to ourselves. Our decoding equipment in the brain tunes in, breaks down the message, analyses the message, understands it and interprets its meaning and then creates a response or answer. This is all helped by the body language or signals, such as smiles or gestures, used by the person who is speaking. When a care worker is speaking with a service user, they are forming a mental picture about what they are being told.

Written communication

The rules that govern writing are very different from those rules for verbal communication. In all health, social care and early years settings, it is very important that written communication is accurate. If inaccuracies occur in formal records, a service user could have the wrong treatment or be given incorrect information, with disastrous results. This could lead to a complaint being made or to court proceedings being taken. False, inaccurate or misleading written records could result in:

- inappropriate actions
- failure to act
- complaints and legal proceedings.

Date	Needs	Aim	Action	Evaluate
20/12/06	Personal hygiene	To wash, and clean teeth	Assisst Mr S to bathroom Use hoist to get him into bath Help to wash back Leave Mr S to wash parts that are possible, and to soak Make sure Mr S can pull alarm cord if needed Use hoist to get Mr S out of bath Provide chair for Mr S to sit at basin to clean teeth	

Part of a care plan for Mr S

When writing information down, it needs to be clear, accurate and legible. Written records are used in care settings for care plans, monitoring a service user's health, menus and personal details, for example. Opposite is an example of part of a care plan for a service user, which involves the use of written information.

Non-verbal communication

Communication can be enhanced through appropriate use of **body language**, which is also called **non-verbal** communication. Body language can give the receiver of the message a context. In other words, it helps the person who is receiving the message to know, for example, whether the person is being welcoming or if they are trying to distance themselves from the situation. Similarly, the care worker can show through their non-verbal communication if they are friendly and responsive to the needs of the service user. Examples of non-verbal communication include:

- smiling
- gestures
- positive positioning
- facial expressions
- touching
- eye contact.

The gestures a person uses can indicate a friendly or unfriendly approach. For example, drumming the fingers or twiddling the thumbs probably conveys impatience. Signalling a child, for example, to come to a care worker using an outstretched arm and a beckoning gesture, could mean the care worker is happy with them and wants them to come closer. Alternatively, the same gesture could mean that a care worker wants to question them about what they were doing. The accompanying facial expression and tone of voice indicates which message is being conveyed.

Care workers need to be aware that a gesture that is acceptable in one culture may be unacceptable in another.

Hand gestures can be involved in the use of Makaton, which is a language programme based on a series of signs that represents language. It follows a specific teaching procedure and is combined with appropriate facial expressions, body language and speech. It is mainly used with people who have learning difficulties.

Every individual likes to have an area around them which is their own and that others do not invade. Positive positioning means ensuring that the service user is comfortable with the distance

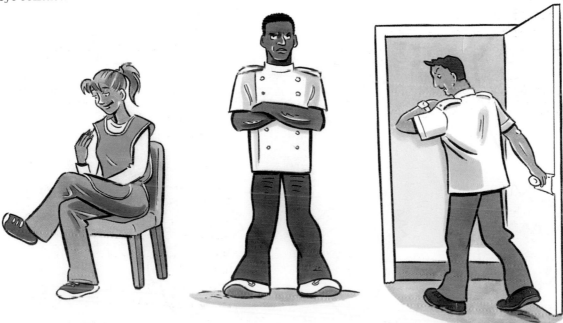

What message is being conveyed by each care worker?

between them and the care worker. For example, if a care worker is conveying a personal piece of information, they may sit or stand very close to the person to whom they are speaking. On the other hand, if they are giving an instruction they could be further apart.

Positioning depends on:

● the person's culture
● the feelings the two people have for one another
● the nature of the information.

Facial expression can communicate complex messages. A face that looks tense and grumpy sends out the message, 'Stay away, you are not welcome'. A forlorn or sad face can illicit sympathy. A happy, smiling face is more likely to draw the service user towards the care worker because it is welcoming, and shows warmth and openness. A smile encourages positive interaction.

Touching, for example shaking hands, can make a service user feel wanted and accepted. However, care workers should be very careful about touching a service user as the action can be misinterpreted and misunderstood. This is particularly so if different genders are involved, for example, a male nursery nurse giving a cuddle to a female child when the child is distressed. It is important to ensure that other staff are present if such a situation arises.

Making eye contact is recognised in western culture as a way of conveying interest in a conversation. It indicates to the listener that they are the central focus of the communication and that other things around are shut out. In some

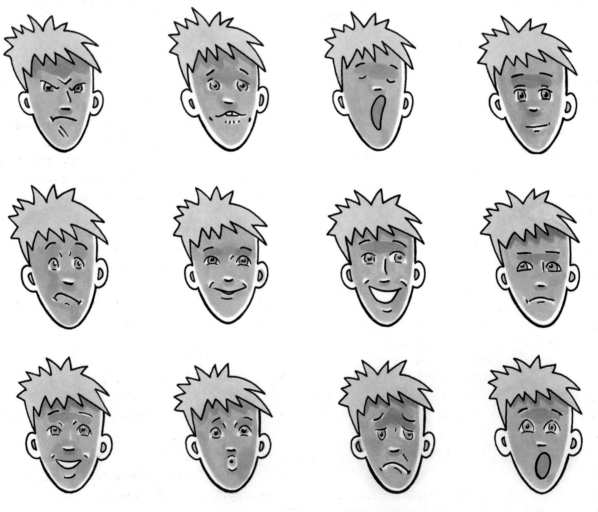

What are these facial expressions showing?

cultures, however, having direct eye contact is considered to be rude and should be avoided.

Computerised communication

Electronic forms of communication are now a well established method of exchanging information for businesses and individuals. Computers not only use the written word, but can also be used to present information in graphics and sound.

In health, social care and early years settings, computers can be used for networking between one organisation and another. For example, a health centre can use the computer to send information about a patient to a consultant at a clinic or to send a prescription to a pharmacy. Similarly, an internal network system can be in place so that employees within one setting can be linked with others to share information. It is very easy for organisations to update their information by using the computer; therefore, it is time- and cost-effective.

Electronic mail (e-mail) can be both formal and informal, depending on its purpose. Sending an e-mail can be advantageous as it is a very quick way of interacting with another person or organisation. Answers can be received in a matter of minutes, rather than having to wait several days for a letter. When sending e-mails that contain confidential information, care has to be taken to ensure that a secure system is in place before the information is sent.

Increasingly, the internet is being used as a source of information for a variety of purposes. The internet can also allow for on-line discussion where service users can voice their opinions or obtain advice in a quick and cost-effective way. Video conferencing is also an easy way to have virtual meetings, with people from different locations communicating exactly as they would had they all been in the same place. Video conferencing can save time, energy and the inconvenience of having to travel, and can be more productive.

In all situations, care must be taken to ensure that the requirements of the Data Protection Act are followed when using the computer. The Act:

- gives responsibilities to those keeping personal information about people
- requires that a service user be given a copy of any information which is kept about them; this is known as 'right of access'
- requires that any inaccurate information about a service user is corrected or deleted
- gives a service user the right to complain to the Data Protection Commissioner if they think someone is keeping data and is not complying with the Act
- allows service users to claim compensation through the courts if they suffer damage through mishandling of information about themselves
- permits a service user to find out from any person or organisation whether information is being kept about them and if they do, to be told the type of information kept and the purposes for which it is kept.

People keeping personal information must give individuals access to their personal information and must correct or delete any information found to be inaccurate. Settings must:

- obtain personal information fairly and openly
- use it only in ways compatible with the purpose for which it was given in the first place
- secure it against unauthorised access or loss
- ensure that it is kept accurate and up-to-date.

A setting must not:

- disclose information to others in a manner incompatible with the purpose for which it was given
- retain information for longer than is necessary for the purpose for which it was given.

Special methods

Any health, social care and early years setting may need to provide for service users who have special communication needs. This could include:

- difficulty in hearing or deafness
- poor sight or blindness
- language difficulty, e.g. not speaking English as a first or preferred language.

Visit a care setting or invite a care worker to your centre (with your tutor's permission) to find out about the different types of communication used in their care setting. Try to obtain some examples of written communications used by the setting.

A variety of organisations can help to provide specialist equipment or specialists to help with such needs, for example, the provision of interpreters, or Makaton and sign language specialists, or materials in Braille.

The purpose of communicating

Communication can have different purposes (see the table below), and in any one form of communication there may be several purposes.

Purpose of communication	Explanation and examples
To give information	Information must be given using language that is clear and accurate and which does not confuse the receiver through over-use of technical terminology.
	Examples: times of appointments, directions, diagnosis of illness, options available for care.
To obtain information	Obtaining information requires skilful use of language and very good listening skills in order to understand what is being said, reading skills to understand written information, or familiarisation with the use of special methods. Accuracy is of prime importance – a mistake could result in the wrong treatment being given or the wrong person being contacted.
	Examples: medical history, who to contact in the case of an emergency, allergies, social history.
To exchange ideas	This involves sharing ideas and usually occurs in oral communication. Being attentive, a good listener and showing an interest in what the other person has to say is important.
	Examples: exchanging views about proposed treatments, options for different types of care, what is in a picture (e.g. child at nursery).
To obtain views	Oral conversation can be the main medium for this although in some circumstances written questionnaires are used to obtain service users' views. If the latter is being used, great care needs to be taken over the preparation of questions to ensure they are not **ambiguous**.
	Examples: views about the way in which a residential home is managed, views relating to the complaints procedure, expressing an opinion about a treatment.
To give instructions To receive instructions	The person giving instructions must use vocabulary that is clear so that the instruction can be followed. Unambiguous communication is essential if others are expected to follow exactly what has been said. Short sentences are best used when verbal instructions are being given.
	Examples: fire evacuation, events, outings, tests (reception classes), taking medication.
To record actions To record medical/personal history	Recording actions could be paper-based or computerised. The purpose is to provide an accurate record of what has been done, what has taken place or perhaps to summarise what has happened in a meeting. Records must be accurate, legible and relevant.
	Examples: care plans, achievements, medical history, daily health monitoring, visitors' log.

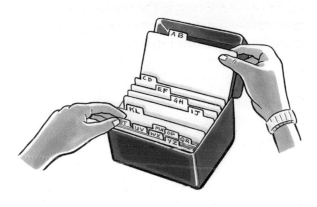

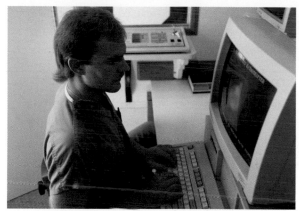

Both written and computerised records can be used

Decoding a message may, therefore, be quite complex, particularly if the service user is emotionally upset, is trying to hide something or has difficulty in expressing themselves.

The purposes of communication are the same whether the information is being exchanged orally, in written or computerised form or by any special methods.

Factors that contribute to establishing effective communication

Effective communication is at the heart of any relationship. It involves a care worker giving undivided attention and conveying acceptance of the service user. This means that care workers need to be aware of and to be able to use skills that will enhance communication, knowing when and how to use each skill.

Skills

In his book, *The Skilled Helper*, Gerard Egan suggested an **acronym** to summarise the components required for effective communication with others. The acronym he used was SOLER, as shown below.

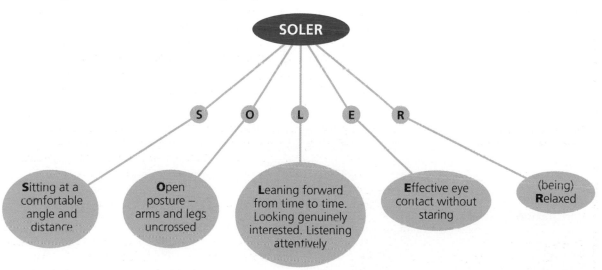

SOLER

S — **S**itting at a comfortable angle and distance

O — **O**pen posture – arms and legs uncrossed

L — **L**eaning forward from time to time. Looking genuinely interested. Listening attentively

E — **E**ffective eye contact without staring

R — (being) **R**elaxed

The components of communication

A number of skills can be used to enhance a conversation. The table opposite lists the skills with some examples.

Environment

Factors such as noise, heating, light, ventilation and seating can have an **enhancing** effect or an **inhibiting** effect on a conversation. The environmental factors shown in the table below must be taken into consideration when having an interaction with a service user.

Forming good relationships between care workers and service users means:

- showing respect and listening carefully
- not gossiping about personal information to others
- establishing a sense of trust with the service user
- using skills appropriate to the conversation
- making sure the environment is well prepared
- making sure the service user's disabilities (if any) have not prevented them from participating.

The care worker and the service user should be able to have direct eye-contact during a conversation. The care worker should have at least a mental plan, if not a written plan, of the desired layout and of the seating arrangements that will enhance the conversation.

Activity

Making environmental arrangements for a conversation

Grace is to have a conversation with the social worker and the team who are responsible for her care in the rehabilitation unit where she is staying. There will be seven people involved in the discussion.

1 Explain how the room should be prepared, making reference to the environmental conditions.

2 Look at the seating arrangements given in the socio-gram below:

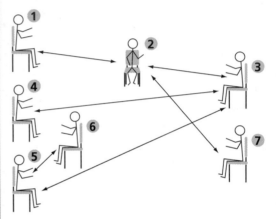

Is this the most effective arrangement?

a) Could all the participants see one another? Give reasons for why or why not.

b) Explain why it is important that all participants should have direct eye-contact.

Noise	Too much noise can prevent the service user from hearing the correct information and could lead to the wrong decision	If it is too quiet the service user may feel too embarrassed to speak
Ventilation	If a room is stuffy, the service user may lack concentration or appear disinterested	If a room is too well ventilated, the service user may lack concentration or fidget
Seating/ Proximity	Can the service user and the care worker see and hear one another easily? Has the care worker allowed the service user their own space?	
Lighting	Bright light may not encourage a service user to share information	Having the light too dim could lead to inaccurate information being recorded
Heating	Too much heat can cause a service user to be drowsy and fall asleep	Too little heat can cause fidgeting and lack of concentration

Skill	Explanation	Example
Closed question	These are questions which require a specific answer. They are a way of gathering facts, but do not provide the opportunity for a service user to express an opinion.	How old are you? What is your weight? How often do you attend the day care centre? Where do you live?
Open question	A care worker can gain insight from the answers given as the question gives the service user the opportunity to provide longer answers.	How do you feel about the actions that have been suggested for your treatment? Why do you like playing in the dressing-up corner? What do you think would help you with this problem?
Clarifying	This is putting your communication into order and making sure that there is no misunderstanding.	Oh, do you mean …? Did you say that you did not like the way you were spoken to? Remind me, what did you say you didn't want to do?
Prompts	A prompt is used to encourage a person to go on with what they are saying or to be more specific.	This is the worst thing that could ever happen to me. (Prompt) Worse in what way? Tell me more about what was actually said by the care assistant.
Summarising	When summarising, the relevant facts are outlined. Sometimes a summary is used to close a discussion and to move a conversation forward. Summarising brings together all the facts that have been scattered throughout the conversation.	It seems from what you have said that you would prefer to attend the day care centre twice each week instead of once? So, you would prefer your daughter not to be allowed to play on the large equipment outside because …?
Paraphrasing	Paraphrasing is to reword what someone has said to show what you have understood by it, and to check that you have understood it correctly. It captures the main points of what they have said.	So you think you would like to try some complementary approaches to care? Do I understand that it is Sid's threatening attitude that is worrying you?
Tone	Tone indicates whether the speaker is being friendly or aggressive. A warm friendly approach is more likely to help build a trusting relationship, whereas a tone that suggests a person is too busy to speak sends the message that they do not value the individual who is on the receiving end.	Hello, come and sit here and tell me how you got on. You'll have to keep that news until later. I've still got to get Dolly up.
Pace	This is the speed at which we speak. When nervous, a person will often speak much too fast. Some people will speak at the same speed all the way through a conversation which makes the dialogue boring! Care workers should be aware that they need to alter the speed at which they speak in order to add interest to a conversation.	Have you heard the news? (fairly rapid speech) They then told me I would need an operation. (fairly slow speech to emphasise the point being made). … and do you know, I then had to do three other exercises … (slightly speeded up to draw attention to the point being made)
Empathy	To empathise is to see a person's world as they see it, to be able to step into their shoes and to see things through their eyes. It is accepting a person 'warts and all' and valuing them as an individual. It does not mean liking the individual or the things they do, but being able to see things from their perspective.	So, when you're on drugs you feel as though you can cope with anything? But how does it feel when they wear off?
Reflection	To reflect is to look back during the conversation and to recap the most important points. By using reflection, the care worker draws the service user back to think about what has been said, but they also move them on to a new focus.	We have talked about what you don't want to happen in your care plan and you have explained why. Can you talk me through what care you think would be appropriate?
Assertiveness	To be assertive is to be focused. Sometimes a service user will want to talk about every illness they have experienced, but there may not be time for this. The care worker will need to firmly draw the service user back to the purpose of the conversation.	I am really interested in hearing about all the different illnesses you have experienced, but can we for the present just concentrate on the one that has brought you to see me?

Social, emotional and physical factors contributing to effective communication

Abraham Maslow (1908–70) developed a theory that human life could be understood in terms of the development of an individual's ability and potential. He suggested that we all have levels of needs which have to be met.

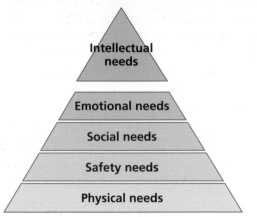

Maslow's hierarchy of needs

Pyramid from top to bottom:
- Intellectual needs
- Emotional needs
- Social needs
- Safety needs
- Physical needs

Care workers will need to be aware of the service user's **p**hysical, **i**ntellectual, **e**motional and **s**ocial needs (PIES). The service user will trust the care worker not to do anything that harms them. Whether they trust the care worker or not will probably be based on the care worker's attitudes and on the previous interactions that the service user has had with the care worker. A lack of clear communication could result in a service user's physical, safety, social, emotional and intellectual needs not being met.

Assessment activity 2.3

Ways of communicating

1 Identify **three** different ways of communicating that could be used in **one** of these settings:
- GP surgery/health centre
- day care centre
- reception class at an infant school
- residential home.

2 Arrange a visit to a care setting to find out about the different ways of communicating, for example:
- written
- non-verbal
- computerised
- verbal
- special methods.

If a visit to a care setting is not possible, you could, with your tutor's permission, arrange for a care worker to visit your centre.

3 Produce materials to explain the purpose of each way of communicating and give some examples, based on the care setting you have chosen.

4 Produce information about the skills that could be used to aid oral communication between care workers and service users in one care setting. Show how these skills could be used to enhance communication between care workers and service users.

5 Produce materials to provide care workers with information about three factors that contribute to establishing effective communication in the care setting chosen. You could choose factors from:
- environmental factors
- social factors
- emotional factors
- physical factors.

Barriers to communication

What can inhibit communication? If two or more people are trying to hold a conversation, it can take only one small point to prevent that conversation from being successful. Barriers or inhibiting factors can include:

- environmental factors
- social factors
- emotional instability
- inappropriate language
- lack of skills
- inappropriate behaviour
- cultural barriers
- use of gestures
- lack of confidentiality
- incorrect positioning.

Environmental barriers

For a conversation to be successful, the service user must feel comfortable. They must also feel relaxed and be able to concentrate on what is being said. If they do not feel comfortable, the service user is likely to be uneasy and distracted.

One environmental factor is noise. For example, if a conversation is being held near an open window where traffic is constantly moving, braking and stopping, a service user may not hear what is being said or could misinterpret the information. This is particularly important if the service user has a hearing impairment as their aid may receive all the background noise.

Similarly, if a room is too quiet, the service user may be reluctant to speak, particularly if in a one-to-one situation with a care worker. Sometimes, very soft and unobtrusive music in the background will help to put a service user at ease.

Social barriers

A social barrier can occur when a service user feels inferior or if they feel that the care worker or other members of the group are 'looking down on them'. In other words, if they are showing that they feel the service user is of less value than themselves or if the service user feels patronised.

Building a professional relationship with a service user takes time and effort. It is important that the care worker knows themselves well and that they are aware of any prejudices they may have. These prejudices can influence a situation and inhibit conversation. The psychologist Sigmund Freud called this process by which feelings become known to others as **transference**. This means that if the care professional or others within the group have unfavourable feelings and attitudes towards those to whom they are speaking, the interaction could become prejudiced.

Barriers can be formed within groups, for example, when:

- the objectives of an interaction are not understood by all participants
- there is a lack of trust between participants
- there is a clash of personalities within the group.

Bruce Tuckman, a theorist on the subject of communication, considers that there are usually four stages in group interactions:

1 Forming – a quietness and waiting period where participants are reluctant to speak

2 Storming – where individuals put forward views and opinions but where sometimes clashes of personality occur

3 Norming – where groups are not quite so tense and really start to share knowledge and experiences

4 Performing – individuals begin to work independently.

If barriers are not to form, discussion within groups must be led very carefully.

Emotional barriers

If a service user is upset, for example because they have received bad news or because they have had a disagreement with someone, emotional barriers will emerge. During an interaction, a service user will need to feel safe and secure. If they feel they are being neglected or misunderstood, they are likely to withdraw and become quiet, or alternatively could become very aggressive. Care workers need to remember that a conversation with a service user is part of their working relationship and that they are not conversing with a friend. It is important that a service user:

● feels that the care worker has empathy and empathetic understanding
● considers that they are being offered **unconditional positive regard**
● knows that the person or persons with whom they are talking are genuine or **congruent**.

Egan (2002) considers that 'empathy is not passive', i.e. the care worker needs to show that a genuine interest is being taken in the service user. Barriers are less likely to form if the care worker, or others involved in an interaction, focuses entirely on what is being said. Having 'unconditional positive regard' means accepting a service user as they are and not as you would like them to be. This means listening carefully to what is being said and responding without prejudice or bias. Being 'congruent' means being sincere, open and honest and that issues are dealt with sensitively, without being judgemental.

If a service user feels emotionally safe, they are more likely to reveal their innermost feelings, being able to talk confidently and without fear.

Inappropriate language

Have you ever been involved in a conversation where the speaker has used so much technical language or used difficult vocabulary that you have felt that they were speaking in an unknown language? This type of behaviour will certainly cause barriers in any interaction. There are, of course, occasions when some technical terms will need to be used, but these should be clarified

within the conversation so that the receiver of the message is not wondering what has been meant, as in the case study below.

Case study

Edna

Edna went for a consultation at the hospital. She was given several diagnostic tests as her skin had turned a dark yellow colour and she was no longer able to eat. Following the diagnosis, a group of specialists involved in the tests and the consultant asked Edna and her husband into the office to discuss the situation. Each used correct and complex technical terminology to explain their findings. Edna listened and didn't understand any of what was being said until a nurse asked, 'Where would you prefer to die? At home or in a hospice?' Edna was so shocked she fainted!

The case study above is an extreme example, but care needs to be taken to ensure that language is appropriate for:

● the age of the service user
● the ability of the service user
● the situation being discussed.

Lack of skills

Look back at the earlier section relating to skills (page 77). From the information given, it is possible to understand which skills enhance communication.

If these skills are not put into practice, it is likely that an interaction will not be as successful as it should be. For example, silence or long pauses should not be viewed with dismay. Service users often need time to think about what has been said and to frame their response. Shyness too can have a detrimental effect on a conversation. A service user who is shy may struggle to express themselves or may be unable to use skills, either because of lack of knowledge or because they have a poor self-image.

As a care professional it is important to use skills effectively. Interactions that demonstrate a lack of skills are those:

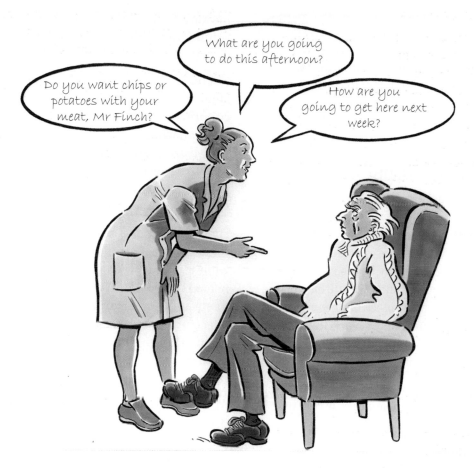

Which question does she want me to answer?

- that use multiple questioning techniques
- that are full of leading questions
- that have sentences that are too long and have no focus
- that use too many closed or monosyllabic questions
- in which listening is not active and there is a lack of genuine interest
- where there is a lack of congruency
- where tone and pace are not used appropriately.

Inappropriate behaviour

Inappropriate behaviour can take many forms:

- shouting, or talking too quietly
- speaking so that the lips and face cannot be seen
- using abusive language
- physically threatening a service user.

Inappropriate behaviour will contribute to a service user not feeling valued. This can result in their behaviour being:

- physically violent
- verbally aggressive
- tearful
- angry
- withdrawn.

Maslow considered that 'the goal of living is self-actualisation'. Look back at Maslow's pyramid of needs (page 22) and you will see that self-actualisation is at the top of the pyramid. If inappropriate behaviour is used, it is unlikely that a service user would be able to achieve their full potential. It also means that there is likely to be a poor relationship between the care worker and the service user or between service user and service user. A relationship without trust can lead to disaster!

Consider this

Why is inappropriate behaviour on the part of a care worker likely to cause a lack of trust?

Lack of confidentiality

If confidentiality is broken, it means that information that was personal and which was entrusted to another has been passed on to other people. This could have happened deliberately as a result of gossiping, or may be the result of unthinking behaviour. Whatever the cause, the realisation that confidentiality has been broken can have a detrimental effect on any future interactions. When this happens, a lack of trust develops between people.

Any interaction must be based on professionalism, where rules are observed and boundaries are set. It is essential that care workers know where the boundaries have been set and that these are not crossed. For example, a care worker should never promise to 'keep a secret', as they never know when other professionals will need to know this information in order to apply positive care. The information may be needed if the service user is intending to harm themselves or others, or if care is being provided by other organisations.

Everyone has the right to expect confidentiality to be maintained. Not to do so can seriously harm relationships.

The effect of culture

Neil Thompson, in his book *Communication and Language*, talks about 'the language game'. He shows that we are all highly skilled and become very adept at handling a variety of different behaviours, recognising which forms of language are appropriate in particular circumstances.

For some professionals, some words have different meanings. For example, a social worker may use the word 'interview' to indicate a formal meeting with a service user, but in a different culture this word could mean 'interrogation'; something which is not so pleasant!

Not understanding that words and body language can have different meanings in other cultures can prove to be a barrier when providing care and when communicating, particularly as we live in a multi-cultural society. Care workers need to be aware and to learn about the language perspectives of others and to appreciate the values, beliefs and practices of other cultures.

For example, talking in a familiar manner to someone of a different gender may be offensive, while touching a person to whom you are not related can be a form of body language that is totally unacceptable. In western culture, having direct eye-contact is considered to be desirable when having a conversation, but in some other cultures such behaviour would be considered rude.

In western society, older men and women may consider that calling them by their first name is disrespectful, being preferred to be called Mr Tate and Mrs Connor, rather than Steve and Mary. Some subjects may also be considered taboo or personal by older adults, such as talking about sexual illness, their income or their savings. Some individuals may have been brought up at a time when challenging authority by asking questions was not permitted. Such people may be reluctant to ask GPs, for example, difficult questions and are less likely to ask questions about their treatment or to express their concerns.

Care must be taken to ensure that service users do not feel that care workers are trying to dominate them or to have power over them. As a result they could act in a defensive manner and be uncooperative.

It is the professional care worker's responsibility to provide support when communicating with service users. Communication is an important aspect of caring, and diversity of language must be respected. In some interactions, a translation of the information that is being shared may be needed.

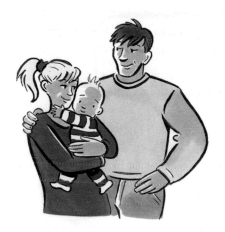
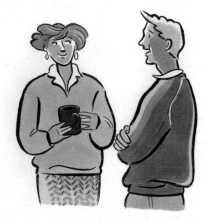
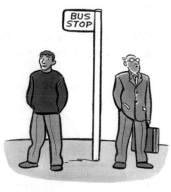

How much space?

The effect of positioning

How close do you like someone to be when they are talking with you? Have you ever had a conversation with someone who stands very near to you and almost puts their face into yours? Unless you know the person very well, you will probably find that this is a very unpleasant experience!

Not giving a service user their own space can inhibit communication. How much space do we need? For example, some people from other cultures prefer to keep a large space around them and may feel threatened if a care worker comes too close.

On the other hand, being too far away can also produce barriers. For example, attempting to give a service user information when you are two metres away would also prove to be a barrier, as confidentiality could not be maintained and it is unlikely that the service user will hear all the information, particularly if they are suffering from a hearing impairment.

For a one-to-one interaction, a 'social zone' is probably the best positioning. It is important, however, that arms and legs are not crossed as this could also be a barrier.

The effect of the use of gestures

Sometimes, gestures can hinder communication between service users. Gestures should be used to aid understanding, but when they are used in a haphazard way and when there are too many of them, this can cause confusion.

It is important to be aware of what is acceptable and what is not acceptable for service users in different cultures. For example, in western cultures, holding the thumb up is a sign that something is good, but in another culture the same sign can be insulting!

The effect of barriers on self-esteem and relationships

Barriers that inhibit communication can have serious effects on self-esteem and relationships. They can affect how an individual feels about themselves and how they see themselves in relation to others.

Relationships with others can also be disadvantaged to such an extent that lack of trust between both parties can lead to feelings of guilt and anger. Michael Argyle, a psychologist, considers that each individual looks at the reactions of others to find out what they themselves are like. This contributes to the formation of self-esteem through self-image. If barriers have come between participant communicators, self-esteem is likely to be low.

As individuals develop, they incorporate more and more roles into their self-image. If the image is threatened as a result of communication barriers, anger, depression or withdrawal is likely

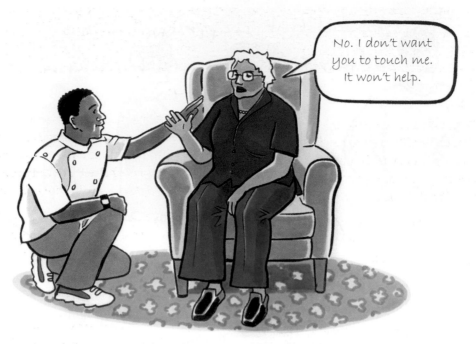

No. I don't want you to touch me. It won't help.

Some actions can have a detrimental effect on self-esteem

to result, as the service user's social role could have been affected.

Adolescents who experience barriers when communicating are likely to exclude those who are 'at fault' and may exclude themselves from the company of the person who has offended. The tendency will be to isolate themselves from friendships, advice and to develop a feeling of hatefulness.

When working with service users, great care should be taken to help them to explore situations in an atmosphere where they will be accepted and helped to move on. They will need to understand the facts and explore their feelings.

Assessment activity 2.4

Barriers to communication

Choose **one** of these care settings:
- GP surgery/health centre
- day care centre
- reception class in a primary school
- residential home.

1 For your chosen care setting, produce materials to show the care workers the different types of barriers that could be experienced when using or working in the care setting. Give examples of barriers to communication. These could include, for example:
- environmental
- social
- use of inappropriate language
- lack of skills
- inappropriate behaviour
- lack of confidentiality
- culture
- positioning
- use of gestures.

2 Produce materials to show the care workers the likely effects of barriers on the service users in your chosen care setting. These could include:
- effects on their relationships
- effects on their self-esteem.

Planning

An interaction will need to be planned. This means that an order will need to be established, a sequence which will ensure that all the information is discussed and that feelings and options are explored. Good planning will involve:

- setting the overall aim for the interaction
- determining the objectives that will provide stepping stones to reach the aim
- considering the factors that are likely to contribute to making the interaction effective
- taking into consideration any special needs that the service user has, for example, having a different language from our own or having a hearing aid
- taking into account the physical, intellectual, emotional and social needs of the service user
- making sure that constraints are minimised
- working out approximate timescales.

Aim

Before beginning on any interaction it is important to decide on the aim. The aim is the overall purpose and outcome required.

Case study

Carmen

Marguerite, a care assistant who works in a residential home for older adults, has been asked by Carmen, a resident who has a mild form of dementia, to help her respond to a letter she has received from her friend, Joan. Carmen is not able to do very much for herself without help.

Carmen's illness is such that she can still recognise people, but she does have short-term memory loss. This often causes her to be distressed, frustrated and even angry if she misplaces her belongings.

The aim of the interaction with Carmen is to help her to organise her response to a letter that she has received.

Objectives

To achieve the aim, Marguerite will need to set **objectives**. These are the stages that she will make within the plan to make sure that the aim is met. Most aims require three or four objectives. The objectives that Marguerite has made are to:

- encourage Carmen to her bedroom so that she is not disturbed while carrying out the task
- help Carmen to find the equipment she will need in order to do the task
- talk to Carmen to help her reply to her correspondence
- help Carmen to address the envelope and to obtain the correct stamps that will be needed.

Factors that contribute to effective communication

Having set the aim and the objectives, the factors that ensure that the communication is effective must be considered. These could include:

- environment
- special needs
- positive positioning
- emotional and social factors
- physical factors
- skills.

These factors have been considered earlier in the unit. Look back to remind yourself of the detail that is involved. In Carmen's interaction, Marguerite has planned to consider:

Environmental factors

- Location: the interaction will need to be carried out in a private place which is familiar to Carmen. This will be her bedroom, where she will have her own things around her. She will be quite free to move around her room as she wishes. In this way, Marguerite and Carmen will be free from interruption. Carmen will also have her own things around her which she can talk about if she wishes.

- Noise: if others are talking to Carmen, it is likely that she will lose her train of thought or that she will talk only when it is absolutely necessary. Due to her mild form of dementia, Carmen will tend to repeat things frequently. In the quiet area of her bedroom, Carmen is less likely to be interrupted and to have distractions.
- Lighting: in the community areas there is fluorescent lighting, but in Carmen's bedroom, lighting is softer as bedside lamps are available as well as a main light. If the day is bright and clear, sunlight will come through the large window so artificial lighting may not be needed at all. The light from the window will be sufficient to read the letter and, if not, either a small light or the main room light can be put on.
- Heating: the central heating is on throughout the home. If the residents are cold, they can either turn the heating up or put on the fire that they each have in their bedrooms. Carmen feels the cold and often likes to sit next to the fire with a blanket around her. If Marguerite holds the interaction in the bedroom, Carmen can snuggle into her blanket by the fire if she feels the need. A small table is kept in the bedroom and this can be moved to wherever Carmen is so that she has something to rest on when writing the letter.

Special needs

Carmen does have special needs. She:

- is unable to concentrate for long periods of time
- has short-term memory loss
- lacks confidence
- occasionally has co-ordination problems.

Marguerite will need to take these into consideration when planning the interaction. She may find that she has to break up the interaction by allowing Carmen to talk about some of the items in her room, for example, the photographs of her family. When planning, Marguerite considers that Carmen may ask her to write a few lines for her if her co-ordination is poor at that time. Marguerite may have to give

confidence to Carmen by praising her when her memory is accurate. By taking such actions, Marguerite is trying to minimise barriers to the interaction.

Positive positioning

Making sure that Carmen is sitting comfortably will be important as this can prevent distraction from occurring. Marguerite knows she will need to place her chair near to Carmen, but with sufficient space between to prevent Carmen feeling crowded. Marguerite also considers when planning that it may also be a good idea if she can see Carmen's facial expressions and have direct eye-contact with her. Being too near could make Carmen feel threatened, but being too far away could cause her to feel rejected. Marguerite will have to make sure that sufficient space is allowed to enable Carmen to look at objects, such as her correspondence and photographs.

Physical, intellectual, emotional and social needs

Making sure that physical, intellectual and social needs are met is an important part of Marguerite's plan for Carmen when considering the interaction. She has shown that she is very much aware of Carmen's lack of concentration and has made provision for this by breaking up the tasks into smaller manageable parts, interspersed with different types of interactions, for example, talking about photographs in Carmen's bedroom.

Carmen's emotional needs will also have to be considered. For example, she will need to feel safe, secure and be able to trust Marguerite. Having the interaction in Carmen's bedroom will help her to feel safe and secure. Marguerite knows that she will need to build a trusting relationship with Carmen. This has already been partially achieved as Carmen has already asked Marguerite to help her with the task of responding to the letter. Marguerite can expand this further by talking to Carmen at an appropriate pace and tone, in a manner that is not patronising. She will also allow time for Carmen to think about her responses and allow her to make choices.

Social factors have been considered in so far as there is less likelihood of interruptions from other residents as the interaction is to be held in Carmen's bedroom.

Physical factors such as seating arrangements, proximity and environmental factors have all been considered.

Minimising constraints

One additional action could be taken to minimise constraints during the interaction. A notice could be placed on the door asking people not to disturb the meeting.

Marguerite intends to arrange the room in order to encourage communication:

- the window will be shut to prevent outside noise from penetrating into the room
- Marguerite's chair will be placed next to Carmen's but with sufficient space between so that Carmen does not feel overpowered
- the fire will be on low so that Carmen is warm

- a table will be placed nearby so that it can be used to put materials on for writing
- there will be no trailing wires across the floor, which is a health and safety requirement.

Timescales

A good plan will give the approximate timescales for action. Marguerite will need to have some idea about how long the preparation will take. She will also need to gauge how long the interaction will take overall and approximately how long the various parts of the interaction will last. To give some idea of the overall timescales, Marguerite will need to produce a plan. The example plan on the next page shows how this could be done.

Stages of an interaction

There are three main stages to any interaction:

- introduction or greeting
- the main content
- winding up, including some reflection

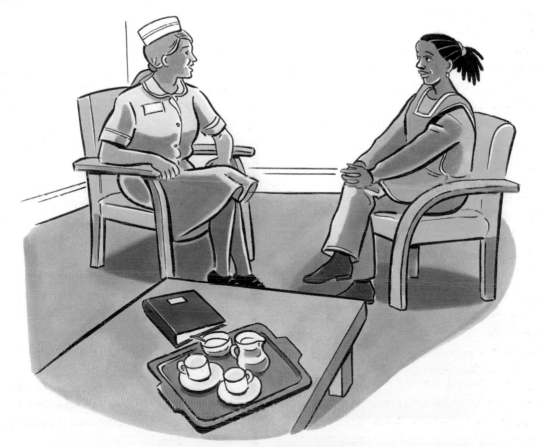

Effective communication is more likely to take place in comfortable surroundings

Date and time	Action	Reason for action
20/12/06 9.30am	Fix a time and place for the meeting	So that everyone is aware of what time and where it will be
21/12/06 9.45am	Prepare room – make environmental checks	To ensure it is laid out to enhance communication and prevent barriers
21/12/06 10.00am	Prepare tea/coffee tray	To make service user welcome...

Working out the order of actions to be carried out with timescales

Introduction

During any introductory session, whatever the topic, the care worker will need to:

- welcome the service user, if not known or if only slightly known – probably extending a hand in the form of a handshake, smiling and making direct eye contact
- inform the service user of their name and enquire how the service user would like to be addressed
- invite the service user to sit down and explain the aim of the interaction.

Carmen is already at the residential home and knows the care assistant well, so in this instance the greeting will be short. Marguerite will need to remind Carmen that they agreed to meet to work out how Carmen could respond to the letter she received.

Marguerite will also need to suggest that they move to Carmen's bedroom, which has been prepared for the interaction.

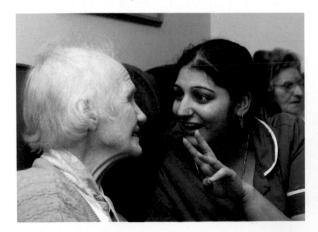

Use a friendly, warm tone for any interaction

Marguerite will need to use a friendly, warm tone and be careful not to overwhelm Carmen by being too loud or confuse her by speaking too quietly. Marguerite knows she will need to speak at an appropriate pace, not speaking too quickly or in a rush, and needs to give Carmen time to think. Carmen would be given Marguerite's complete attention, showing that she is interested in her and values her as an individual.

Activity

Communicating with a service user in a residential home

As a care assistant you are working with Pat, who is a resident at Hedge End Residential Home. Pat wants some help to plan a short walk for herself.

1 Write two closed questions that could be used while working with Pat during the introduction to the interaction.

2 Write two open questions that could be used when working with Pat during the initial stage of the interaction.

3 Give some ideas of the body language that would be appropriate to use while working with Pat at the introductory stage of the activity. Explain the reasons for the use of each.

4 Prepare a transcript of the conversation during the first contact with the Pat. Indicate:
- closed questions
- open questions
- an example of reflection.

5 What other factors would you take into consideration when interacting with Pat to make sure the communication is as effective as possible?

Main contact

The main part of the conversation can take place immediately following the introduction or initial contact. The care worker will have decided before starting the conversation what the main purpose is to be, for example to:

- obtain information
- give information
- exchange views
- reflect on the past
- help with a task
- explore a topic.

Use of skills

In this part of the conversation, Marguerite is likely to use more open questions so that the service user can expand the information she is giving. Some closed questions will be used in order to gather specific information.

When planning the interaction, a 'skills checklist' will need to be prepared. This can be used to make sure that all the necessary skills that are relevant to the interaction are included. Such a list will also help to focus the mind on the order or sequence of the content. For example, the checklist produced by Marguerite for her interaction with Carmen could look like the one below.

Example skills checklist	
1 Use of open questions	☐
2 Use of closed questions	☐
3 Simple words used to convey meaning	☐
4 Speaking slowly and clearly to make sure Carmen has understood	☐
4 Clarifying points made	☐
5 Use of reflective listening	☐
6 Use of summarising techniques	☐
7 Prompts and probes	☐

Skills such as clarifying, reflecting and summarising will be used, as will appropriate body language. Sometimes a conversation will need some help to 'move it along', as the person speaking may have run out of steam or be stuck on a particular thought. Examples of phrases that can be used to help a conversation along are:

- Please continue
- Do tell me more
- So ...
- Uh-hmm
- I see.

Carmen may have given quite a lot of information and may have included some ideas and thoughts that are muddled or confusing. If this happens, Marguerite may need to clarify (check) what the service user is actually saying or wants. Examples of clarifying are:

- So do you mean ...?
- Do I understand that you ...?

Whether a conversation is in a group or on a one-to-one basis, care workers may need to summarise. This means to bring together all that has been said in a short sentence or two which 'sums up' a particular part of the conversation. Examples of summarising could be:

- Just to make sure that I have understood what you have agreed ...
- You seem to prefer ...

At the top of the next page is an example of part of a main contact that Marguerite might plan to have with Carmen.

From this planned outline transcript of the main part of the conversation between Marguerite and Carmen, it is possible to see that the care assistant has used a wide range of skills to encourage Carmen. She starts the conversation with a closed question, to help her focus on the task to be done. Later in the conversation, she uses open questions to try to draw out ideas from Carmen. During the conversation, she plans to try to help Carmen to feel relaxed by leaning slightly forward when speaking and through showing a genuine interest in what she is saying. She will actively listen and used reflection to show that she is listening by repeating some of the things said in a different way.

Marguerite: Are you going to show me the letter that you want to answer, Carmen?

Carmen: Yes, here it is. I can't remember who it's from.

Marguerite: Shall we look at the end of the letter? What is the signature, Carmen?

Carmen: Oh, it's from Joan. That's right, I wanted to write back to her.

Marguerite: Shall we do that next then, Carmen?

Carmen: Yes, will you help me? Oh! Where have I put my pen?

Marguerite: Shall we do it together, Carmen? Your pen is on the writing table.

Carmen: Yes, so it is, and there's the card I want to write on as well!

Marguerite: You put your address in here. You can copy it from this piece of paper where it's printed, at the top. Good, that's fine. Now what do you think you should say in your letter?

Carmen: I want to tell her about that concert we had here last week. The music was so good.

Marguerite: The concert last week that had all the old songs in it?

Carmen: Yes, I enjoyed that. I knew most of the songs. We used to sing them when we were younger.

Marguerite: OK, let's see if we can get that down. What do you think you should write? ... Shall I read it back for you?

Carmen: Have you seen this photo? It's Joan when she was younger.

Marguerite: Where was that taken, Carmen?

Carmen: It was when we went to the beach five years ago. It was a lovely day.

Marguerite: What shall we write next then, Carmen?

Carmen: I would like her to come and see me.

Marguerite: Do you mean you would like her to come here to see you?

Carmen: Yes, I wonder if she could come next week?

Marguerite: Why don't you ask her to visit you?

Carmen: That's a good idea. I'll ask her to come next week. How shall I put it?

Marguerite: Would next week be too soon as she isn't likely to receive the letter until Friday? Why don't we think about asking her on the 28th when we have that special sing-along? Why don't you write ...

Activity

Communicating with Carmen

1 Read the transcript of the conversation above again. Select three closed questions and explain why they have been used.

2 From the transcript, select an example of reflection and give its purpose.

3 From the transcript, select two open questions. What is their purpose in this particular conversation?

6 Continue the conversation between Marguerite and Carmen. Make sure you use at least two closed questions, two open questions and include an example of clarifying or summarising.

Winding up the conversation

Bringing a conversation to a close successfully requires careful thought and the use of appropriate skills. The service user should feel that the conversation has reached a natural conclusion.

How a person ends a conversation can have a positive or negative effect on a service user and this has consequences on the relationship with that service user in the future. For example, if a conversation is ended abruptly, the service user may feel guilty because they have done something wrong and then they are not likely to communicate willingly with the care worker again.

A conversation is often ended by one of the participants giving a signal that they are ready to stop talking. This could be in the form of a sigh or increasingly long pauses or body language such

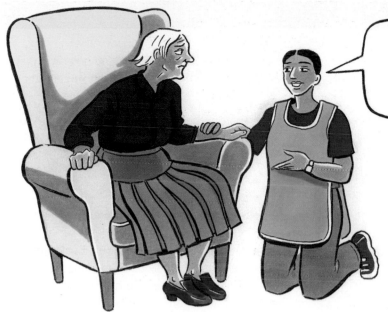

I'm glad you've talked about how unhappy you've been feeling. Now we can try to work at making things better.

Bringing a conversation to a close successfully requires careful thought and the use of appropriate skills

as restlessness, less eye-contact or even physically moving away from the other person.

It is important that these signals are noted and appropriate action taken to end the conversation. It can be very annoying when the signals are ignored and a person carries on talking, being insensitive to the body language that is being displayed.

Phrases that can help with the ending of a conversation include:

- I very much enjoyed talking to you ...
- I hope we meet again ...
- If you need help with other letters, let me know ...
- Let me know if you get a reply ...

Any phrases that are used should be accompanied by a smile and a tone of voice that indicates that you are being sincere.

Conversations are built around the use of complex behaviour. This involves anticipation of our own behaviour and the behaviour of others. We have to:

- plan what we are going to say
- try to understand what others are saying
- know how to finish.

Activity

Winding up the conversation with Carmen

Marguerite has helped Carmen to write her letter to Joan. Marguerite has addressed the envelope for Carmen as Carmen felt that she was unable to do this.

1 Make a transcript of the conversation that Marguerite might have with Carmen to end their conversation.

2 Why is it important to end communication with service users in a positive way?

Assessment activity 2.5

Plan an interaction

Raj

Raj is 35 years old. He moved from India to England a few years ago with his family. He is a supervisor in a large factory shop. He has diabetes and has regular check-ups with his GP. The practice nurse sees Raj every six months to give him advice on his diet. Raj and his family live in a village in the south of England. They do not have any transport of their own.

Cecelia

Cecelia is married to Raj. She is 28 years old. She has one child. Cecelia works as a care assistant for the local council for three days each week at the day care centre.

Patel

Patel is 5 years old. He is the son of Raj and Cecelia. Patel has just started at the local primary school. He is in the reception class.

Amir

Amir is 80 years old. He is Raj's father. Amir has very little short-term memory and needs looking after. He has decided that looking after him is too much for his daughter-in-law and is considering moving to a residential home.

Activity

Choose **one** of the case studies above and prepare a plan for an interaction between you and the service user.

1 Prepare a checklist of skills that you think you will use during the interaction.

2 Prepare a plan showing:
- the aim of the interaction
- the objectives
- factors that will contribute to the effectiveness of the interaction
- any special needs that should be considered
- the physical, intellectual and emotional needs of the service user and how these could affect the interaction
- how you will minimise constraints
- the timescales for each part of the plan
- reasons for the actions taken within the plan.

3 Make a plan of the seating arrangements for the interaction and explain why it is suitable.

4 Make an outline transcript for the interaction to include each of the main stages, for example, the:
- introduction
- main content
- reflection and winding up.

The one-to-one interaction that you have with the service user may have a single purpose or it may have a combination of purposes. These could include, for example:

- obtaining information
- giving information
- exchanging ideas or opinions
- reflecting on the past
- exploring a topic.

The plan you have already drawn up will clearly indicate the aim or purpose of the interaction. The outline transaction you have prepared will have determined the way in which you hope to shape the interaction, but obviously you will not have been able to prepare for the whole conversation, as much will depend on the answers given by the service user.

During the interaction remember to:

- keep calm
- show interest
- help the service user to feel valued
- try to develop an atmosphere where there is congruency
- be prepared for the unexpected!

You will need to arrange for a tutor to carry out an assessment of the interaction. They will be checking on the skills you have used and the level of competency achieved. An example of an assessment observation sheet or witness testimony is given on the next page.

Evaluation

What is evaluating?

Evaluating is:

- thinking about what we have done within the interaction and how we have done it
- asking ourselves whether good relationships were established and how this was achieved
- considering the skills used and the reasons why they were used
- questioning which factors influenced the interaction and whether they enhanced or inhibited the communication
- considering whether the aim was achieved fully or whether it was only partially achieved
- making judgements about the effectiveness of the planning
- thinking about any improvements we could have made and, if so, what these could have been.

When evaluating, we use skills such as those listed in the table below.

To help when evaluating, we may decide to use the help of others, for example:

- the assessor/tutor
- our peers, e.g. those people who are in our group or class.

Skills used in evaluating	Examples
Reflection	Thinking about what we have done against theory, and making judgements about the standard achieved
Analysis	Examining what we have done in detail, making judgements about the outcomes
Drawing conclusions	Making a decision about how well we have completed the tasks or skills. This is done against criteria which can be measured, for example, how well did the skills match those suggested by theorists?
Planning	How to improve the tasks or skills by making realistic suggestions

Record of performance assessment

Candidate: _____ Date: _____

Environment: _____

Basic skills demonstrated	Comment/level achieved	Signature/date
Positioning		
Tone of voice/pace		
Vocabulary		
Use of open questions		
Use of body language		
Skills in communication used: Clarifying Summarising Paraphrasing Prompts/probes		
Any others used		
Method of managing the situation		
Effectiveness/benefits to the service user		
Seating arrangements		
Improvements that could be made		
Strengths		

Tutor's signature: _____ Date: _____

Candidate's signature: _____ Date: _____

An example of an assessment observation sheet

The feedback we receive from others can be used to help guide our thoughts about any improvements that we may want to make for future communication with service users.

What happens when we reflect?

When we reflect, we think about the whole conversation we have had from start to finish. Below is an example of reflection by Marguerite, who communicated with Carmen at the residential home. She is thinking about, or reflecting on, the first part of the conversation she had with Carmen.

> 'My introduction was clear and my tone of voice was friendly and welcoming. I established a good relationship with Carmen. I think this was because I smiled at her and reminded her that we were meeting to write a response to the letter she had received. I am pleased that I arranged the seats so that they were side by side and not facing one another. I think this helped Carmen to feel more relaxed. I needed to put Carmen at ease and to focus her mind on what we were intending to do, as with her mild form of dementia Carmen finds concentrating difficult.'

In this example Marguerite is thinking about her aims and objectives, what she actually did and how well she did it. She is going over in her mind what actually took place. It often helps if we make notes at this stage to remind ourselves of what we did.

How do we analyse?

Once Marguerite has thought through and clearly remembered all the parts of the communication she had with Carmen, she will begin to analyse her thoughts. That is, she will think about particular things she said and/or the skills she used and will make **judgements** (decisions) about how well she used them. For example, she may want to make judgements about the skills she used and how she used them. An example of an analysis of the skills Marguerite used follows.

> 'I think my tone of voice was appropriate because I did not have a raised voice, neither was it too quiet so that Carmen couldn't hear. I made frequent eye-contact so that Carmen knew I was interested in what she had to say and that I was focusing on her and not thinking about other things. I used quite a number of open questions, for example, one I used was, "What do you think you should write?" This gave Carmen the chance to talk about her feelings. I also used reflective comments to show Carmen that I was actively listening. For example, "... so you liked the concert we had the other day". I did summarise during the conversation because at one stage Carmen was jumping from topic to topic and I wanted to make sure that I had understood her correctly. I said, "So you would like her to come next week ...?" '

Marguerite has considered the skills she used in her conversation with Carmen and she has analysed which skills she used and has given examples to illustrate the points she was making. She had information and/or knowledge about communication skills and how they should be used and so she could make judgements about the quality of those she used. She was able to think about the skills against the theory she had learned. Thinking about each component part within the task or activity is part of the analysing process.

What is drawing conclusions?

When making decisions we should be making 'informed judgements', that is, measuring something against the knowledge we have of the subject.

If we are making decisions and explaining them, we will be making 'reasoned judgements' as we will be examining the facts and knowledge supplied by others who may be experts, and we will make decisions against the facts, opinions and views of others. This could be the views of theorists, other people who have knowledge and opinions of the subject, or we could be using the feedback we have received from the assessor or from peers. Additionally we could include our own opinions. At the top of the next page is an example of Marguerite drawing conclusions from her conversation with Carmen.

'In my opinion, I used prompts very successfully as Carmen moved the conversation forward as a result of my saying, "So, what do you think you should write?" If I had not done this, it is likely that Carmen would have continued to talk around the subject without making any decisions. In her feedback, my assessor confirmed that this was appropriate.

I was not afraid of silence. Carmen had one long silence during the conversation. I think she was thinking back over past times she had spent with Joan. Jan Sutton and William Stewart in their book *Learning to Counsel* state, "Silence can be threatening but it can also be constructive." In Carmen's case I think it was constructive because she was recalling memories of pleasurable activities, which helped her to arrive at a decision.'

In this example, Marguerite is expressing her own opinions and referring to the opinions of others. She is considering the skills she used and their purpose, and discussing the reasons for points in the conversation. In a full evaluation Marguerite would discuss a range of skills used, drawing conclusions about their effectiveness.

How to plan for improvements

Having drawn conclusions, good practice is to think about the ways that the interaction could be improved, for example in the use of skills, in the planning or when considering seating arrangements. For example, we may consider the points under the headings in the table below.

Planning for improvement

If we do not think about how the interaction could be improved, it is unlikely that the skills used will get any better. Care workers should always think about their own professional development or, in other words, how to do things better. When planning for such improvements, it is necessary to think about:

- what needs improving
- the order in which the improvements should take place
- the timescales.

Using the checklist in assessment of own skills

Earlier, you were given information about producing a checklist of skills to use during the interaction. This list will be very useful during the evaluation, as you will be able to look at the skills you planned to use and which skills you actually used. You might also like to think about why you used them (purpose) and how effective they were; in other words, did they help to achieve the outcome?

The contribution of others in assessing own skills

Having a person who is observing during the communication is always helpful. The person who is observing, perhaps your assessor or one of your peers, will not be actively involved in the interaction and is, therefore, more likely to record which skills were used and whether they achieved their purpose. To do this effectively, observers will need a document on which to record their observations. Videoing the communication is also a very good idea, as long as you have obtained permission from the participants. A video can be played back and the pause button used to help consider each skill used and its effectiveness. This is very helpful when trying to evaluate your own performance.

Purpose	Did the skills used enable the purpose of the communication to be achieved?
Reasons for use	What were the reasons for using the skills chosen? Were there other skills that would have been more suitable?
Effectiveness	Did the skills used enable both yourself and the service user to understand and have a meaningful exchange of information?
Achievement of outcomes	Did the skills allow the outcomes to be achieved? Could the service user have benefited if something had been done differently?

Assessment activity 2.6

Interact with a service user

Choose **one** person from those listed in Assessment activity 2.5:

1 Greet the person you have chosen to have an interaction with and interact with them for **10 minutes**, establishing and maintaining effective communication.

2 Evaluate the way in which you contributed to the interaction. The following questions may help you to do this task:

- How did the interaction achieve its aim?
- What was the quality of my own performance?
- Did I establish a good relationship with the service user?
- What skills did I use? How effective were the skills I used?
- What factors affected the interaction? Did these enhance or inhibit the interaction?
- Could my planning have been improved before the interaction?
- What improvements could I make?
- How does my evaluation compare with the evaluations of the assessor and others about my performance?

Glossary

Acronym: word formed from the initial letters of other words

Ambiguous: having more than one meaning

Analyse: to explain or consider in detail

Assertive: being able to voice one's rights or opinions; being focused

Authoritarian: to tell others, to allow no choice

Autocratic: ruling by one's own power

Body language: conveying meaning without speech

Care values: derived from human rights; how we would like others to care for us

Characteristics: distinctive qualities

Clarity: clearness

Cognitive: activity of the brain; thinking

Complex: complicated, needing simplification

Congruent: agreeing, friendly

Contextualised: placed so that clues can be gained

Democratic: collective power

Empathy: to see as though through the eyes of another; complete understanding

Enhancing: providing greater benefit

Gender: femaleness/maleness

Holistic approach: one that views the subject as a whole, not its parts

Inhibiting: suppressing or restraining

Interaction: making a connection with another person or persons, e.g. by talking

Interpret: to translate; to make sense of something

Judgements: decisions made based on facts

Life stages: different time periods of our life

Non-verbal: without words being spoken

Objectives: the steps taken to achieve an aim

Partnership: working together

Patronise: to act in a superior manner; to be condescending; to act pleasantly to someone you think is inferior to you

Social co-ordination: being able to form relationships with others from different ages and backgrounds

Socially constructed: put together from a social perspective

Socialisation: the way we are influenced as we develop

Stereotype: to judge someone by certain characteristics without knowing them

Transferrence: the movement of ideas/feelings from one place/person to another (Freud)

Unconditional positive regard: acceptance of a person for who they are

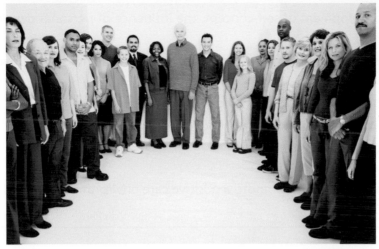

What makes us what we are?

Introduction

Why do we need to study people's behaviour? The answer is that, if we intend working in health and social care settings, we will be very close to vulnerable people who need to feel respected and worthy of respect. When people feel 'at risk', they often become aggressive or defensive, behaving in a way that is threatening to the professional care worker.

Care workers need to be aware of how to manage challenging behaviour and offer support. So they need to have a sound knowledge and understanding of developmental theories of self-concept and personal development. They need to know about special conditions and illnesses that can affect behaviour.

Managing challenging behaviour can include adapting the care setting to be user-friendly and calming. Promoting a positive environment for service users encourages good physical health, promotes good mental health and makes service users more able to interact with others.

Behavioural awareness is one of the best skills that can be learned for any situation where people are the focal point.

In this unit you will learn

Learning outcomes

You will learn to:

- investigate the development of self-concept, the influence of personal development and relationships of children
- describe illnesses and conditions that affect the behaviour of children and ways of providing support
- explain the factors that affect the behaviour of service users in care settings
- explain ways of providing support to service users
- explain how to manage challenging behaviour in a care setting and provide a safe and positive environment
- plan and demonstrate how to promote a positive care environment for service users.

Factors that influence other people's reactions

Murphy (1974) describes **self-concept** as 'the individual as known to the individual'. It is our sense of who we are, the picture we have of ourselves.

Everything that you considered in this activity has been evaluated through how you have been reflected back to yourself through other people's actions. Cooley (1902) called this 'the looking-glass self'. If someone tells you something good about yourself enough times, you believe them, particularly if they are people whose opinions you value. This works with negative aspects of your self-concept too – the 'naughty' girl, the 'uncooperative' boy or even the person who is 'useless at maths'!

Our self-concept is important because it affects all our relationships and interactions with others. We need to have a good opinion of ourselves in order to enjoy good relationships with others. If we have a poor self-concept, it is likely to affect our behaviour, e.g. we could become withdrawn from others, may not achieve in examinations and may become a bully towards others. Having a high self-concept is, therefore, a very important feature of development.

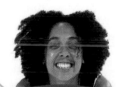

Self-esteem
An evaluation of how we see ourselves, including how much we like ourselves

Ideal self
The sort of person we would like to be

Self-concept

Self-image
Our description of who we are, which includes knowledge from our social roles, e.g. mother, father, aunt; the personality traits we have, e.g. whether we are clever, have a sense of humour; how we see our appearance, e.g. brunette, tall, fat

Self-concept

Consider this

Why do you value yourself or why do you not value yourself? How has this affected your behaviour?

Self-concept develops as a person grows. Babies do not distinguish themselves from their mother or primary carer. It is not until an infant is around 18 months old that they begin to realise that they exist as a separate entity from anyone else.

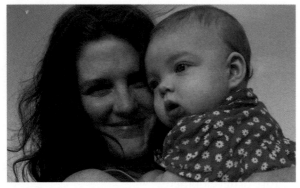

Babies do not distinguish themselves from their mother

As we grow older, we adapt to become part of different groups (in work and leisure) and take on the values held by those groups, because we need to feel that we belong. When this happens, we feel comfortable and secure enough to allow other people's perspectives of us to have an influence on the way we see ourselves.

Psychologists such as Argyle (1983) believe that childhood has the greatest impact on self-concept. Argyle believes there are four major influences on self-concept:

- the reaction of other people towards us
- comparison with other people
- social roles and identification.

Own personal identification and identification with others

Our personal identification splits 'self' into two parts, as shown below.

When these two parts are combined, we become aware that although our values, beliefs and regard for ourselves may change, depending on how others react to us, there is a continuity of identity throughout our lives.

According to Sigmund Freud, children learn a sense of who they are through a process of identification, e.g. around the age of 5–6, children identify with their same-sex parent. Freud felt that this was a most natural development and it was necessary in order for a child to develop normally into adulthood.

Comparisons with other people's roles

It is human nature to compare ourselves with other people. Parts of our self-concept will only make sense if they are considered in relation to other people.

People choose their own targets for comparison. Consider a group of new mothers meeting

Self

The **existential 'I'**
How we identify all our physical characteristics and abilities such as green eyes, brown hair, ability to walk, talk, sleep, etc. Our awareness of our own ability, i.e. we are able to perform actions based on our own decisions.

The **categorical 'me'**
Qualities and characteristics that define us as individuals, influenced by social factors and interaction with others.

Our personal identification

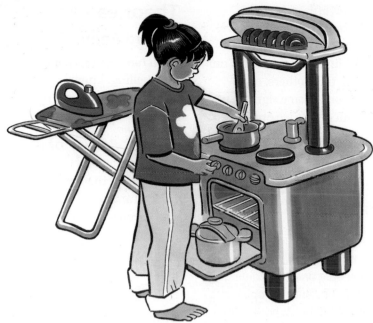

I do the same things that Mummy does

together and discussing their new babies. They will probably compare the babies' weights, the length of time they sleep, whether they have reached any developmental milestones and also how they, as mothers, are coping with the change to their lives. Some new mothers will go away feeling quite proud of their child's development, while other mothers will start to worry that their baby is not 'normal'.

A child's self-concept can be affected when their abilities are compared with those of another child, e.g. if one boy's football skills are compared with another. Rosenberg (1956) studied a group of adolescents and found that children who were able to compare themselves favourably with other people had a higher self-esteem.

We create a personal and social hierarchy of people we know, depending on the role they have and how we value them, fitting ourselves into that hierarchy.

Consider this

Who do you compare yourself with? Why?

Current and past role models

A social role is one where we relate to others in some way. As individuals we have a number of social roles at any one time, as the table below shows. Children have fewer social roles than adults.

Person	Possible social roles
Father	Family member Participant in a sports team
Mother	Relating to husband and children Member of a charity group
Neighbour	Having friends and doing things together Neighbourhood Watch member
Aunt	Supporting nieces and nephews and taking an interest in what they do Organising local history group

If we had the experience of meeting others and interacting with others when we were children, e.g. attending playgroup or attending sports clubs, we will probably have a positive self-concept and be quite confident. We will have had the opportunity of comparing ourselves with others, however simplistic the comparison.

How other people react towards us is very significant in relation to how we view ourselves. As young children, we look to and admire our parents and this is a very important aspect of our development. Later, as we meet others, e.g. teachers and peers, they too become significant and influence our self-concept, as we **emulate** the characteristics that we like for ourselves. The effect of parenting on self-esteem lasts throughout life.

Case study

Amber

Amber is 5 and lives with her mother and two older brothers. Amber cried a great deal during her first few months and constantly disrupted family life. As a result, her father left home and her mother blamed Amber for this.

As a toddler, Amber spent a lot of time playing on her own as her mother was too depressed to play with her. As a result she is a quiet, withdrawn child who does not speak very much to others in the reception class.

Amber's mother compares her with her brothers, whom she praises a lot. She often tells Amber that she is a nuisance and that having to look after her prevents her from having any life of her own.

Amber's father takes both boys to football matches at the weekend, but Amber is not invited to go with them. Amber's brothers often tease her and tell her that it's her fault that their father left and that he doesn't want to know her.

At school, Amber does not make any effort to make friends and spends a lot of time just day-dreaming.

1 Explain the factors that have influenced Amber's development of self-concept.

2 How do you think Amber identifies herself? What has influenced this?

3 How do you think Amber compares herself to others? What has influenced this?

4 What past and present role models does Amber have to model her own behaviour on? Explain why this is.

Theories

Gerard Egan

Egan has developed a three-stage model of counselling, known as the 'skilled helper model', to help people to help themselves to find solutions to problems.

Stage 1: Review of present situation

Service users and children are encouraged to think about their problem and develop a deeper understanding of it. In Egan's model, counsellors and parents use skills of listening, **paraphrasing**, **reflecting** and summarising. Silence is often used to allow the service user or child to think about their situation and to focus on a specific issue of concern.

Stage 2: Development of new or preferred scenario

This is about helping service users to identify what it is they want or need in order to deal more effectively with the problem. The skills Egan recommends here are:

- challenging
- immediacy
- counsellor self-disclosure
- identifying patterns and themes
- giving information.

Stage 3: Moving into action

The service user is helped to think about ways of dealing with the problem, based on the knowledge and understanding gained from the previous two stages. The counsellor and the service user will explore a variety of ways of achieving the goals that have been set.

A plan of action is discussed and formed. In this way, the counsellor can provide support and can evaluate any goals that are set. The skills used at this stage are:

- goal setting
- making choices
- creative thinking
- giving encouragement
- evaluating.

For more about Egan's theory, see Unit 3.4, pages 128-9.

Activity

Amber

Amber is unhappy about her life and talks to her reception class teacher about some of her problems.

1 Work in pairs to role play this situation. One should be the teacher and the other should be Amber. Apply Egan's three stage process of counselling to the discussion.

2 Write your own scenario about a child aged 4–7 who is upset about what is happening to her.

3 Change roles and apply the three stages of Egan's theory to the discussion you have with the child as her teacher.

4 Give a comprehensive account of the theories of Egan showing how his theories apply to either Amber or your own case study.

Carl Rogers

Carl Rogers believed that all individuals are able to 'self-direct' – to shape and direct their own lives. He developed a 'person-centred' approach, believing that the best expert on any individual was that individual themselves, not others.

The main focus of Rogers' theory is our individual view of self, for which there are two main sources of information:

- personal experience
- evaluation of self by others.

All children need to experience positive regard from their parents – they need to feel valued by their parents, not to be continually told they are in the wrong. They also have the need for positive *self-regard* – they need to value themselves. This is known as congruence and is an indicator of having high self-esteem.

How a child feels they are regarded by others can affect their self-concept. For example, Rogers believed that children learn that to obtain love and approval from others, particularly their parents, they have to behave in a certain way. As a result, children believe that love and praise will be withheld until they achieve certain standards of behaviour. Rogers calls this **conditional positive regard**. A child who learns to behave in ways that are approved by parents and significant others will gain approval and **self-worth**. Conditions of worth are **internalised**. If they match with the child's experiences and values, then the child will have a positive self-concept. If they do not match, the child will try to suppress their own feelings to ensure that they gain approval from others. This can lead to a poor self-esteem and a low concept of self-worth.

Rogers believes that a child needs to experience **unconditional positive regard** – total acceptance and non-judgemental support. Then positive self-regard will develop independently.

Theory into practice

Try to observe a child either in their own home or in a care and education setting for fifteen minutes. Record what they do. How would Rogers interpret their behaviour?

Theory of 'life stages': Erikson

Erikson believed that our personality continues to develop throughout life. He thought that development:

- has a biological basis, e.g. that the life stages are genetic and universal and affect a person's behaviour
- is influenced by our interaction with our environment, enabling us to pass through the stages of development
- is part of psychosocial development.

Erikson's life stage	Crisis	Significant relationships	Outcomes
0–1 years	Trust vs mistrust	Mother	Trust in people, or mistrust of others
2 years	Autonomy vs shame and doubt	Parents	Self control vs fear
3–5 years	Initiative vs guilt	Family	High or low self-esteem
6–11 years	Industry vs inferiority	Friends	Success or failure
Adolescence	Identity vs role confusion	Peer groups	Sense of identity or lack of identity
Early adulthood	Intimacy vs isolation	Same and opposite sex relationships and friendships	Ability to have deep relationships or failure to love others
Middle age	Generativity vs stagnation	Marriage	Wider interests and personal growth or self-concern
Old age	Integrity vs despair	All people	Sense of fulfilment or lack of fulfilment with life

Erikson suggested that we pass through eight stages of development, each one characterised by a psychosocial crisis which adapts our behaviour. He considered that we never fully resolve these crises, but retain an element of both the adaptive (positive) and the maladaptive (negative) features of each stage. For healthy development of self, the adaptive quality needs to outweigh the maladaptive quality. Unsatisfactory experiences can be compensated for in later life, although it becomes increasingly difficult to do so. Likewise, positive early experiences can be reversed by later bad experiences.

Consider this

Look back to the activity relating to Amber. How would Erikson interpret her behaviour?

Piaget

Piaget is a theorist who has researched how infants and young children organise their thoughts or perceptions and link them to behaviour. Piaget based his research on how children develop their thinking, having made observations through watching them when playing, interacting with others and when being involved in solitary play.

Piaget thinks of early concepts as being **schemas**, which are bits of information clustered together to fit into a whole piece. This is like a jigsaw puzzle, as the young child has lots of small pieces of information that when fitted together gives a whole picture about a topic.

An example of a schema is when a baby experiences moving a leg 'up' and then 'down'. Up and down are very important schemas which cluster together.

Piaget considers that the development of a child's thinking and ideas occur in the same **sequence** within each stage. The exact age may vary but Piaget believes that the sequence is always the same. The sequence is:

- 0 – 18 months: the sensori motor stage
- 18 months – 7 years: developing operations stage
- 7 – 12 years: concrete operations stage
- 12 years – adulthood: formal operations stage

Infants explore and recognise people and objects through:

- their senses
- their own activity
- their own movements.

The sensori motor stage

It is through these patterns or schemas that an infant can increase their co-ordination. For example, a baby of around 4 ½ months can reach out for a favourite toy, grasp it, and put the toy into their mouth. This is tracking, reaching, grasping and sucking.

An infant only sees things from their own point of view and focuses on only one aspect of what is happening. Piaget called this being **intellectually egocentric**.

It is not until the end of the first year that an infant will understand that people and objects are permanent and constant; that is, they go on existing even when they cannot be seen.

Developing operations stage

A young child will begin to use symbolic behaviour which includes language, drawings (without shape or form) and pretend play. As these are **internalised**, the child begins to think. In this process, the child is recalling past thoughts and ideas and past experiences, and is able to anticipate the future. By being able to do this the child will be able to develop concepts (ideas) and will begin to think about time and space. For example, they may make reference to people who are not present and they may try to share with others what they know and what they feel. It must be remembered, however, that children still focus on one aspect of any event.

Concrete operations stage

At this stage children and adolescents begin to have some understanding of mass, number, area, quantity, volume and weight.

They begin to understand that things are not always as they look, but they still have great difficulty in thinking about the abstract. To do this, they will need to be given practical work to help them understand numbers and concepts in mathematics.

Children who are at this stage of their development have the ability to take into consideration more than one aspect of an object or an event. In other words, they no longer concentrate on just one thing at a time but can manage several different things. They also realise that there may be more than one correct solution to a problem and have the ability to think about an issue or problem.

Formal operations stage

When children have reached this stage in their development they understand abstract concepts such as 'fairness'. They also have the ability to form hypotheses and to solve problems. Children are able to speak about things in an abstract form; they do not have to have the object or event present.

Piaget's ideas have been improved upon by other theorists and he has been criticised for some of his ideas.

Consider this

Look back to the activity relating to Amber. How would Piaget interpret her behaviour?

Find out more information about Piaget to help you with your answer.

Assessment activity 3.1

Development of self-concept

Amir

Amir is 12 and has grown up in a large, happy family. He has thrived at school and has plenty of friends. Amir's family is the only ethnic minority family in his neighbourhood. Sometimes he is shouted at by white youths who make abusive remarks about his ethnicity. Sometimes Amir feels as though he has to make twice as much effort as anyone else to be accepted outside of school.

Joy

Joy has been in residential care since she was 3 years old and is now 5. She finds it difficult to make friends as she doesn't always feel confident. She often feels that she is less important than other children who live at home with their parents.

Marcus

Marcus lives with his mother in an inner-city area. He is 8 years of age. His father has been in prison since Marcus was 3 and so in his early life he spent a great deal of time with his mother. His mother works between 6.00 p.m. and 8.00 p.m. each evening and so Marcus is left on his own. He often goes out with friends and roams around the streets. Sometimes they get bored and play pranks on people or vandalise the local play area.

1 Use the case studies and at least two other sources of evidence to explain the factors that have influenced the development of either Amir's or Joy's self-concept. Include information about:
   - own personal identification
   - comparison made with other people's roles
   - current and past role models.

2 Give a comprehensive account of the work of **two** of the following theorists, showing how their theories relate to Amir's, Joy's and Marcus' development and relationship with others: Argyle, Piaget, Rogers and Erikson.

Make sure you include the factors that influence personal identification and relationships giving at least **two** examples to illustrate the points you make.

Try to make significant connections between theory and application of knowledge to the development and relationships of children.

Illnesses and conditions

Attention Deficit Hyperactivity Disorder (ADHD)

ADHD is a condition which can cause havoc for the sufferer and those around them. The key characteristics are shown in the diagram below.

> The National Institute for Clinical Excellence (NICE) estimates that as many as 500,000 children in the UK (1 in 20) may have ADHD. Of these, 100,000 may be seriously affected.

Impulsivity
Blurting out answers before the question is complete
Unable to wait for turn
Interrupting or intruding on others

Key characteristics of ADHD

Hyperactivity
Constant fidgeting with hands/feet; squirming in seat
Leaving seat when expected to remain there
Running about excessively and inappropriately
Difficulty in playing quietly
Always 'on the go'
Talking excessively

Inattention
Poor attention to detail; frequent careless mistakes in schoolwork or other activities
Difficulty in sustaining attention
Appearing not to listen when spoken to directly
Not following instructions or finishing tasks
Difficulty organising tasks and activities
Avoiding or disliking tasks that require sustained mental effort
Losing things
Easily distracted
Forgetful in daily activities

Key characteristics of ADHD

Case study

James

James, aged 10, has seven doses of Ritalin a day to control his behaviour. On one of his first days at primary school, he stripped naked and was chased round the school by two teachers. 'He would crawl over desks, and start climbing on equipment in the classroom,' says the headteacher. 'Then at one point he opened the window and stood on the ledge. The whole school was in a panic.'

1 Identify aspects of James' behaviour which you think show signs of ADHD.

2 If you were asked to observe James with a view to giving a diagnosis, what other symptoms would you look for?

Ways in which behaviour is affected by ADHD

A child with ADHD may 'act out' a lot. They often take the role of the 'class clown' having learned that this brings rewards in the form of admiration from others, whereas very little else they do or say is met with positively. They may also be aggressive.

Ways of providing support for children with ADHD

Psychosocial support A major goal is to make the child's day as predictable as possible so they can do things for themselves as much as possible. This also helps the child to learn to be calm and have self-control.

- The most important thing is to set clear boundaries and make sure they are enforced fairly and consistently.
- Establish a routine with the child that is followed faithfully each day. Create a daily timetable including visual items, e.g. pictures of clocks with the hands set to times when an activity is scheduled to begin.
- Follow the old adage 'a place for everything and everything in its place', e.g. a special hook for holding outdoor clothing and school bags and special places for school books, PE kit and other equipment.

Consider this

Refer to the case study on the previous page. If you were in charge of James, what kind of rewards would you set up to encourage positive behaviour? How often would you give these? How would you monitor the effectiveness of the interventions being used?

- Talk to teachers and teaching assistants to ensure that the child writes down instructions in a special notebook which can be checked regularly.
- Reward good behaviour! Look for positive behaviour (no matter how small) and reward it. A reward can be as simple as a smile and a 'well-done' or you can use strategies such as star charts.

Medical support The medication most commonly used to treat ADHD is one of a group of stimulant-based chemicals which has the effect of improving behaviour and reducing symptoms. Research has shown, however, that a combination of drug treatment and psychosocial support is more effective than either alone.

Theory into practice

Try to arrange to interview the head of Special Educational Needs in a school about their experience of working with children with ADHD to find out how ADHD affects people in their everyday lives.

Learning difficulties

This term refers to conditions where a person has difficulties with understanding, learning and remembering new things, with social skills, such as communication, and with tasks such as self-care.

The most reliable method of diagnosis is using an intelligence quotient (IQ) test. This involves individuals answering a series of questions measuring ability at mental arithmetic, logic and linguistic skills. A numerical score is allocated, with 100 representing the average of the whole population. A score of lower than 70 represents a learning difficulty (see the table below).

IQ range	Diagnosis
50-70	Mild learning difficulty
36-49	Moderate learning difficulty
20-35	Severe learning difficulty
Below 20	Profound learning difficulty

Conditions causing learning difficulties include the following.

Down's syndrome One of the most common birth defects, in which children have an average IQ of 50. The life expectancy for a child born today with Down's syndrome is approximately 55. Characteristic features include a sloping forehead, protruding tongue, short stubby limbs, a slightly flattened nose, and a distinctive fold to the eyelids. Physical problems include:

- defects of the eyes, ears or heart
- gastrointestinal tract problems – vomiting, diarrhoea, constipation, small bowel obstruction
- sleep problems.

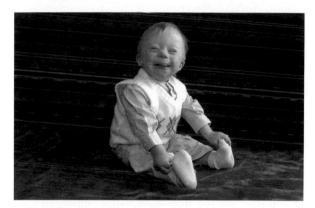

A child with Down's syndrome

Phenylketonuria (PKU) This is a genetic disorder, which if untreated can lead to seizures and severe learning disabilities. With early detection, a special diet can be provided to prevent serious learning difficulties developing. Physical features include microcephaly (a small head), prominent cheek and upper jaw bones and decreased body growth.

Foetal alcohol syndrome This is caused by heavy alcohol consumption during pregnancy, which damages the developing foetus. Research shows that the number of abnormalities increases dramatically with the number of fluid ounces of alcohol consumed daily. Abnormalities include:

- decreased alertness
- hyperactivity
- low IQ

- heart defects
- motor problems
- facial abnormalities.

Cerebral palsy This is a physical disability which affects the brain and body causing severe difficulties in walking, talking and providing self-care throughout life. Learning disabilities, ADHD and epilepsy are all associated with this condition. Although many children with cerebral palsy have a high IQ, about a third have a severe learning disability.

Although not classed as a learning difficulty asthma can have the same effects as some learning difficulties, e.g. acting up, misbehaviour, etc., and many of the ways of providing support apply to asthma as well. (See Unit 16, pages 216-7).

Ways in which behaviour is affected

Aggression and acting out To a child with a learning difficulty, the world can sometimes appear to be a bewildering and unpredictable place, with arbitrary rules that do not always make sense. Frustration can result from difficulties with understanding abstract concepts such as kindness, politeness, concern for others, empathy, waiting in turn and other social skills. This can turn to anger and aggressive behaviour. The child may be attention-seeking, annoying or destructive. If too much attention is given to these antisocial behaviours, the child will learn to perform them more frequently.

Mental health

Depression is a mental health problem common in varying degrees in the general population. It consists of low mood, sadness, loss of energy, eating too much or too little, altered sleep patterns and a lack of interest in activities that usually bring pleasure. In children with learning difficulties, it may not always be easy to recognise signs of depression (see the diagram at the top of the next page).

Ways of providing support

Although some people can manage to work through feelings of sadness and loss, some required professional intervention in the form of

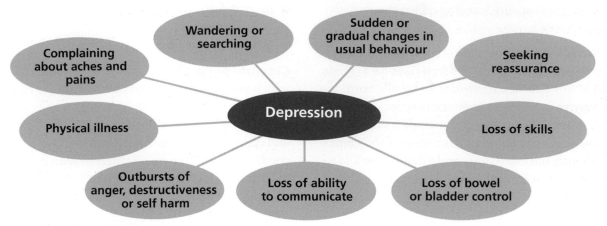

Signs of depression

counselling. The child would be helped to identify the causes of their unhappy feelings and learn to come to terms with them.

It may be helpful to talk to someone outside the family about issues that are causing concern: it is often easier to open up to a kind stranger than to someone we know well. Specialist counselling services are provided by MIND, MENCAP and CRUSE, amongst many.

In certain cases, the cause of a depressive episode may by biological, such as an underactive thyroid gland, or severe hormonal changes,

causing disruption to the child's body chemistry. In this instance, medication would be needed to restore the body's balance. A GP can prescribe appropriate medication.

A helpful strategy to deal with aggression is to provide support by **reinforcing** positive and helpful behaviours.

Psychosomatic illnesses

Sometimes physical illness can be caused by a mental or emotional disturbance. Such illnesses are known as psychosomatic illnesses. For example, a tension headache is not caused by damage to part of the brain but by constriction of blood vessels and muscles as we become stressed. Because the cause is psychological and the result is physical, this is called a psychosomatic headache.

Stress can cause psychosomatic illnesses. Certain types of asthma may be psychosomatic if the attack is brought on by psychological distress.

Ways in which behaviour is affected

A child can be affected by a psychosomatic illness in the same way as by a physical illness, experiencing headache, stomach ache, vomiting and other aches and pains. The child will feel unwell, possibly afraid, grizzly and in need of tender loving care.

Young children may show physical signs of stress such as trembling, shaking and crying or they may have a flushed or pale face, damp palms and forehead and difficulties in breathing.

Case study

Sanjay

Sanjay's family are entertaining some important visitors for lunch. Just as the visitors arrive Sanjay begins to throw a tantrum. His mother hastily takes him out into the kitchen so the visitors and other family members are not embarrassed, and gives him a packet of crisps and a chocolate bar to calm him down. As a result, Sanjay doesn't eat his meal, gets bored and begins to misbehave.

1 What has Sanjay learned from his mother's actions?

2 How do you think he will behave in future?

3 What other antisocial or annoying behaviours do you think could be learned and strengthened if they are reinforced?

4 What could Sanjay's mum have done instead?

If a physical cause is ruled out, it is important to manage the condition in a different way, as in the case of Scott, below.

Case study

Scott

Scott, aged 10, complained over a period of more than a year of severe stomach aches, which often resulted in vomiting. Having visited a doctor, it was found that there was no physical basis for his symptoms, but it was noted that he had virtually no free time, spending long hours playing soccer and practising the trombone, and often staying up until midnight to complete his homework. Scott's parents began to think his complaints were imagined. (Cited in *The Child Study Centre*, Vol. 6, No. 3, January/February 2002 – see page 282 for web address)

How could Scott's parents be advised to make lifestyle changes that would reduce the stress in his life and help his symptoms disappear?

Ways of providing support

It is important to take symptoms seriously and not dismiss them as being 'all in the mind'. Some practical strategies include:

- encouraging the child to talk about their feelings. For very young children, drawing or using dolls can be a good way of expressing feelings non-verbally
- trying to identify triggers that precede an outbreak of symptoms and making changes to minimise their occurrence
- asking teachers and others involved in the child's care if they are aware of anything troubling the child at playgroup or school
- helping the child to gain control by teaching them techniques of relaxation to use when they feel symptoms beginning or anxiety building up.

Assessment activity 3.2

Case study A

Erin is 8 years old and has ADHD. She has lots of behaviour problems, for example, she cannot concentrate for very long, is hyperactive and is unable to organise her thoughts into any correct sequence. She is causing his parents lots of problems, because although she is taking medication, she is still causing them embarrassment particularly when out on social occasions.

Case study B

Rebekah is 5 years old and has been diagnosed as having learning difficulties. Rebekah has started to attend a special school. Recently, she has begun to cry when leaving her mother, and when her mother meets her from school Rebekah clings to her. At home she has stopped playing with her toys and has lost interest in the television programmes she used to enjoy. The GP thinks that she is suffering from stress and anxiety.

Case study C

Ben, who is 4 years old, has autism. He has never bonded very well with either of his parents and

does not communicate with them. He often appears not to be interested in what is going on around him and when his mother tries to play with him he will sometimes join in but will not communicate with her. At playgroup he plays by himself, although sometimes he does watch what the other children are doing.

1 Choose **two** of the case studies above and investigate the condition. Write a comprehensive and detailed account of the symptoms and signs which causes the condition. Explain at least **two ways** in which both children's behaviour may be affected.

2 Explain and justify **two ways** in which each child could be provided with support. Choose **two** from:
   - counselling
   - education
   - interventions
   - psychosocial.

3 Explain, and use examples to show, how each type of support would help the children.

Factors affecting the behaviour of adolescents

The challenge of change and transitions

Adolescence is a time when an individual's self-concept undergoes dramatic change, including:

- physical changes, which bring about an altered body image and affects one's sense of self
- intellectual development, which allows the adolescent to become aware of what is possible as well as what currently exists
- emotional development, which involves increasing emotional independence.

The individual is also involved in making decisions about careers, values and sexual behaviour.

Erik Erikson (see pages 107–8) described adolescence as the key time for self-identity to form. It is a life stage characterised by role confusion, which can involve:

- negative identity (e.g. delinquency, which permits some sense of control)
- lack of intimacy (the person avoids close personal relationships, but may hero-worship a celebrity)
- time perspective (the thought of adulthood provokes anxiety and the person avoids making plans)
- industry (e.g. compulsive overworking or difficulty in concentrating).

Relationships

During adolescence, relationships with parents and peers change. The peer group takes on increasing importance from around the age of thirteen and helps the youngster to experiment with a variety of different identities in the search for a new, stable, personal identity which can be taken on into adulthood. This may involve adopting particular forms of dress (e.g. Goths) or taking on a new set of values and beliefs. Many adolescents question their parents' values and norms and become vegetarian or take on causes such as environmentalism. Experimentation is a key feature, and one's choice of peer group often influences the type and extent of experimentation, e.g. sexual activity and the use of alcohol and other substances.

Peer groups also serve a positive function – they allow adolescents to interact with members of the other sex in a non-intimate way. For those who are left out of such cliques or do not have a strong friendship group, however, the outcome is not too bright. The following example illustrates the pain and anxiety that can arise in such situations:

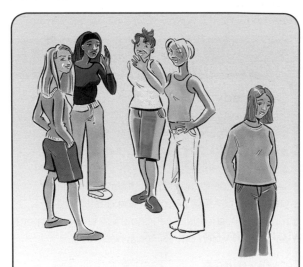

'Have you ever felt like some one is always calling you and hating you all the time well if your one of the few then join the club at skool i use to b one of the "populars" its so weird how they du sections bout it anyways and i had a fight with another girl got knocked out in hospital and every 1 disliked me cuz of it so it carried on n my best friends stood by me but then it got persinal i got phone calls with girls from my skool pertending to be my teachers and i was always grounded my mum went into school when she saw bruses all over my arms it isnt happening no more but theres still name calling ans little things wt sud i do?'

(Source: Girland.com.)

The outcome for some adolescents who experience relationship or adjustment problems can be very negative. One research study carried out in America found that sixty-three per cent of high-school students interviewed had considered suicide and eleven per cent had attempted it.

Attachment and loss

John Bowlby researched the relationship between the helpless infant and its major care-giver and found that a secure **attachment**, particularly in infancy and the first 3–5 years of life, is essential for healthy personality growth and development.

This need for attachment is still important in adolescence, where new attachments are typically formed with opposite sex partners.

- Those who were securely attached in infancy and early childhood tend to be good at forming new relationships and can develop close relationships where there is an element of individuality and an ability to give and take. They tend to negotiate adolescence easily.
- Those who were insecurely attached tend to be dependent, clingy and jealous. Or they may put up invisible barriers to stop people getting to know them well, or alternate between being over-friendly and angry and aggressive, pushing people away. Relationships with parents can become strained, there may be conflict at home and they are more likely to attach themselves to a delinquent peer group.

Motivational factors

Motivation is an inner drive to perform a particular behaviour with the aim of achieving a goal. All behaviour is motivated by something.

In adolescence, individuals are beginning to learn the self-discipline to continue working at something that may not have immediate rewards in order to achieve a longer-term goal. Some become excellent students, in order, for example, to obtain a later reward of good GCSE grades or a place at university with the long-term goal of obtaining a satisfying job. Others do not have the ability to plan so far ahead, so for them motivational factors may be much more immediate, such as earning money to buy the latest pair of trainers. For others still, the motivation may be to be popular or to belong to a particular 'in-crowd'.

For those working or living with adolescents, finding out what motivates them is essential in offering support and guidance.

Case study

Nehal

Nehal has just turned 15 and attends a comprehensive school in a fairly affluent town. She joined the school later than her contemporaries, in Year 8, and found it quite hard to make friends. A rather quiet, thoughtful girl, she was unhappy for the first six months. Then she fell in with a crowd of outgoing girls who were popular with the boys but rather disliked by other girls, both in her year and in the higher years. She began going out with a boy three years older than her. Her mother was concerned that Nehal's whole personality seemed to be changing. She was obsessed with having the latest designer clothing and judged other girls on their attractiveness and popularity. She spent less and less time on her schoolwork and increasing amounts of time with her friends and boyfriend.

1 What do you think is motivating Nehal at the moment?

2 Are her goals short- or long-term?

3 What are the influences on her self-concept and self-esteem?

4 What advice would you give to her mother?

Authority and autonomy

Adolescence is typically a period when the individual wants more and more freedom (**autonomy**) and tries to break away from parental and other types of authority.

Developing autonomy means being able to make one's own decisions, do things for oneself and make life choices that were not available in childhood but are a necessary part of growing into a well-functioning adult.

The psychologist Diana Baumrind has researched the parenting styles which help in this process.

- Parents who show a democratic parenting style consult their offspring and explain reasons for their decision-making. Relationships are more harmonious and the adolescent displays less deviant or rebellious behaviour, finding it easier to achieve autonomy and move into the adult role.
- Authoritarian parents insist on absolute obedience without consultation and without giving reasons for their decisions. Their teenagers are more likely to rebel and associate with deviant peer groups. They are possibly trying to reject their parents' values and norms.
- Parents who are laissez-faire (very laid back) and set few boundaries for their children are

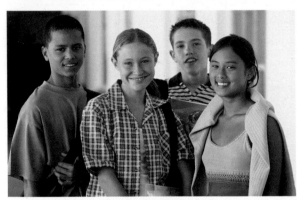
Adolescence is a key time for self-identity to form

also likely to have adolescents who find it difficult to develop autonomy.

Personal responsibility

This is the awareness that we must live with the consequences of our decisions and actions. Young children are frequently heard to say in an aggrieved tone, 'It wasn't me!', or, 'It wasn't my fault – she made me do it.' This denial of personal responsibility for one's actions in adolescence is a sign of immaturity that youngsters must work to overcome.

This is particularly so in the world of employment, where being late for work, for example, or not doing one's job properly could result in being sacked from the job. Those who are able to develop autonomy also tend to be better at taking on personal responsibility.

Substance abuse

The use of illegal drugs can result in dramatic behaviour changes in adolescents and can include any or all of the following: paranoia, depression, lethargy, violence, school refusal, school exclusion and poor self-esteem.

Two common substances that can be abused are given in the table below, with the associated signs and symptoms.

Drug	Signs and symptoms
Alcohol – beer, wine, whisky, gin, vodka, alcopops	Odour on the breath Intoxication Difficulty in focusing: glazed appearance of the eyes Uncharacteristically passive behaviour; or combative and argumentative behaviour Deterioration in care for personal appearance and hygiene Reduced interest in, and motivation for, school work and/or part-time work Unexplained bruises and accidents Irritability Loss of memory (blackouts) Changes in peer-group associations and friendships Impaired interpersonal relationships, e.g. alienation from close family members
Marijuana – skunk, weed, puff, blow	Rapid, loud talking and burst of laughter are early effects Later affects include becoming sleepy Forgetfulness in conversation Inflammation in whites of eyes, pupils unlikely to be dilated Distorted sense of time passage – tendency to over-estimate time intervals Use or possession of paraphernalia including roach clip, packs of rolling papers, pipes or bongs

Other substances that can be abused are: PCP, anti-depressants, tranquillisers, stimulants, narcotics, hallucinogens.

> ## Consider this
>
> *Why do you think adolescents abuse substances? How much do peers influence this? Does personality play a part?*

Personality disorders

Personality disorders are psychological disorders which are long-term and affect almost every aspect of a person's life. They range from mild, where people can live a more or less normal life most of the time (although traits of the disorder will be exhibited more severely at times of stress), to severe, where the disorder seriously affects emotional and psychological functioning. Features common to all personality disorders include:

- disturbances in self-image
- difficulty with successful interpersonal relationships
- absence of an ability to experience a range of appropriate emotions
- distortions in perception of oneself, others and the world.

Physical and psychological boundaries

Adolescents need boundaries, though they will change and become wider and more flexible with time. For example, the physical boundaries set for a 14-year-old may include permission to travel to a local shopping centre or a nearby city provided certain guidelines are adhered to (e.g. phoning home periodically to reassure parents/carers that all is going well). As the adolescent grows older, they become responsible for setting their own physical boundaries.

Although the adolescent may appear to rely on friends more than family members for emotional and social support, it is very important that the home provides a predictable and stable environment. This psychological boundary allows them to experiment and develop without their lives becoming too chaotic. It also allows for a safe haven to retreat to when life gets difficult.

Environment

The environment may influence activities an adolescent engages in and their choice of peer group. Those living and attending school in impoverished areas may encounter poor housing, boarded-up shops covered in graffiti, poor street-lighting and areas which appear unsafe because of the presence gangs of youngsters who may appear threatening. Those who are inclined towards a negative identity may be attracted by this type of environment, while others may feel threatened by it and thus restrict, or have parents restrict, their physical movement. By contrast, those living in more spacious, pleasant suburban or rural environments may feel more comfortable and find it less easy to join 'gangs'. These factors will affect aspects of self-concept (e.g. seeing oneself as 'hard' because of living in a run-down neighbourhood).

Factors affecting the behaviour of adults

Family relationships

As adults, we leave our parents' home to live alone, with friends or with a partner. This is a time when many of the worries of the adult world rest on our shoulders, and it can be a scary time. Our parents become a less integral part of our lives and their place is taken by friends, partners and, for some of us, children.

Erikson views this stage of life as one where we are looking to establish a sense of intimacy by forming close and meaningful relationships with others yet at the same time maintaining the hard-won sense of identity established during adolescence.

Important relationships at this stage of life include romantic and sexual ones with a partner. We are no longer dependent upon our parents but are in charge of our own lives and families, financially independent and making our own decisions.

In the early stages of adulthood this can be a very exciting time, but these new relationships also require a considerable amount of adjustment which is not always easy. For example, finding the right balance between meeting the needs of one's partner, satisfying one's own needs and still remaining close to parents can be quite tricky. Mother-in-law jokes highlight some of the conflicts that can arise in trying to get this balance right!

For those who do not create close, intimate relationships, a sense of isolation can occur and life can seem psychologically meaningless. These negative feelings can result in an increased vulnerability to stress and depression.

Many find the new role of parent immensely satisfying and adapt well to sharing attention between partner, parents and child. For others, however, the birth of a child can cause friction in a partnership. Help from one's own parents can be either a blessing or a nuisance, depending on how it is offered and perceived. If 'help' is perceived as being interference, conflict may arise, which can put a strain on relationships.

Work

Having a full-time job, where money is earned to pay for life's necessities (mortgage or rent, bills, food, etc.) is a major difference between adolescence and adulthood. Work is no longer a short-term motivating factor but a lifelong pursuit. People who have a satisfying occupation which has stable and positive prospects get a sense of fulfilment from it. Work may form an important part of their self-concept. Others, often those in manual occupations, may see work as simply a means to an end and not derive much satisfaction from it.

Whatever the type of occupation, there is a considerable amount of adaptation required to adjust to the restrictions of work. Holidays are not so frequent or long, and there may be financial penalties associated with being ill (such as losing pay).

Class, education and culture

There has always been a **social class** divide in the UK. This is closely related to employment and education. People who go to university usually have jobs that are well-paid, interesting and with good career prospects, while others go straight from school into a job, or move into the work environment via an apprenticeship or vocational course. Generally speaking, those with jobs classified as professional or managerial (e.g. doctors, lawyers, teachers) have a better lifestyle than those in skilled, semi-skilled or manual jobs.

While skilled employees who learn a trade such as plumbing, electrical work or car maintenance, etc. tend to earn a good living and are able to afford a high standard of living, those who take up unskilled work are frequently destined to do the same type of job for years with little prospect of change in terms of job content or responsibilities (e.g. working on a factory assembly line).

The job we do and the 'class' to which we feel we belong can have a strong influence on self-concept. Those who are born into a middle-class environment but do not go to university and take up manual work may well feel inferior to their contemporaries who have entered higher status occupations such as medicine. Such negative feelings can lead to bitterness, low self-esteem and even depression.

Closely linked to class issues are those relating to culture. The experiences of different cultural groups in our society are evident in employment statistics. A survey followed the employment of 140,000 people in England and Wales over thirty years from the 1960s onwards. It found that:

- Fifty-six per cent of people from Indian working-class families took up professional or managerial roles in adulthood, compared with only forty-three per cent of those from white, non-immigrant families.

- Among youngsters from Caribbean families, the figure was forty-five per cent.
- People of Pakistani or Bangladeshi origin have a much higher chance of either spending long periods being unemployed or only achieving low-paid, unskilled or semi-skilled employment.

Religion is an important aspect of culture, and the survey found that Jews and Hindus had a greater chance of **upward mobility** than Christians, whereas Muslims and Sikhs had a lower chance of worldly success.

Current life stage

According to the psychologist Levinson, adulthood can be divided into five stages, as shown at the bottom of the page.

Personality disorders

During adulthood, at times of severe stress, the symptoms of a personality disorder may be worsened. A disorder known as Adjustment Disorder can be mistaken for a personality disorder and is believed by some to be the basis of the mid-life crisis. This disorder is characterised by an extreme stress reaction which is out of proportion to what would be expected from such a stressor, accompanied by significant impairment of social, occupational or educational functioning. Triggers for such a reaction can be marriage, becoming a parent or failure to reach the goals one had set for occupational success.

Attachment and loss

Loss of, or separation from, a loved one (a parent, partner or friend) can trigger an episode of depression in someone who was insecurely attached in early life. Children leaving home can lead to 'empty nest syndrome' where a parent can feel desolate and grief stricken. People who were securely attached in childhood can manage loss more easily. Secure attachment to a partner can act as a buffer against loss and depression.

Role identification

The importance of roles in the development of self-concept was discussed on pages 103–6. Loss of a role (e.g. of the role of breadwinner through redundancy) can cause a loss of self-esteem and lead to insecurity and, sometimes, depression.

Environment

Our environment affects us in both positive and negative ways. People living in towns or suburban areas of cities tend to have better facilities (transport, health care, housing, shops, leisure facilities, etc.) than those in rural locations or inner-city locations.

Factors affecting the behaviour of older people

There is little agreement about what 'old age' actually means, and it can be defined in different ways, as shown at top of the next page.

17–22: Early adulthood transition	22–28: The novice phase	28–33: The age-30 transition	33–40: The settling down stage	40–45: The mid-life transition
People are trying out aspects of identity developed during adolescence.	People are concerned with occupational choice, lifestyle, values and relationships, and may be influenced by older people they admire and want to be like.	People are concerned with making seriously committed decisions. This can cause stress and self doubt yet they realise that commitment is necessary at this life stage.	People make a much fuller commitment to occupational and lifestyle choices. Their sense of identity is now of themselves as responsible adults.	Or the mid-life crisis. People are represented, often humorously, as adults reverting to childish or adolescent behaviours (e.g. suddenly wearing jeans and going to rock concerts) as though to deny the reality of their age.

Levinson's stages of adulthood

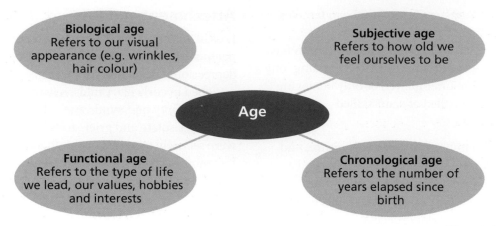

Ways of defining age

Physical factors

As we grow older, certain physical changes are inevitable. See 'Physical and mental degeneration' on page 123.

Psychological factors

A major change during this stage of life concerns one's psychological functioning. This includes aspects such as self-concept and self-esteem, which are discussed below, as well as cognitive aspects such as weakening memory and a less sharp intellect.

Social factors

The social life of older people often shrinks after retirement, especially following bereavement, during periods of illness and as the individual approaches death. See 'Disengagement from mainstream society' and 'Withdrawal', right.

Environmental factors

Environment is important for older people who lack mobility and need easy access to good quality health care and leisure activities. Poor environmental facilities can restrict their lives. People living in 'environmental poverty' fare much worse than people living in areas which are well served by transport systems.

Current life stage

Erikson sees a positive outcome to this stage being the achievement of 'integrity' – being able to look back and reflect on life with a sense of achievement. This involves being able to come to terms with disappointments and failures. If this is not achieved, the person may be bitter and distressed that time is running out. It is then hard to accept one's impending death with a sense of peace, and the person may feel angry and helpless.

Disengagement from mainstream society

As people get older, they begin to withdraw from social life. Many of their roles will have been taken on by younger people, e.g. they may no longer be a breadwinner but dependent on a state pension. The role of parent is no longer relevant and, if infirm, the individual may take on the role of a dependent, with their children caring for them. Social and leisure activities may be reduced as a result of reduced finance or decreased mobility, poor health or a general loss of interest in matters outside the immediate family.

Withdrawal

With disengagement comes increasing withdrawal from the outside world of church, community, workplace and so on, and a tendency to remain at home with family members. This is accompanied by an increasing preoccupation with thinking about oneself, including mulling over old memories. This seems to be a natural part of preparation for the inevitability of dying.

Sense of impending death

Although withdrawal can lead to an acceptance of impending death, people with terminal illnesses can find it hard to accept the reality of dying and experience denial, anger and grief.

Loss of a sense of 'self' and the absence of a role to play

Retirement and change of role can lead to a huge sense of loss. For those who identify strongly with their occupational role, retirement can cause anger, bitterness, resentment and a dramatic drop in self-esteem – even leading to depression. People can be helped to accept the changes involved in retirement if they have enriching leisure activities or are offered a pre-retirement programme. These usually consist of discussions and advice on aspects to do with social life, health, relationships and financial aspects of retirement.

Physical and mental degeneration

Physical degeneration

Regardless of how old we feel ourselves to be, our bodies undergo changes as we age, particularly beyond the age of 60, including:

- decrease in height, reduced muscle mass, reduced total body weight, and reduced organ size, e.g. the bladder
- slower reaction time and less effective immune system, so wounds heal more slowly
- more brittle bones, which break more easily, and weaker muscles
- loss of some hearing and sight when the ear drum and lens of the eye lose elasticity.

Circulatory problems can also occur due to loss of elasticity of blood vessels.

Physical decline is not, however, inevitable. Research has shown that keeping healthy and taking regular exercise slows down the loss of bodily functions.

Mental degeneration

Loss of sharpness in cognitive capacities, such as memory, the ability to think and solve intellectual problems, is not inevitable. Individuals who remain intellectually active (e.g. by reading, doing crossword puzzles, keeping up with the news) tend to suffer no noticeable mental degeneration.

As knowledge increases across the life span, so does crystallised intelligence, which includes:

- how to reason
- language skills
- an understanding of technology.

Fluid intelligence is the ability we have to apply our understanding of the world to new problems and solve them. Research shows that this type of intelligence is at its peak between the ages of 20 and 30, but then declines as we age. This may be an inevitable part of the neurological changes associated with ageing, or it might simply be that while we don't practise new skills on a regular basis, we do continue to read a daily newspaper and add to our crystallised intelligence.

Assessment activity 3.3

Case study A

Al is nearly 16 years old. He has become very moody recently and rarely speaks to his parents. He ignores the advice they give him about his future and does very little revision for his examinations. Instead, he prefers to go out with a group of mates who are older than himself. He smokes and drinks alcohol and is sometimes so ill that he is unable to get up the next morning to go to school. Al's parents are very worried about him.

Case study B

Barbara is 32 years old. She is married to Tony, who is 35 years old, and they have two young children, Alicia aged 4 and Marcia who is 2 years old. As a result of having the children Barbara has put on quite a lot of weight and is disgusted by her appearance as she is not very tall.

Tony has a job teaching in the local college. He and Barbara are both really happy that they have been able to have a family and want to provide as much as possible for their children. To help with this Barbara has a part-time job, and the money she earns is put aside for holidays and special occasions.

The family has a lot of outgoings as they are buying their house in a nice rural area and have an expensive car, so they have to take care with how they spend their money. This means that Barbara cannot visit her mother often as she lives nearly a hundred miles away. This also means that the children do not see one of their grandparents very often. Barbara is worried as her mother, who is 65 years old, seems to have memory problems, which are getting worse.

Case study C

Bart is 71 years old. He retired five years ago as he had a mild heart attack. His wife looks after him at home, but Bart feels that his life will never be the same again. He cannot do any strenuous exercise and is afraid to go out very far unless his wife is with him. This has become more difficult recently as his wife has mobility problems, which means that walking any great distance is impossible.

Bart and his wife have become somewhat isolated from their friends and relatives and are very much dependent on one another.

1 Using the information from the three case studies, explain:
   - four factors that affect the behaviour of Al
   - four factors that affect the behaviour of Barbara
   - four factors that affect the behaviour of Bart.

All service users are individuals, and their individual needs have to be taken into account. Those who are involved in the decision-making process will have to help them to decide on the most appropriate form of support for them.

Support

There are different ways to support service users, each appropriate in particular circumstances, as the diagram below shows.

Counselling

Counselling is not about giving advice. The main aims are to:

- empower the service user – the key to the whole process, giving them autonomy and responsibility for changes to their behaviour or attitudes
- help them have a greater sense of self-understanding
- enable them to live in a more satisfying and resourceful way
- establish a greater sense of well-being in the service user
- ensure that these are lasting.

Care workers should always use active listening when communicating with a service user, but counselling is a specialised skill which needs to be

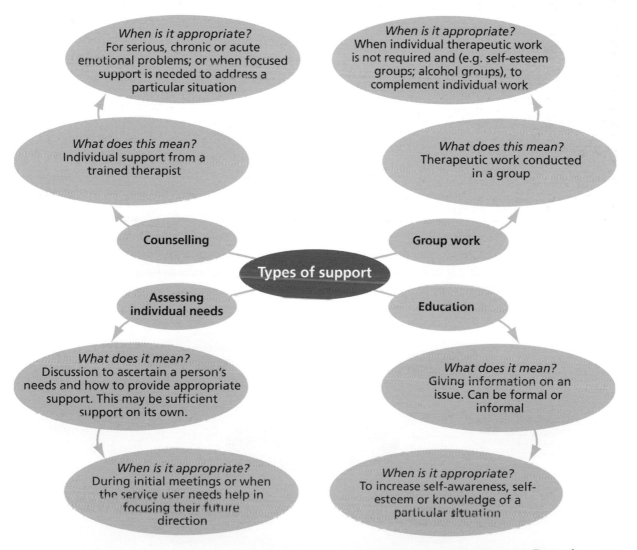

When is it appropriate?
For serious, chronic or acute emotional problems; or when focused support is needed to address a particular situation

When is it appropriate?
When individual therapeutic work is not required and (e.g. self-esteem groups; alcohol groups), to complement individual work

What does this mean?
Individual support from a trained therapist

What does this mean?
Therapeutic work conducted in a group

Counselling

Group work

Types of support

Assessing individual needs

Education

What does it mean?
Discussion to ascertain a person's needs and how to provide appropriate support. This may be sufficient support on its own.

What does it mean?
Giving information on an issue. Can be formal or informal

When is it appropriate?
During initial meetings or when the service user needs help in focusing their future direction

When is it appropriate?
To increase self-awareness, self-esteem or knowledge of a particular situation

Types of support

learned. Counselling sessions should, therefore, only be practised by a qualified counsellor who will abide by a code of ethics and practice. Counsellors often need to refer clients on to other professionals.

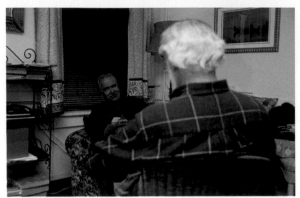
A one-to-one counselling situation

The essential qualities of the counselling relationship include:

- not making judgements about the service user
- helping them to feel valued as a person
- showing respect for them and their values
- making them feel safe
- mutual negotiation between service user and the counsellor about what they want to achieve and how they will go about achieving it.

These factors apply to all types of counselling.

Counsellors base their approaches on different theorists, for example, Egan, Freud or Rogers. The purpose of counselling is to provide the opportunity for the service user to work towards living in a more satisfying and resourceful way.

It can involve working with pairs, individually or with groups of people.

Theory into practice

If you were going through a difficult time, what skills and qualities would you want from a person who was helping you?

Assessing individual needs

In psychiatry, assessment is:

- the measurement of the service user's ability to function independently
- the comparison of that ability with the level of change in behaviour needed to achieve true sufficiency.

Care workers must, therefore, have an understanding of what is expected in the 'norms' of development in order to know whether there is a deficiency. The care worker will then have to determine whether the needs are:

- primary problems – 'actual' needs, often very apparent to the observer
- secondary problems – those which might occur and are far more difficult to assess. These problems often depend on influences over which the service user has no control.

One service user's needs are quite different from another, because we are individuals living in our own particular surroundings. We have some common needs, such as basic physical needs, for example, food, warmth and shelter; security needs; and emotional needs.

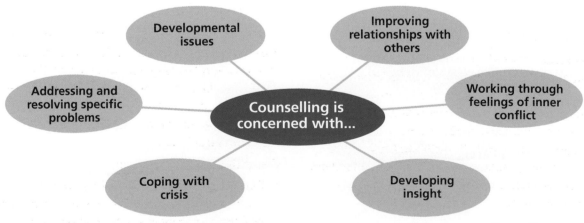

Developmental issues

Improving relationships with others

Addressing and resolving specific problems

Counselling is concerned with...

Working through feelings of inner conflict

Coping with crisis

Developing insight

Counselling concerns

Consider this

Remind yourself of Maslow's hierarchy of needs in Unit 2, page 80. Where do you think you fit on the hierarchy? Why? Should the triangle be open-ended?

Some people survive by reaching only the second or third level of Maslow's hierarchy with very few people actually achieving the top level of self-actualisation.

The only real way to assess an individual's needs is to talk with them, or more importantly, to listen to them. Once their needs have been identified, you need to write them down and, with them, work out the best way to meet these needs.

The principles of assessment are given in the table below.

Principle of assessment	What does this mean?
Be person-centred	Consider the whole person, not just the parts that are not functioning according to the norm
View the person to be assessed in their family situation	Look at the needs of others in the family as well as those of the person with the disability
Apply the care values	Treat the person who is being assessed and their family with respect and dignity, making sure that their confidentiality is maintained and that equal opportunity, rights and beliefs are promoted
Identify the service user's weaknesses as well as their strengths	Try to build on the strengths of the service user to assist with any weaknesses that exist
Based on evidence which is clear	Base decisions on information gained through questioning and observation

Case study

Sam

Sam is 18 and finds he cannot cope with living on his own. He has a bedsit which he cannot keep tidy and he is disorganised with his money. He is suffering from stress. He cannot sleep properly and he keeps taking time off work. His GP decides that Sam requires additional help.

1 Explain how counselling could help Sam.

2 What do you understand by the term 'assessing need'?

3 Work with another person and prepare part of a counselling session, with one person being the counsellor and the other taking Sam's role. Assess Sam's needs and prepare the first part of a counselling session.

4 Role-play the part of the counselling session to others and obtain feedback.

Group work

Whereas counselling is often carried out on a one-to-one basis, group work includes more than three people meeting together to support each other through a common situation, e.g. alcohol addiction, a phobia or bereavement. These groups will generally be facilitated by a skilled and trained practitioner, but the group members work through the problems brought by their fellow members.

In group work, members set their own agenda, are encouraged to feed back their own feelings about what others say and do, respect fellow group members and uphold confidentiality. It is an opportunity to interact with others and try out new experiences in a safe environment where they won't feel judged.

Group therapy has advantages:

- Participants can work out their problems/needs in the presence of others, e.g. emotional problems or problems with relationships.

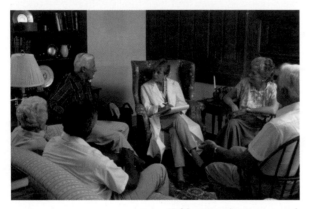

Experiential groups
Participants rely on experiencing, not just talking about, their needs

Encounter groups
Encourage therapy and self-growth through disclosure and interaction

Types of group therapy

Self-help groups
People who share a common problem are brought together to share information and to support each other

Family therapy
Can be used to deal with behaviour problems caused by poor relationships within a family

Types of group therapy

- They can gain comfort from others within the group.
- They may receive therapeutic benefit from listening, observing and watching others.

Taking part in group work

Education

Education is giving people information to help them deal effectively with a situation. They may be unaware of support that is available or of the situation they could find themselves in, e.g. teenage pregnancy is often the result of a naivety about sex.

Education can be used to:

- teach about an illness and its causes, helping the person to cope and manage the problem. Family members can also receive education to help them to a better understanding of the illness and to know how to provide support
- prevent future behavioural problems, e.g. emotional deprivation can be discussed and facts given by showing parents how to

contribute positively towards a child's development
- teach family members how to maintain a healthy family relationship – how to manage controllable factors, such as environment, that may be contributing to behavioural problems.

Often the subjects that service users need educating on are sensitive and may be connected with sex, financial worries, family problems, emotional issues or health, but people also need information regarding day-to-day topics.

Activity

Beatrice

Beatrice has an alcohol problem and has finally recognised that she needs help. She telephones the alcohol helpline and is invited to attend a group meeting with people who have similar problems.

1 Explain what is meant by the term 'group therapy'.

2 How could Beatrice benefit from attending an 'encounter group'?

3 Explain how education could help a service user.

Theories of counselling skills
Gerard Egan

The theories of Gerard Egan were discussed in Unit 3.1. Look back and remind yourself of the overview of his theories.

Stage 1 What is happening?	Stage 2 What do I want instead?	Stage 3 How could I get what I want?
Review of present situation Story Blind spots Leverage	*Development of new or preferred scenario* Possibilities Change agenda Commitment Action leading to valued outcomes	*Action strategies* Possible actions Best fit Plan

Egan's 'skilled helper' model

The main goal of Egan's three-stage model is to help people to help themselves. It is about empowering a person to move towards outcomes of their own choosing. It works best when working on issues in the recent past or in the present.

Egan's model shares Carl Rogers' core conditions of genuineness, respect and empathy. Egan also advocates active listening and that the model should be flexibly used and moved backwards and forwards in order to meet the service user's needs.

This model helps the service user to consider three main questions, which correspond to the three stages, as shown in the flow chart above.

Stage 1

Often, on deeper exploration, it becomes clear that something quite different is at the root of their problem. The helper will identify the story, challenge any blind spots by looking at the problem from different perspectives, then focus and prioritise to identify any aspect of the problem that the client can move on from, and make a difference.

Stage 2

All too often people will say that they are unhappy with their lives and want to change. However, all they are really aware of is what they don't want. An individual cannot move forward until they know where they are going. Here, participants can be creative and imaginative. The question can be asked, 'If you were to walk out the door and everything was perfect, what would it be like?' Moving on from this point questions

become more specific, e.g. the participant can be asked, 'How achievable is this? Can you set specific targets for this?'

> Non-achievable targets are not motivating in the long term and so targets need to be SMART:

- **S**pecific – not vague
- **M**easurable – so progress can be seen
- **A**chievable – not too ambitious
- **R**ealistic – able to be achieved with the time and resources available
- **T**imed – target dates to be met.

Stage 3

At this stage the goals are set using questions such as, 'How will things be different?', 'What will be the benefits?', 'Are there any disadvantages?' The main questions are, 'How can these goals be achieved?', 'What could help?', 'Are there different ways of reaching a solution?' The most appropriate strategy for the service user is selected, together with the available resources. The chosen strategy will then be broken into achievable steps for the service user to work on and to be supported through.

One important aspect of Egan's model is that the service user can move up and down through the stages to meet their individual needs, which should always be central to the counselling provided.

Ellen Noonan

Ellen Noonan promoted of the use of **psychotherapy**, which involves discussion of the service user's thoughts, behaviour and everyday functioning. This is broken down into shared goals and solutions that can be carried out, usually in the time between sessions.

Psychotherapy is based on the idea that psychological problems depend on a person's life experiences and the ability to shape their ways of thinking. It is about guiding the service user to their correct goal and supporting them along the way, rather than doing the work for them. Psychotherapy can help with a number of problems, such as anxiety, phobias, depression and relationship problems.

Ellen Noonan and those who adopt her theory prefer to see service users in their own homes, whenever possible, because:

● the service user will feel more comfortable in their own environment and be more likely to speak freely
● the person providing support can gain more personal knowledge of the service user from the things the service user has around them, e.g. books and pictures.

She does not judge people before she gets to know them, but tries to treat each service user equally and individually.

Seeing beyond the external reality is important in Ellen Noonan's theory. She wants to get in touch with the person's inner feelings. Her theory is based on psychoanalytic theory, particularly the work of Klein and the belief that the mind consists of :

● the conscious mind – the thoughts we are aware of

● the unconscious mind – the thoughts we are not aware of, but which direct our behaviour.

The unconscious mind is a far more powerful influence on us than our conscious mind. We repress into our unconscious the feelings and experiences that we cannot cope with. Although we do not have to confront these feelings and emotions, they continue to influence our behaviour. Counselling consists of trying to understand how our unconscious mind directs and shapes our current behaviours and emotions.

Diagnosis of a service user's problems is not based on the medical model of labelling a set of symptoms. Instead it is part of the therapeutic process by which the counsellor and client are able to identify the symptoms and place them in their context. By working through the cause of the symptoms, the client is able to resolve the problem and move on.

Ellen Noonan's theory is specifically about working with young people. Teenagers often have problems with self-identity. If a young person has been brought up with feelings of anxiety or abandonment, these difficulties can interfere with their mental well-being. A counsellor works with a young person by:

● recognising that the relationship between counsellor and client is more important than any insight or interpretation of behaviour. Counsellors need to provide the space for a positive relationship to develop

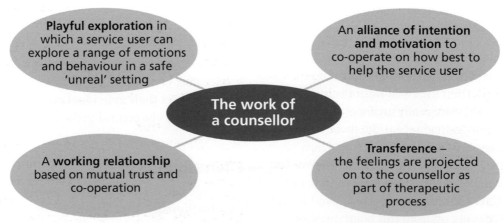

Noonan's four facets of a counsellor's work

- maintaining boundaries and standing back in order to get an overall perspective on the whole person and their difficulties
- working in the client's emotional space, without becoming over-involved. This means that they should be empathetic without adopting the emotional state of the client.

Ellen Noonan has done much work on counselling young people and whilst the principles of respect, honesty and acceptance will remain the same whatever the perspective of the theorist, it is clear that often young people have their own issues to contend with. This is a situation recognised by Noonan and addressed in her book *Counselling Young People*.

Theory of group work: Gaie Houston

The basis for running a group should be that participants will benefit more from sharing their experiences and will be better able to work collaboratively than alone. For many therapists, group work has the added benefit of ensuring that the counsellor is not the most important person in the process of change. The leader's role is not to 'lead' but is more about being non-directive and equal to those who are participating.

Houston is a very influential Gestalt therapist. Gestalt is a school of psychology that believes that patterns and themes are important and that 'the whole is more than the sum of its parts'. It is a process theory based on individual experiences. Houston suggests that group work can have great impact when organised well.

> ## Consider this
>
> *Why do you think treating the whole person is better than treating just the parts that appear to be troubled?*

A Gestalt group has a set process:

1 Starting

2 Experimentation

3 Ending.

Starting
Houston suggests that all groups are started by a sharing of objectives. Often this is done through the purpose of the group itself. However, the objectives of each individual member need to be included in the shared and agreed purpose of the group. This allows group members to feel as though they own the group-work process.

Ground rules have to be agreed between group members, including:

- to listen, and not to interrupt
- to use 'I' statements to express themselves, rather than judgements of others
- to report emotions before judgements
- to agree the amount of participation for each group member
- how decisions will be made.

Experimentation
The middle phase is characterised by active experimentation. Group members are encouraged to share individual objectives at the start of each session and to explore issues raised by the group. Group members may have to be

taught how to communicate, listen, give and receive feedback effectively. This is done through group work activities.

Ending

Ending the group is as important as any other stage and Houston suggests that great care needs to be given to this part of the process. Ending needs to be conducted properly in order to achieve closure, so that all participants have the tools and insights they need in order to move on. Often, sharing personal objectives with the group followed by 'circle time' where each group member states what they have gained from individuals within the group and their hopes and fears for the future, is a good way to mark closure of the group.

Other theorists

There is a vast number of theorists who have made a contribution to the way in which behaviour is understood. Below is a table which outlines the ideas of some theorists who have created positive and constructive ideas on what influences behaviour. These views and opinions can be very helpful when working in health, social care and early years settings.

Approaches	Which theorist?
Psychodynamic approaches	The founder of **psychoanalysis** is Sigmund Freud (1856-1939), followed by C G Jung, Wilhelm Reich, Melanie Klein, etc. Approaches used by Freud include transactional analysis and gestalt therapy.
Humanistic approaches	Carl Rogers (1902–1987) was the founder of the **person-centred approach**, but others include Abraham Maslow and Rollo May. Many modern approaches incorporate Rogers' ideas, particularly in education, where the theme is a person-centred or student-centred approach.
Behavioural approaches	The Russian psychologist, I P Pavlov (1849-1946), and the American psychologist, J B Watson (1878–1958), together with B F Skinner (1904–1990), are the founders of **behaviourism**. Their work acknowledges the role of behaviour in the learning process, and their approaches are deeply embedded in 'learning theories'.
Cognitive approaches	Aaron Beck (b.1921) and Albert Ellis (b.1913) separately developed cognitive approaches to mental distress and change, known as **cognitive approaches** or **rational emotive therapy**. This approach is often used in health care settings where time-limited helping work is undertaken. Other cognitive approaches have an impact on the treatment of severely disturbed people who are experiencing mental health problems

Activity

1 Investigate the work of **three** theorists, giving examples to explain in detail how their theories could be applied to counselling, or support given in settings.

Formulate individual action plans

Individual action plans are often used by professionals to assess the current situation of the service user, and to direct future work. They involve discussion and negotiation in setting realistic short-term targets in order to reach longer-term goals.

The format of an individual action plan varies between care settings. However, they all contain similar information.

- At the beginning of the action plan the current situation is identified, including any presenting issues or problems.
- Long-term problems or issues may also be discussed and progress towards resolving these issues may be noted.

Individual Action Plan		
Name:		
Issue:		
What are the options?		
Goal to be achieved:		
Targets:	**By whom:**	**By when:**
Date, time and place of review:		
Signed (client): _____ **Date:** _____		
Signed (staff): _____ **Date:** _____		

An individual action plan

- The position that the service user would like to reach is the aim or goal of the care work. In some cases this may involve a discussion of a very long-term goal, e.g. independent living, and in some cases may be a shorter-term target, e.g. managing money on a daily basis.

Theory into practice

What considerations would you need to take account of when drawing up an action plan?

You will probably have included some of the following:

- What are the service user's needs?
- What is the behaviour that is being dealt with?
- What are the possible strategies available?
- Have staff been trained in the strategies required or will we need outside help?
- How much time is needed?
- What is the outcome or goal?

An individual action plan must include the short-term targets or actions required to reach the goal. Targets should SMART. They should be broken down into small steps and the service user should discuss and record the actions to be taken in order to meet the targets. Any support needed by the service user to meet their targets should be identified as part of an individual action plan.

All individual action plans must contain a section in which the service user and a care worker evaluate the progress made towards the targets. This will involve reflection about whether the targets are still appropriate or whether the service user needs additional support. The service user is encouraged to set new targets with the care worker.

Assessment activity 3.4

Ways of providing support

Debbie-Anne is 35. She has had two partners and is currently living with her third, Matt. This relationship is having difficulties and Debbie-Anne has frequently visited her GP complaining that she is not able to sleep, she cannot cope with her two children, Erin 5 and Bonnie 2. She also has money worries and is getting very behind with the rent and other bills. Debbie-Anne suspects that Matt is having an affair and this leads to lots of rows which frighten the children. She admits that she and Matt have taken 'soft' drugs at times. Her stepson Aaron, who is 16, spends most evening out with his friends and often comes back to the house at 2.00 a.m. Debbie-Anne is sure he is going to be caught by the police for some sort of criminal activity.

1 Using the theories of **three** theorists, explain the ways of providing support for Debbie-Anne and her family. Include information on:

- counselling
- assessing individual needs
- group work
- education.

Make sure you make significant connections between the ways of support and the three theorists.

2 For Debbie-Anne or one other member of the family, draw up an individual action plan in detail. The action plan should include:
- information about how the plan will provide support
- the stages within the plan.

Give examples to illustrate the points you make. Try to show connections between theory and practice.

Working with challenging behaviour can be difficult, both mentally and physically. At some point, in any care setting, there will be small outbursts of challenging behaviour, e.g. in a reception class between children or in a residential home between residents. Providing a safe environment helps to prevent some forms of challenging behaviour, but not all.

Ways to manage

Effective behaviour management does *not* mean using physical force, humiliation or subterfuge.

Confront the problem, not the individual

Care workers need to identify the behaviour that is causing the problem and deal with it. They have to make sure that they confront the problem, not the individual. This is sometimes difficult to do. For example, if a client throws a plate of food across the room, the first reaction will possibly be, 'What have they done now? This is the last straw. Someone get them out of my sight before I wallop them!' This is a natural reaction. However, care workers need to be detached and investigate the reason for the behaviour. Often this type of behaviour is attention-seeking and by dealing with the problem rather than the person, the person has time to 'cool off', become calm and more objective, enabling the care worker to ascertain the cause of the action.

> ### Key point
> Behaviours can be bad, people are not.

Addressing the problem means that:

- the care worker can break the problem down into manageable parts
- the care worker is less likely to show prejudice against the individual

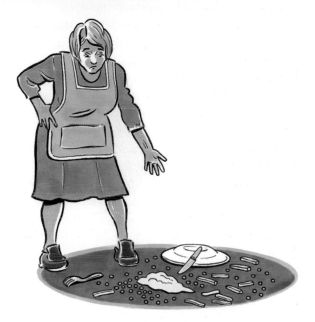

Whatever has Angie done now?

- the person who demonstrated challenging behaviour may be prevented from having to 'live up to the reputation'.

For example, if a child is being naughty, then the parent or carer should tell the child that *what they are doing* is naughty, not that *they* are naughty, which could lower their self-esteem and may also lead to a self-fulfilling prophecy.

Motivational factors

Negotiating and discussing provides motivation for the service user as they are actively involved in the process. Negative behaviour causes tension, and discussing feelings and problems is a way of removing tension from the situation.

Working with the service user is likely to improve relationships as the care worker and service user are sharing and learning to trust one another. Communication skills are likely to be improved as the care worker will be using several open questions which allow the service user to express their feelings and concerns. Negotiating is, therefore, a way of enabling the service user to come to an agreement with the care worker. The decision-making is their own and is more likely to be honoured.

The reason behind the behaviour is the key issue. By understanding why a person has done something, it is possible to remove any triggers that might set off a similar reaction.

> ## Consider this
>
> *Discuss with a partner how you have behaved since you got up this morning. Give reasons for each action. Is there anything you have done for absolutely no reason?*

Some actions are taken purely out of routine, e.g. 'I went to a certain room *because* that's where the nurse would be.' Other behaviours may be a consequence of the actions of others or something outside of our personal control, e.g. 'I dropped my trays on the floor *because* I was rushing and didn't collect them together properly.' There is always a 'because' for our behaviours, either a positive or a negative reason. Helping a person to think about 'why' or 'because' will help to stimulate motivation.

Providing the service user with a distraction is another way of managing challenging behaviour. It diverts their negative energy into something productive. It brings calm to the situation, e.g. a service user who has attempted to hurt another person could be asked to help the care worker lay the table in the dining room. The care worker will then have the opportunity to talk to the service user and to discover the reason and help them to see alternative approaches to the problem.

> ## Activity
>
> Menza pushed Moira away from the chair which she was about to sit in. She was extremely angry and threw her cup of tea over Moira.
>
> 1 List three reasons why Menza may have demonstrated challenging behaviour.
> 2 Describe the action that the care worker could take to motivate a change from challenging to desirable behaviour. (Remember, do not bribe.)
> 3 Work with a partner and role-play how to manage the challenging behaviour shown by Menza.

Shared responsibility

Taking part of the blame oneself as a care worker is part of shared responsibility, e.g. 'If only I had thought about that, Brandon, I could have prevented you from feeling ...'

Care workers also need to give service users a shared ownership of their behaviour. As a result of discussion and negotiation, they could share responsibility with the service user by saying, 'If you start feeling like this, let me know before it boils over', or, 'If I see you starting to behave inappropriately, I'll give you a sign so you can stop.' It is always easier to conquer challenging behaviour when support is available.

Ground rules

In order to behave appropriately, service users need to know what the rules are. Rules:

- help care workers to set structure and discipline
- give service users boundaries (what is and what is not acceptable)
- show service users that challenging behaviour is not tolerated and this will help them to direct their behaviour differently.

Service users need to be given space and time to make the right decisions and to behave in the correct way.

It is important to make sure that everyone knows the ground rules and the consequences of breaking them. It is a good idea to draw up these rules together giving service users some shared responsibility.

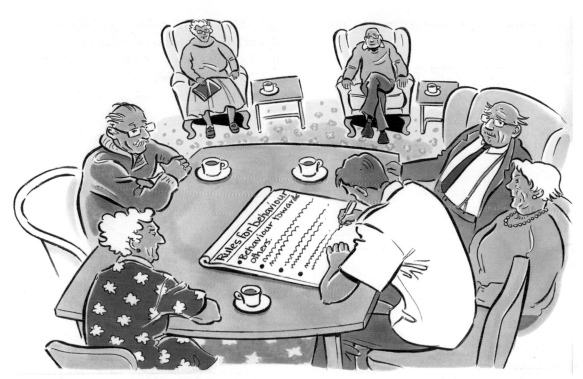

To behave appropriately, service users need to know what the rules are

Reinforce own personal, professional boundaries

When dealing with behavioural issues, care workers must always remember that they are professionals, although there will be an element of friendliness in their relationship with the service user.

Care workers do not have to accept challenging behaviour. It is essential for them to remain objective and detached at all times, and to tell service users when their behaviour is not acceptable. Part of professionalism is being clear about what is expected and the consequences that could result otherwise. Care must be taken not to interpret the challenging behaviour personally.

Behaviour that is sometimes challenged by care workers and sometimes ignored is unlikely to change. If the care setting does not allow any

threatening behaviour, this rule has to be upheld, no matter what justification there might have been for the behaviour in the first place. It is important to ensure that fairness and consistency are shown at all times.

Discourage physical harm to self and others

If there is any chance that a behaviour may harm the care worker, the service user or others, the care worker's first action must be to remove that possibility. This may mean removing the perpetrator to another area, moving everyone else out, or removing any objects that could cause harm. Alternatively, it may mean calling in assistance from elsewhere.

The safety of everyone must be the care worker's chief concern. It is important to give a service user freedom, but not at the cost of someone else getting hurt. In extreme situations, 'restraints' can be used, but only in specific care settings where the service users are considered to be dangerous.

Negative behaviour can be intimidating, both to the care worker and to other service users. Remember that the service user displaying aggression may also be scared and, therefore, every effort must be made to restore calm and dignity.

Provide positive role models

A positive role model is a model for appropriate behaviour. The most powerful way to express the desired way to behave is to display that behaviour.

It is important to provide service users with positive role models and encourage them to have respect for one another and for care workers. Positive role models in care workers encourage service users to share their thoughts and opinions and to discuss their feelings. A service user may admire the way a care worker or another service user conducts themselves and this may encourage them to act in a similar way.

Positive behavioural role models are achieved through being polite, respecting colleagues and service users, considering and acting on individual needs, giving praise when something has gone well, and generally creating an atmosphere of calm and positivity.

It is important not to behave badly as a care worker, as this will also be modelled!

Offer clear goals and regular feedback

If a service user is prone to challenging behaviour, it is important to set goals and to give feedback. This can help a service user to work on a particular aspect of their behaviour. Setting goals gives service users the opportunity to be slightly challenged. By achieving their goals, they are likely to grow in confidence, and this will help them to move forward.

If behaviour is challenging, there is little point in criticising it without discussing how it could be made better. To tell a service user, 'Your behaviour is appalling', is pointless as it neither tells the perpetrator what aspect of their behaviour is unacceptable nor what they can do to make it better. It would be far better to say, 'I was really disappointed to hear you using that language to Eric because it was really insulting. You know that we don't tolerate those words

here. I don't want to hear you using those words again.' Remember also to give praise if they manage to refrain from using bad language, e.g. 'I'm so proud of you using appropriate language all afternoon. Well done.'

Notice there are lots of active 'I' messages with the 'you' being more passive. This serves to keep the control of the situation with the care worker.

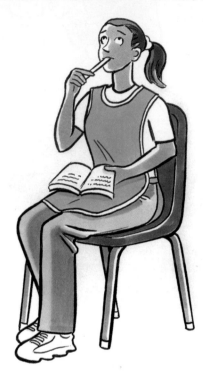

Hmm! What are my goals?

Discussion and negotiation

The use of 'I' messages is also useful when discussing and negotiating acceptable behaviour as it allows the service user to have an input whilst not losing sight of who is in charge. If people have a say in how they behave and what the rules are to be, they are far more likely to keep to them. Negotiation gives people ownership, increases self-esteem and makes co-operation far easier. So, although it may seem like an extra task at times, it is a valuable exercise. Remember, however, that negotiation is not just giving in to everyone's demands.

Always treat the service user with respect and dignity. Encourage them to explore the issues surrounding their challenging behaviour and, through this discussion, negotiate the ways by which they can improve their behaviour.

How to provide a safe and positive environment

Physical conditions

Surroundings can affect the way we feel and behave. Research suggests use of colour for different effects (yellow for learning, green for relaxing, etc.) and of Feng Shui to decide the best positions for objects.

> ### Consider this
>
> *Look at the rooms below. Which would you prefer to be in?*

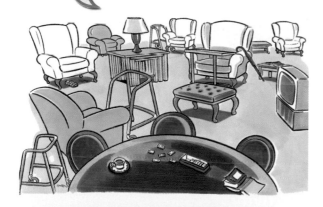

> ### Theory into practice
>
> Design a playroom for a nursery school explaining why the furniture and equipment have been placed in specific positions.

The physical environment should be pleasant, comfortable and effective in layout for its use. The position of doors and windows is very important. Sitting service users between the care worker and the door is potentially dangerous. Doors that open inwards present a hazard as an aggressive service user can trap a care worker inside the room by easily blocking the door. Moveable furniture can be hazardous. Blocked fire exits can cause injuries or loss of life.

Provide clear channels of communication

Care workers must make sure that clear channels of communication are known to service users and that they can speak easily and freely to those who can help them. Knowing this will have a positive psychological effect on service users and will probably help to build confidence.

Having effective skills in communication is important for all care workers. They must be able to demonstrate the skills shown below to enhance communication with service users.

Patronising language, invasion of personal space, tiredness and boredom all inhibit communication and should be avoided. Look back at Unit 2 for further details about skills that promote trust and value individuals.

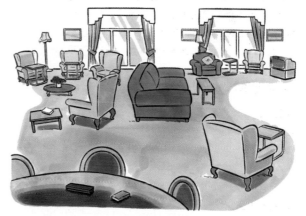

Positive integration of carers and service users

This is about how care workers interact with service users and with other care workers. Remaining professional at all times is essential, but this does not mean being aloof and unapproachable. Being able to interact with service users, and respecting their needs and feelings, are important if trusting relationships are to be established. When confronted with challenging behaviour, they should try to view it from the service user's perspective, which will make it easier to deal with. However, this will only be possible if care workers have given themselves the opportunity to get to know the service users as individuals.

Factors to consider	Reasons
Ambience	The general atmosphere of a setting sets the tone for all interactions, e.g. happy, comfortable, uncaring, cold. An ambience of aggression or negativity will impact on all forms of behaviour. Consider carefully what sort of atmosphere is required. Ambience is created by decoration, pictures, noise levels and patterns.
Attitudes	Positive attitudes are an important feature of all care environments. If care workers do not hold positive attitudes and do not believe that all service users deserve to be treated with dignity and respect, then the care provided by the setting will not be effective. Attitudes can be encouraged through shared aims of the service, identified through recruitment and modelled by all workers.
Identify and address consequences of 'negative' behaviour	Clearly-published rules and sanctions should be available to all service users. This helps to remind them of acceptable behaviour and also acts as a protection for more vulnerable service users.

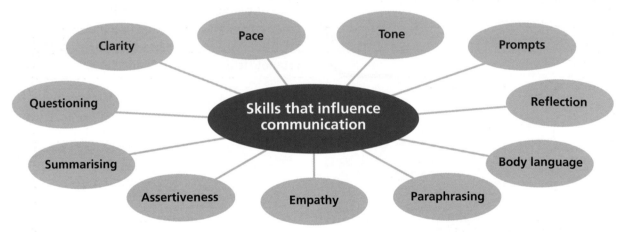

Skills that influence communication

When a new service user arrives, you need to take time to make sure they feel comfortable with the people with whom they are learning or living. The care worker will need to find out about the interests of the service user and their disposition and introduce them to others who will be sharing their environment.

Formulate personal action plans

Personal action plans were discussed at the end of Unit 3.4. Look back and refresh your memory.

Individual action plans set targets and goals to meet individual needs. Below is an example of an action plan for Reena.

Activity

Hedgerow Residential Home

Guiseppe and Tony enjoy playing cards in the evening and this is their after-tea routine. Joe has recently arrived at the home and wants to join in. Guiseppe was quite rude to him and the care worker when asked if Joe could take part. He used bad language, upset the table and stormed off.

1 Why do you think Guiseppe behaved like this?

2 How could the care workers have prepared the residents for Joe's arrival?

3 How could the care workers have prepared Joe better when he arrived?

Case study

Reena

Reena is 16 and suffers from depression. She lives in a children's home because she lost both parents in a car crash and has no other family or relatives to care for her. She is very aggressive, verbally abusive and shouts a lot.

The staff have drawn up an individual action plan for Reena.

From the action plan above it is possible to see that clear targets have been set, who is going to supervise each task and the date when the action plan will be reviewed.

Individual Action Plan

Name: Reena

Issue/aim: To reduce her depression

Objectives: Planning activities that will help Reena to cope.
Managing her money.

What are the options? Medication
Church-based activities – Reena likes church
Practical shopping and managing money

Goal to be achieved: To be able to live independently

Targets:	By whom:	By when:
Approach Reena – try to find something in common, build a realationship with her	Care Assistant	2 weeks
Take Reena to church	Care Assistant	Sunday morning
Take her to and fetch her from the Church Youth Club	Care Assistant	Friday evening
Sit down and work out allowance – what is needed, how much there is to spend	Care Assistant	Saturday morning

Date, time and place of review: 10 August 2006

Signed (client): RB   **Date:** 01/06/06

Signed (staff): AIF   **Date:** 01/06/06

An individual action plan for Reena

Assessment activity 3.5

Managing challenging behaviour

For a section in a resource pack that is being prepared by Hedgerow Residential Home, you have been asked to prepare materials that could be used to train staff in different ways of managing challenging behaviour.

1 Produce handouts that can be kept in the resource pack to explain different ways of managing challenging behaviour. You must include:
   - how to confront the problem, not the individual
   - motivational factors
   - shared responsibility
   - ground rules
   - how to reinforce own personal professional boundaries
   - how to discourage physical harm to self and others
   - how to provide positive role models
   - how to offer clear goals and regular feedback
   - discussion and negotiation.

2 Explain the consequences of negative behaviour.

3 Visit a care setting or ask a care worker to visit your centre. Find out the different types of challenging behaviour experienced by the setting. Use the information to illustrate how challenging behaviour is dealt with by care settings.

4 Explain how a care setting promotes a positive care environment for service users. Discuss in-depth how the physical and psychological environment can influence the behaviour of service users.

Try to make significant connections between theory and practice.

Settings will find that they are required to manage challenging behaviour in a variety of ways, as shown in the diagram below.

Service users may seek support for a number of reasons, including:

- feeling stressed or anxious
- being unable to make a decision
- having difficulty finding a solution to a problem
- experiencing mood or behaviour changes
- being unable to cope with life
- not achieving their potential
- harming themselves and not understanding why.

Care workers need to keep records of the actions taken, the decisions made and the goals and targets set. In some settings this is a legal requirement. The Data Protection Act (1998) gives service users the right to access information held about them on computers and in some instances also hand-written records. If records are kept, therefore, they should be written and stored in line with the Act. It is vital that the person making and storing the records keeps up-to-date with legal requirements.

It is important to prepare for a meeting with a service user who has presented challenging behaviour. Meetings can be very useful to assess, negotiate and discuss, to review progress or just to share information. They can influence a service user by motivating them to move forward and achieve more or they can disengage the service user and cause them to **regress** or to give up.

Remember that a positive care environment does not just happen, it must be planned. When planning, it is important to consider the factors in the table opposite.

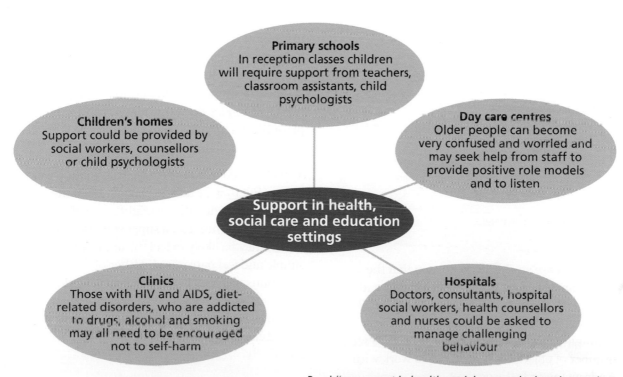

Providing support in health, social care and education settings

Factor to be considered	How to plan
Aim	What do we hope to achieve by having the meeting? How does the meeting fit with the overall care of the service user? What is the long-term goal?
Objectives	These are the stepping stones that will provide a way to achieve the aim, a set of targets that help the service user to reach the required outcome.
Time-scales	Planning will involve working out how long the meeting will last and the time-scale for the course of action that is planned. If not done, the meeting could be vague and have no specific purpose. The person leading the meeting should consider when the review should take place. In other words, what time-frame is reasonable to expect the service user to achieve the goal set?

Case study

Andrew

Andrew is 5 and is in the reception class of primary school. He is always aggressive and demanding, particularly when he does not get what he wants. His behaviour needs to improve. The classroom assistant has been asked to look after Andrew and help him with his problems for a maximum of one hour each day.

Aim: To provide a safe and positive environment that will be conducive to improving Andew's behaviour

Objectives:
● To work with Andrew on a one-to-one basis on daily activities
● To actively listen to what he has to say
● To provide praise when something he does is good
● To confront the problem not the individual
● To set ground rules
● To remain calm and positive when he presents challenging behaviour
● To offer an alternative when he presents challenging behaviour, giving him an alternative to think about

Time-scale: Four weeks

From the case study, it can be seen that the classroom assistant has, in consultation with the teacher, thought through the overall aim. She has thought about the different ways of managing challenging behaviour and has set a number of objectives to help her to work with Andrew towards the goal set.

Consider this

Liz, aged 71, has thrown a cup of tea over another resident three times in the last two days. What would be your aim in managing her challenging behaviour? What objectives would you set?

Skills

Are any specific skills required for the activity you are planning to manage? Do you need a range of skills? Which skills are needed? (See next page.)

Do you have enough qualified staff to care for the number of service users who will attend the meeting or to cope with service users who are not involved? Do you need to bring in any specialist staff, e.g. a support worker or an advocate? You need to consider these questions early in the planning stage so that you can arrange what is needed in good time.

You also need to consider the skills of the service users. Will they be able to participate in the activity independently or might some of them require assistance, e.g. a support worker? Or would they be likely to feel the activity is too simple and feel patronised? Either of these situations will lead to challenging behaviour because the service users will feel disrespected and undervalued if they do not consider that their needs are being recognised and met effectively.

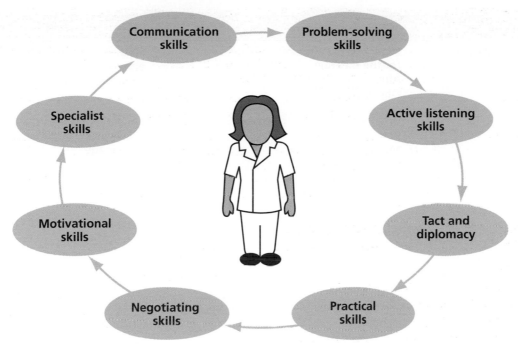

A variety of skills could be required

Environment

When looking at the environment, it is important to consider whether it is appropriate for the user group. Older service users would not feel comfortable in a room decorated with children's pictures.

You should also check that the environment is clean and tidy. Service users will feel far more respected and inclined to keep an area tidy and clean if they are presented with a clean and tidy environment. If, for example, your work involved organising and running a youth club and the members arrive to a room with overflowing bins and used cups on the tables, how likely do you think they would be to clear away after themselves and throw away their rubbish? If half the equipment is broken or has bits missing, how inclined will members be towards looking after it or trying to use it?

Approaches

What approach is to be used? The meeting you are planning might be formal or informal. It could involve training service users in new skills, developing current skills or having a role that enables the service user to approach you for advice and guidance or as a listening ear. The group or individual may have been referred for assessment and, if this is the case, plans will need to be detailed to ensure that assessment is fair and reliable. Most service users like to have a person who is in authority whom they can trust. They also expect that person to have knowledge in their problem area. You need to take all these points into consideration when producing the plan.

Prepare the physical and psychological environment

Types of environment

The environment must be appropriate, both physically and psychologically.

Physically, the room needs to be large enough for the meeting to ensure that it adheres to health and safety regulations. If a one-to-one meeting is intended, the room should not be too large, as the person could feel uncomfortable. You should ensure that emergency exits are not blocked and that there is sufficient ventilation and lighting. If the individual, or any group member, has special needs, such as using a wheelchair, they should be able to move around comfortably and participate fully in the session.

Time-scale	Action to be taken	Reason for action
Monday 10.00 a.m.	Work out the aim and objectives for the meeting: **Aim:** **Objectives:**	So that I have something to aim for and I know what steps I will need to take to achieve it.
10.20 a.m.	What skills am I going to need? **Communication:** **Motivational:** **Goal setting:** **Discussion and negotiation:**	Thinking about the skills that will be necessary to enable me to manage.
10.40 a.m.	Environment: **Where?** **Time?** **Points to remember?**	So that...

Example of a plan

From a psychological perspective, it is important that planning should ensure that the environment is appropriate to the age and needs of the service users. In other words, they should feel as if this room was intended for them. This may mean adding a few items that will make them feel more comfortable, e.g. some older people prefer to use cups and saucers rather than mugs. The type of chairs to be used, their height and positioning are extremely important. If it is a one-to-one meeting, the chairs might be better placed side by side; if a group meeting is being planned, a circle arrangement may be preferable.

Lighting needs to be appropriate for the occasion. If a service user is having a counselling session, shining a bright light directly on them is not going to help them to talk about their needs and the things that are worrying them. If a service user is trying to obtain some information from a care worker, being able to see them as they speak and the body language that they are using could help to convey meaning.

Noise

If it is noisy when a care worker is giving information, the service user may not hear exactly what is being said and may receive incorrect information. This could lead to the service user making the wrong decision. It is important, therefore, that external noise is kept to a minimum when having conversations.

On the other hand, if it is very quiet in the room, a service user may be reluctant to exchange ideas with a care worker, because they may be afraid that everyone in the room will be listening to what they have to say.

It will be important that others are informed not to interrupt the meeting. This can be done by placing a notice on the door, particularly if confidential information is to be discussed.

Consider this

How can poor lighting affect the communication with a service user who is being shown information in a leaflet about the treatment that is being proposed?

Consider this

How can noise affect a service user who is attending a day centre for the first time and who is listening to a care worker explain what happens at the day centre?

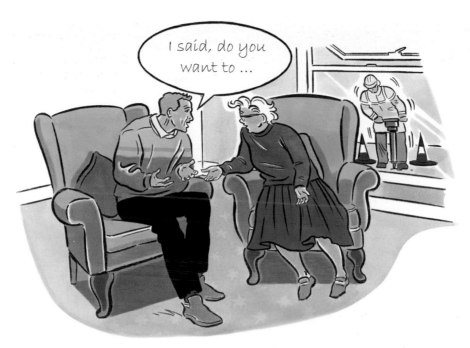

Could you hear what was being said in this situation?

Temperature

A room that is too hot or too cold can cause lack of concentration and loss of interest. Lack of ventilation could cause the person to become drowsy and they may even fall sleep. Make sure that the room is at an ideal temperature: around 18–21° C is best.

> ### Consider this
>
> *When communicating, how can too much heat and little ventilation affect a service user in a residential home?*

Support

Make sure there is sufficient support available. There should be at least one other person in the vicinity for safety reasons. If the service user's behaviour became very aggressive you may need help to remove them from the room or to distract them. It is possible that support for individual service users may be required, so that they can gain as much as possible from the session, e.g. an advocate. A colleague who knows the members

of the group could be present to help in practical ways, such as giving out teas or helping to jot down notes, or they could encourage service users to participate.

Remember to value support workers. They must know the plans and what is expected of them. They should have joint ownership of the plan.

Implementation of clear policies

Everyone who works in the setting should be clear about the policies that apply. This means following the ground rules set out in policies such as confidentiality, health and safety, and equal opportunities. There may be other policies in force. For example, if a policy states that no food is allowed in certain rooms and the meeting is to be held in one of these rooms, then the policy must be observed.

When setting the ground rules for the meeting, stating why certain procedures are being used or why a certain action is not possible will enable all participants to understand and co-operate and may avoid challenging behaviour.

Recording method

For legal reasons, you will need to keep records relating to the meeting. The records you keep will

Individual Meeting Plan		
Name:		
Aim:		
Objectives:		
What information is required?		
Megan's response:		
Issues/Difficulties: **Goals:**	**By whom:**	**By when:**
Date, time and place of meeting:		
Signed: _____ **Date:** _____		
Staff: _____ **Date:** _____		

An individual meeting plan (adapted from the individual action plan on page 141)

depend on the type of meeting that is to be held. An individual action plan could be used if you and the service user are meeting to decide why a certain action happened and how to deal with it. Similarly, if you are discussing information needed by the service user, such a document could be used or adapted, as above.

The records kept must clearly respond to those permitted by the Data Protection Act. These will be confidential documents which must be treated as such with regard to access and storage. They must be clearly written, non-biased and available to the service user should they request to see them.

Activity

Piers has agreed to have a meeting with Margot, his key worker, to discuss his complaints about the food served at meal times and about the way the TV is turned over to other channels without asking those who are watching.

1 Explain how you would prepare the meeting room for Piers and Margot.

2 Draw a diagram of the room layout.

3 How would you organise support?

4 Design a document that would be suitable for recording the meeting.

Demonstrating managing and coping skills

Strategies for managing challenging behaviour were given in Unit 3.5. Look back and remind yourself of the strategies that can be used.

Preparation will be needed for the meeting. This will include:

- a plan showing the time scales that you will use, both for the preparation and the meeting
- a checklist of the preparation to be completed, e.g. at least two physical, two psychological

and two environmental checks that will be carried out
- the recording documentation to be used
- the content of the meeting, e.g. an outline transcript of the initial meeting, the main content and how you propose to wind up.

Ideas for the plan have been given earlier in this section. Below is an example of a checklist that could be produced.

Remember to work out an outline script for the three stages involved in the meeting. For example, what might be said in:

- the initial contact
- the main content
- the winding up session.

This script could be very useful when carrying out the evaluation of the meeting as you will be able to show where you have used, for example, managing and coping skills, and where you used open questions.

To demonstrate your managing and coping skills, you will need to arrange for your tutor or supervisor to be present to record their observations. You may also wish to involve your peers as they will be able to provide feedback which could be used when evaluating. Both tutor and peers will need to be as unobtrusive as possible.

Factors	How checking will take place	Reasons
Physical 1	Room available	To make sure we are not interrupted
Physical 2		
Other physical		
Environmental 1	Is the lighting adequate?	So that we can see one another without difficulty
Environmental 2		
Other environmental		
Psychological 1	The ambience of the room	Making sure it is age-appropriate
Psychological 2		
Other psychological		
Skills to be used	Set ground rules Remind about policies Effective communication Motivational factors	So the service user knows that swearing is not acceptable
Approaches to be used	Egan's model …	Moving through the three stages will help to cover the information and to set goals
Recording documentation		

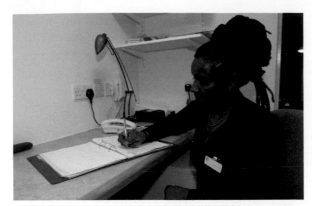
How am I going to do this?

Evaluation

What is evaluation? It is:

- thinking about what we have done and how we have done it
- considering the skills we have used and the reasons why we used them
- asking ourselves questions about how effective we have been when using these skills and whether we achieved the outcomes we wanted. Did we achieve the aims and objectives we set? How well did we meet them?
- thinking about any improvements we could make.

When evaluating, we use the skills set out in the table below.

What happens when we reflect?

When we reflect, we think about the whole meeting with the service user, from start to finish. Here is an example of reflection by Stuart who has had a meeting with Bret at the day care centre. He is thinking or reflecting on the first part of the conversation he had with Bret:

> 'My introduction was clear and my tone of voice was friendly and welcoming. I established a good relationship with Bret. I think this was because I smiled at him and led him towards a chair, asking where he preferred to sit. I also offered him some refreshment which helped to make the meeting feel less formal. I am pleased that I arranged the seats so that they were side by side and not facing one another. I think this helped Bret to feel more relaxed. I needed to put him at ease so that I could collect accurate information about why he was behaving towards the two residents in an aggressive manner. My aim was to find out what emotions Bret was experiencing.'

In this example Stuart is thinking about his aims and objectives, what he actually did and how well he did it. He is going over in his mind what actually took place at the beginning of the meeting. It often helps if we look back at the outline script at this stage to remind us of what we planned to do.

How do we analyse?

When Stuart has thought through and clearly remembered all the parts of the meeting he had with Bret, he will begin to analyse; that is, he will think about particular things he has done and/or the skills he has used and how well he has used them. To do this, Stuart will need to make judgements. For example, he may want to make judgements about the skills and approaches he used and how he used them. Stuart's analysis of the skills he used follows at the top of the next page.

Skills	Examples
Reflection	Thinking about what we have done and how it was completed
Analysis	Examining what we have done in detail. What were the advantages? What did not work so well? Why?
Drawing conclusions	Making a decision about how well we have completed the tasks or skills. Using theory to make judgements against.
Planning	How well did we plan? Did we plan for contingency arrangements? How to improve tasks or skills

'I think my tone of voice was appropriate because I did not have a raised voice, neither was it too quiet so that Bret couldn't hear. I made frequent eye-contact so that Bret knew I was interested in what he had to say and that I was focusing on him. I used quite a number of open questions, e.g. one I used was, "Why do you think you did that?" This gave Bret the chance to think and talk about his feelings. I also used reflective comments to show Bret that I was actively listening, e.g. "So you didn't like the way he spoke to you at lunch time last week?" I did summarise during the conversation because at one stage Bret was jumping from topic to topic and I wanted to make sure that I had understood him correctly. I said, "So have I understood correctly, you did this because you felt he was patronising you when ..."'

Stuart has considered the skills he used in his conversation with Bret, analysed them and given examples to illustrate the points he was making. He had theoretical knowledge about managing skills and communication skills and how they should be used, so he could make decisions. He was able to think about the skills against the 'theory' he had learned. Thinking about each component part within the task or activity is part of the analysing process. For example, Stuart states:

'I managed to prevent Bret from getting angry by taking shared responsibility. I did this by saying, "I wish I had known that was the reason for your behaviour, as I could have taken quite a different role at the time." This helped Bret to realise that the fault was not entirely his own and therefore, he became more trusting in the conversation.'

What is drawing conclusions?

When we make decisions, we are making 'informed judgements'. That is, measuring something against the knowledge we have of the subject, in this case managing challenging behaviour.

When we make decisions and explain them, we are making 'reasoned judgements' as we are examining the facts and knowledge supplied by others who may be experts and we make decisions based on this. Facts and knowledge could be the views of theorists or other people who have knowledge and opinions of the subject; or we could be using the feedback we have received from our assessor or peers or we could include our own opinions. Here is an example of Stuart's conclusions from his conversation with Bret:

'In my opinion I used prompts very successfully as Bret moved the conversation forward as a result of my saying, "So, what would you like to see happening next? It's a difficult choice to make." If I had not done this, it is likely that Bret would have continued to talk around the subject without making any decisions. In his feedback my assessor confirmed that this was appropriate.

I was not afraid of silence. Bret had one long silence during the conversation. I think he was thinking back over what he had done and why. Jan Sutton and William Stewart in their book *Learning to Counsel* state, "Silence can be threatening but it can also be constructive." In Brett's case I think it was constructive because he was recalling memory of actions that had taken place, which helped him to arrive at a decision.'

In this example, Stuart is expressing his own opinions and referring to the opinions of others. He is considering the skills he used and their purpose and discussing the reasons for points in the conversation. In a full evaluation, Stuart would discuss a range of skills used, drawing conclusions about their effectiveness.

What are the reasons for evaluating and improving own performance?

Having drawn conclusions, good practice is to think about the ways we could improve our own performance when managing challenging behaviour. For example, we may consider:

- *purpose* – did the skills used enable the purpose of the communication to be achieved?
- *reasons for use* – what were the reasons for using the skills chosen? Were there other skills that would have been more suitable?
- *effectiveness* – did the skills used enable both yourself and the service user to understand and have a meaningful exchange of information?

- *achievement of outcomes* – did the skills allow the outcomes to be achieved? Could the service user have benefited if something had been done differently?

If listening skills were demonstrated during the meeting, then our evaluation of the meeting is more likely to be accurate. Active listening is when we not only give our undivided attention to the speaker, but we actively try to determine what they are saying to us. This often reaches beyond the words they are using and is learned more from their body language, including eye-contact and positive body language. They will empathise with the client. In other words, according to Egan's theories, the service user will be accepted with unconditional positive regard – they will be accepted and supported in a non-judgemental way.

The benefits of this type of approach for the service user will be of very great value. They will realise that they are accepted, but that their behaviour was not. They will feel valued and this will contribute to their self-esteem and make them more confident. Feelings of guilt are likely to be reduced. Sharing the responsibility for what has happened will have created a sense of trust and self-worth and enabled the service user to face up to the difficulties of their behaviour without loss of face or embarrassment. According to Egan, congruence will enable the service user to feel accepted even if the behaviour displayed does not

Assessment activity 3.6

Promoting a positive environment

Liam

Liam has asked for a meeting with you because he feels that he is not liked by the other residents at the residential home. He lost his temper and shouted at Fran because she was sitting in his chair. On another occasion, he threw his plate of sandwiches at Marcus because he was making a noise when swallowing his food.

1 Make a plan for the preparation and holding of the meeting. Include:
- aim
- objectives
- timescales
- skills to be used
- approaches to be used.

Give reasons for each aspect of the plan.

2 Prepare a checklist to help you prepare for the meeting. Include at least:
- two physical checks that you will make
- two psychological checks you will make
- two environmental checks that you will make.

3 Develop the recording document you will use during the meeting.

4 Record an outline script showing the conversation that is likely to occur during:
- initial contact
- main conversation
- winding up.

5 Demonstrate managing and coping skills during the meeting with Liam. (Remember to arrange for your tutor or supervisor to observe you and to record your level of competency.)

6 Evaluate the meeting to include:
- aim
- objectives
- timescales
- skills
- approaches used
- own performance
- benefits to the service user.

Glossary

Attachment: the bond formed e.g. between an infant and its primary care-giver (usually the mother)

Autonomy: personal freedom; independance

Categorical: relating to a category; putting ourselves into a category

Conditional positive regard: love and approval given if certain conditions are met, e.g. good behaviour, i.e. in a judgemental way

Emulate: to copy

Existential: relating to existence, especially human existence

Internalise: to incorporate within the self as a conscious or subconscious guiding principle through learning or socialisation

Paraphrasing: expressing what something means, using other words

Psychosocial:

Psychotherapy: therapy using mental processes (the mind)

Reflecting: thinking over what someone has said

Reinforce: to reward e.g. a behaviour or response (e.g. with praise) so that it is more likely to occur again

Regress: to go backwards, i.e. in terms of behaviour/ thoughts

Schema: a pattern imposed on a complex experience that helps to explain it

Self-concept: our sense of who we are; the picture we have of ourselves

Self-esteem: how we feel about ourselves

Self-worth: how we value ourselves

Sequence: a following of one thing after another

Social class: one way of grouping people within society according to wealth, income and occupation

Unconditional positive regard: love and approval given without conditions, i.e. in a non-judgemental way

Upward mobility: the movement through society from a lower to a higher social level

Unit 4 Applied practical care in care settings

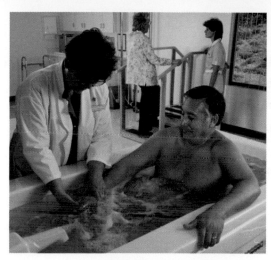

Practical care should respect the service user

Introduction

Have you ever received practical care? What do you remember about it? Did you still feel in control, or did you think that the carers were disregarding what you wanted?

Care workers should provide the highest possible standard of care while making sure service users' choices and opinions are taken into consideration. They need to achieve a balance between giving the care needed and allowing service users to do as much as possible for themselves.

Care workers will need to understand legislation and the influence it has on care settings, particularly in relation to accessing and storage of records. They will also need to be aware of the different types of records that are kept by care settings, and their purposes. Protecting service users through the accurate completion of records is also an important part of their work, not only from the service users' perspective but also from other care workers' point of view. Poor records could result in incorrect treatment or the wrong person being contacted!

Preventing the spread of infection is an important responsibility. A service user does not want to end up with a condition that they did not have before they entered the care setting! Providing a safe environment is also essential as people who receive practical care are often **vulnerable**. Care workers will need to demonstrate a range of skills to put the service user at ease. These will be demonstrated by:

- **monitoring** and supporting a service user when taking their temperature and pulse
- providing first aid
- moving and handling service users who want to change position
- making a bed
- producing a snack
- serving a meal or snack.

Bringing together knowledge and skills to provide a competent approach to practical caring will give you confidence for future work in health, social care or early years settings.

In this unit you will learn

Learning outcomes

You will learn to:

- complete records accurately and to recognise the impact of legislation on care settings
- investigate how to care for service users who have infections
- recognise how to assist individuals who wish to change position
- provide basic health support for service users
- make a bed using the correct techniques
- produce a snack showing understanding of dietary requirements
- evaluate the practical care you have provided.

Legislation

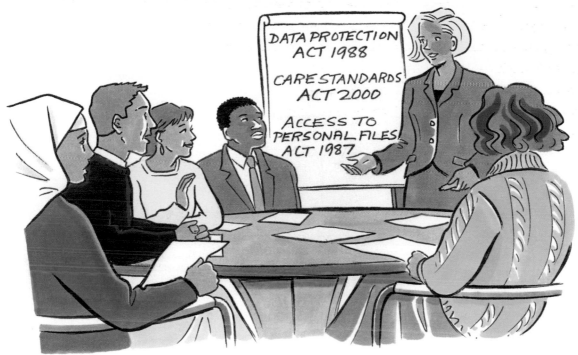

Legislation and regulations underpin all practical care

Being aware of **legislation** that affects care settings is the baseline of any practical care. You will need to know:

- what legislation affects the care setting
- the impact of the legislation, e.g. how it will affect day-to-day work
- the purpose of the relevant legislation
- what you must do to comply with the legislation.

Legislation is the law and must be followed. Having a role in a care setting, whether as an employee or doing work experience, means you have obligations and responsibilities. All care workers have a duty to know about and to follow the legislation that affects the work they do.

Each local authority is required to issue guidelines relating to the registration of care settings in their area. Some of the key requirements that all owners/managers have to fulfil are outlined in the table on the next page.

As a result of Acts of Parliament, most local authorities require residential and nursing homes to maintain certain records. Common records that a nursing or residential home might keep are:

- admission records
- daily statements of service users' health
- care plans
- monitoring records
- progress reports
- visitors log
- accident/incidence report.

Requirement of local authority	Evidence
Suitability and fitness	Could they carry out the care they said they could, e.g. provide 24-hour nursing care and support?
Suitability of premises	Were the buildings designed to cope with the type of care provided, e.g. did they have lifts to move service users from one floor to another?
Number of staff	Were they able to employ sufficient staff to carry out the caring role, e.g. night care staff?
Level of service	Could they provide the necessary level of care? A service user who has mild mobility problems would probably require level 1 care but a service user who cannot move from a bed to a chair unaided would require level 3 care.

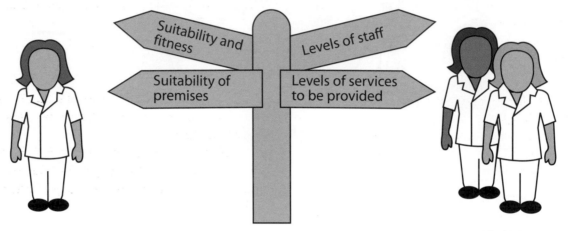

Can we cope with this level of care?

Consider this

What do you think were the effects of Acts of Parliament on service users?

What is the impact of legislation on care settings?

Legislation means that settings must keep records or they could be given written warnings and be closed down by inspectors who check that all procedures are in place.

Data Protection Act 1998

The Data Protection Act 1998 *must* be **implemented** by all health, social care and early years settings. This piece of legislation covers how to deal with confidential information. The Act replaces the Data Protection Act 1984. The new Act was implemented in care settings from March 2000. It sets rules for processing personal information and relates mainly to those records held on computer. The Data Protection Act 1998 covers:

- financial information
- credit information
- membership of organisations
- health records
- social service records.

The main principles of the Data Protection Act 1998 are summarised in the table opposite.

Principle of the Data Protection Act 1998	What it means
Information must be secure	Access to information must be limited to professional care workers who have been given a password. Written information must also be stored securely, e.g. under lock and key
Information must not be kept longer than necessary	A disposal date for records is required of organisations. Service users' records must be destroyed within a few years of them having received the service. Records of adoption can be kept for as long as 100 years
Information must be sufficient, relevant and not excessive	Only information needed by an organisation should be kept, nothing more, nothing less
Information must be accurate and up-to-date	Facts should be checked before they are recorded. If a service user's details change they should be amended as soon as possible
Information cannot be transferred from one country to another without sufficient protection	This is not likely to apply to health, social care and early years organisations. However, if information is transferred to another country it must be sufficiently protected
Information must have limited purpose	An organisation must have a lawful reason to hold the data, e.g. to monitor the services provided

What is the impact of this legislation on care settings?

An organisation must have a **nominated controller**. The controller is responsible for ensuring that:

- information kept about service users is reviewed regularly, i.e. about every six weeks
- information that is no longer relevant is removed from records
- written records filed in secure filing cabinets
- only one supervisor for each shift has a key to the filing cabinets
- any of the staff who add to the records explain to the supervisor what they want to add and are given the relevant piece of paper only, not the whole file.

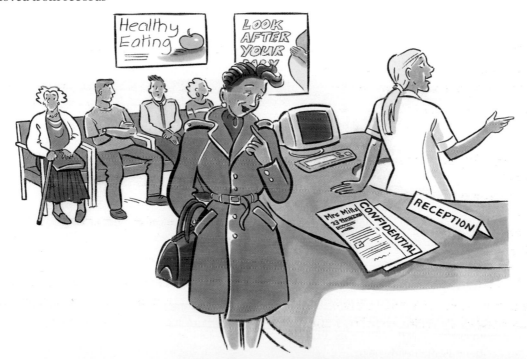

The controller must ensure that confidential material is not left in public areas

The Data Protection Act 1998

Melissa is the controller of records at Patchway Playgroup. The information kept about the children who attend is reviewed every two months. Information that is irrelevant is deleted.

Any written records that the playgroup has are kept locked away in secure filing cabinets and only the supervisor for each shift has access to them. If anything needs to be added to the files, only the supervisor is allowed to do this. The supervisor is only given the relevant piece of paper on which to make the addition, not the whole file.

1 How is the Patchway Playgroup complying with the Data Protection Act 1998?

2 What would happen if the playgroup did not comply with the Data Protection Act 1998?

3 What are the benefits to the service user of the Data Protection Act?

Theory into practice

Find out how the Data Protection Act 1998 affects the practice of a particular care setting.

Care Standards Act 2000

The Care Standards Act 2000 **subsumes** the Registered Homes Act 1984 and attempts to **standardise** the level of care given to service users in any residential care setting. It clearly sets out the **minimum** standards service users can expect when in residential care. The Act emphasises that residential homes and nursing homes must cater for the different individual needs of each service user. For example, a service user who is assessed and is considered to be at a level 3 need should be cared for at that level.

As a result of the Care Standards Act 2000, the National Care Standards Commission (a non-governmental public body) was created. Its purpose is to regulate social and health care services previously not regulated by the local authority. It also includes the regulation of **domiciliary** care agencies, fostering agencies and residential family centres. The Care Standards Act 2000 states that, in residential and nursing homes, service users:

- must be consulted about their choice of home, e.g. they can choose the type of care they would like to have
- must be consulted about personal health care, e.g. what services they would like and what type of support they would find suitable

Case study

Assessing Molly

Molly had been living in her own home until she fell and broke her hip. Before the accident, Molly had been fully supported by a health care assistant who got her up in the morning and put her to bed at night. She had a care assistant who came three times each week and helped with cleaning and meals-on-wheels provided lunches at a small cost.

The fall caused Molly to break her hip and, as a result, she developed severe **incontinence** problems. Molly's memory is also not very good and she forgets when she has washed or eaten. Molly has been assessed as needing level 3 care since her accident as she needs help:

- with mobility
- to eat and drink
- to maintain hygiene.

Molly wanted to go to the same residential home as her friend.

1 What type of care would be best for Molly after her accident?

2 How would the care setting chosen attend to each of Molly's needs?

3 How has the Care Standards Act provided a minimum standard of care for Molly?

- must have an acceptable daily life and social activities, e.g. mental stimulation must be provided in the form of activities and social activities
- are entitled to have a complaints procedure in place and to be protected, e.g. they must know who to complain to, and how, when they are dissatisfied
- are entitled to have an environment that is acceptable, e.g. an en-suite facility
- should have sufficient staffing to meet their needs, e.g. staff who are qualified to meet the standard of care they need and sufficient numbers of staff.

The Act also states that residential and nursing homes should have the required standard of management and administration, e.g. a structure that ensures smooth running with identified personnel.

These standards are measurable and the regulators, such as inspectors, look for evidence of these.

What is the impact of this legislation on care settings?

Places in nursing homes are very hard to find, so while service users have the right to choose, this does not often happen. Nursing homes are very expensive so most people have to have an 'assessment of need' before social services agree to pay the costs. Some service users are private payers. Most nursing and residential homes will have a mixture of people who are paying privately and those who are being fully or partly paid for by social services.

The service users in nursing and residential homes are given a choice of GP. It is probable that the home will have an identified GP, but some individuals choose to remain with the GP they had previously.

Most residential and nursing homes will have a complaints procedure in place and a Mission Statement. A copy of these is placed in a folder in each service user's room so that the service user and their relatives can read the complaints procedures.

Hill Tops Mission Statement

To make a complaint:
- Talk through the complaint with your key carer.
- Write down your complaint and put it in an envelope
- Head the envelope to...

Mission statements show how to register a complaint

All staff who work in residential and nursing homes are either trained or are being trained. Anyone who starts work as a care assistant or a health care assistant has to achieve the Foundation Standards, set by the Care Act 2000, within six weeks of starting at the home. Health care assistants usually follow NVQ courses.

Theory into practice

Try to visit a nursing or residential home. Using a questionnaire or interview questions, find out how their practice has been affected by the Care Standards Act 2000. Alternatively, you could ask a care professional to visit your centre to find out the information.

Access to Personal Files Act 1987

Service users now have the right to access their own health records. If they request to see their medical records, any information relating to another person (a third party) is removed before they see them. The service user has the right to write to their GP and request copies of their medical records.

Nursing homes are also inspected at registration by inspection officers employed by the local NHS trust. Although they have the right to see the day-to-day records relating to care, they do not have the right to see medical records unless the inspector is a qualified medical practitioner.

What is the impact of this legislation on care settings?

If a service user wants to complain about any medical treatment they are receiving, it is good practice that staff remind them that they can send for their medical records.

Inspection officers are able to access records relating to day-to-day care.

Activity

Brendan F

Mr F lives in a nursing home. He has an eye problem and is taken to see a specialist at the hospital. The specialist thinks that the problem has been caused by watching too much television and that his eyes are watering as a result.

Mr F and his relatives, when told of the specialist's opinions, refuse to believe this is the cause, as Mr F hardly ever watches television. Mr F has been confined to his room for some time and he does not have a TV in his room. The matron of the nursing home reminds Mr F and his relatives that they could request to see the medical records if they wish.

All reference to any other persons was removed from the file and Mr F was given access to the file. As a result, he decided to seek a second opinion.

1 Explain how the Access to Records Act 1987 has helped Mr F.

2 Why do you think that any references to third parties were removed from the record before Mr F was given the file?

3 Why did the matron remind Mr F and his relatives that he had the right to see his file?

Types of records

Records are kept by all organisations that provide health, social care or early years services. These records are only as good as the information placed on them. If the information on the records is inaccurate, then the incorrect treatment could

---

Case study

Sheema

When Sheema was in her early 80s, she spent several weeks in hospital. She was quite ill and had received a variety of medication to try to improve her heart condition. After five weeks, Sheema's relatives noticed that the medication had been stopped and that her condition was worsening. They persuaded Sheema to ask for her medical records.

The staff kept saying that they would have the records 'ready by the next day' but, when requested the next day, they were still not ready. Eventually, Sheema's records were reluctantly produced. Sheema noticed that a decision had been made by the staff to stop her medication without consulting her. Sheema asked for an enquiry about why this had happened. The medication was restarted immediately.

1 How were the staff at the hospital not respecting the Access to Personal Files Act?

2 Why did Sheema and not the next of kin ask for the records?

3 What might have happened if Sheema had not seen her records?

4 Find out what impact the Access to Personal Files Act 1987 has on service users in a day care centre or a playgroup?

---

be given or the wrong person contacted in an emergency.

The case study at the top of the next page is an example of how information had been placed on the wrong record. This incorrect information caused a great deal of unnecessary pain and upset to everyone involved.

All records contribute to the quality care of the service user. All professional care workers have a responsibility to communicate effectively in their written records as they work closely with service users, relatives and others.

Case study

Angela

Angela was sleeping peacefully when the telephone rang at about 2.30 a.m. It was the hospital calling asking her to come to the hospital straight away as her father had been admitted and had died. Angela was very upset and cried all the way to the hospital. She was met on the ward by a nurse who told her that she was very sorry but her father had died from heart failure as he was being admitted.

Angela asked where her mother was. The nurse said, 'She is sitting in the little room over there having a cigarette.'

Angela knew immediately it was not her mother as she absolutely hated any form of smoking. When she looked into the room it was not her mother!

Admission records

All organisations which provide health, social care or early years services are required to keep a record of who has been admitted. Such records include details of the service user's name and address, place from where they were admitted (e.g. hospital), name, address and telephone number of next of kin, and the date of admission. Many have other details and most will have a space for the date of discharge or death.

An admission form is a very important document as it contains all the relevant information about a service user's history. The Data Protection Act 1998 requires admission forms to be filled in by a trained, senior person and to be kept for one year after the last entry.

The purpose of an admission record is to provide a quick reference to the service user's personal data. This document can be used to check next of kin or who to contact in an emergency (e.g. if a service user needs hospital treatment). Details include the service user's religious beliefs, their GP and their dentist. Notes are also made of their personal interests, food preferences and of any

other services they may require. An example of an admission form is given on the next page.

Theory into practice

Visit a setting, or ask a professional care worker to visit your centre, to find out about the type of admission form that is used and who would complete the form.

Design an admission form of your own.

Daily statement of service users' health

Statements must be kept by residential and nursing homes of service users' health on a daily basis. By law, one record of a service user's health must be entered every twenty-four hours. Most residential and nursing homes enter a record for health at least every twenty-four hours. One is usually made during the day and the other is taken late evening. A record of a service user's health could include:

- pulse rate
- temperature
- a general statement about well-being.

If a service user had a urinary infection, urine samples would also be taken. For some service users, their food intake and stools would also be monitored, particularly if there were a digestive or bowel problem.

Monitoring records

Records taken to show statements of service users' health are monitored by those who take the measurements. For example, in a nursing home a health care assistant may monitor the records, while in a hospital a nurse may carry out this procedure. Monitoring involves checking whether pulse and temperature and any other measurements that are taken are **consistent**. For example:

- normal pulse rate
- normal temperature.

Portway Nursing Home

Name: Mrs Irene Ashelford

DOB: 16/08/1923

Address: 33 Icen Way, Powerstock, Dorset
DT1 4QS

Tel no: 01305 567904

Marital status: Widow

Religion: Salvation Army

Lives alone: Yes

Property brought in, e.g. valuables:
3 necklaces, 2 watches, 8 brooches

Next of kin: Mrs Anita Thorne

Relationship: Daughter

Address: 24 Castle Close, Donnington

Tel no: 01435 798234

Room: Permanent

Type of admission:
Referral from hospital

Reason for admission:
Unable to move without help (broken hip), incontinent

Confirmed diagnosis:
Report from hospital

Service user aware of diagnosis: Yes

Past medical history:
One previous fall resulting in breakage of left hip. Currently incontinent

Contact in an emergency:
Anita Thorne

Work tel no: 01235 278056

Personal health

Mental state: Some confusion, but only at times. Not constantly confused

Allergies: Plasters

Dentures: Yes, upper plate

Dentist: Mr Bray, Bridport

Next appointment: 10 July, 10.00 a.m.

Vision: Needs glasses for reading

Hearing: No hearing aid, normal

Urinary: Incontinent

Bowel: Constipation

Sleep pattern:
Likes to go to bed at 9.00 p.m. Prefers to get up at 8.00 a.m. Wakes up during the night – likes a drink (tea)

Medication: Atenatol – 25mg – 1 per day
Ramprill – 10mg – 2 per day
Aspirin – 100mg – 1 per day

Details taken by: Marcia Day

Date: 10/06/05

Nutritional state

Overweight – height 5'4"; weight 10st 3lb
Eating normally with help

Dietary preferences:
Meat, eggs, cheese. Not a vegetarian
Prefers coffee, sherry

Mobility:
Unable to walk/recovering from broken hip. Unable to move in bed, will need assistance. Needs hoist to help lift. Will need help with dressing, eating, hygiene routines

Additional notes:
Has some private financial cover. Level 3 care assessment

Additional requirements:
Hairdresser weekly

Leisure activities:
Reading – novels, rug making, bingo, board games

An example of an admission form

When taking a service user's pulse and temperature, the person who is monitoring will want to check:

- that the morning and the evening readings are consistent
- whether the measurements differ from the norm
- how much difference there is from the norm
- what measures could be taken to bring the measurements nearer to the norm.

Monitoring health and accurately recording the service user's measurements are an important part of a professional care worker's role. If changes in the service user's health are not noted, they could be extremely ill and at worst they could die.

Assessment

An assessment of need involves finding out what the service user's needs may be and who is best suited to meet these needs. Wherever possible, an assessment of need takes place before admission to a residential home or nursing home, but for other providers of health, social care or early years service this may not be possible.

Professional care workers who can make a complete assessment of need are:

- social workers
- GPs
- occupational therapists.

Professionals who contribute to the overall assessment include:

- nurses
- physiotherapists

- dieticians
- midwives
- community nurses
- district nurses.

Assessment involves:

- meeting and talking with the service user to find out what they perceive as their needs
- talking with relatives to try to establish how they view the needs of the service user
- observing the service user, perhaps while they carry out several everyday tasks, to find out what they can or cannot do
- checking the service user's history and notes relevant to the assessment of need
- discussing possible options available with the service user and taking into consideration their wishes.

The assessment cycle has a definite pattern or sequence. The diagram below shows the cycle of the **care management process**.

- **Assessing** – finding out about the needs of service users.
- **Planning** – working with the service user to plan which professional care workers and which services will be involved in their care and at which stages.
- **Implementing** – putting the plan into action, checking to see that quality care is provided.
- **Monitoring** – checking that the plan is being carried out to the specifications given and that it meets the needs of the service user.
- **Evaluating** – considering the benefits to the service user, checking that the plan still meets the service user's needs, considering any changes that may need to be made.

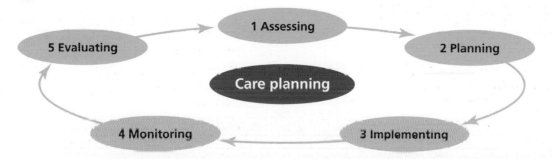

The care management process

Care plans

Each service user has an **individualised** care plan prepared for them and is consulted on its development. If a person is in a residential home, the plan might cover their personal needs and care. If a service user is a resident of a nursing home or in hospital, the care plan may use the 'nursing model'. This model has twelve areas of daily living to help plan care and was originally drawn up by Roper, Logan and Tierney.

Whichever model is used to develop a care plan, it should contain information about:

- mobility
- equipment needed
- personal support required
- medication
- wounds and dressings
- hygiene and personal needs
- eating, drinking and feeding needs
- need for a safe environment.

Information in a care plan includes what is needed for the effective day-to-day care of the person. This includes the service user's preferences, e.g. if a user has mobility difficulties, whether they would rather be given assistance to reach the bathroom to have a bath or be taken by wheelchair.

Progress reports

The purpose of a progress report is to check if the service user is improving, remaining in the same condition or **deteriorating**. It is individual to the service user and monitors how well or not they

Date	Need	Aim	Action	Evaluation
	Move from chair in bedroom to dining room	To help Fred move from his room to the dining room where he likes to eat	1 Discuss what is involved with Fred to find out his preferences 2 Collect wheelchair 3 Put brake on and adjust foot rests 4 With help, move Fred to wheelchair 5 Adjust foot rests and make sure Fred is comfortable 6 Push Fred to dining room	If Fred is moved from bed to a chair near to lunch time, move straight into wheelchair Organise moving Fred earlier so that lunch is not late

Part of a care plan for Fred, who has difficulty with mobility

Date	Progress	Signature
28/06/06	Tea: Mrs A ate two dessertspoons of jelly and ice cream	J Berry
29/06/06	Lunch: Mrs A ate diced vegetables and very small pieces of lamb	J Berry

Part of a progress report for Mrs A who has been on a semi-liquid diet for a month

are making progress in a particular area for a specific area of need. Not all service users will have a separate progress report. It could be part of their care plan where it would be recorded within the monitoring and evaluation sections.

From the progress report above, you can see how the progress Mrs A is making with eating more solid food is recorded.

Visitors log

The visitors log records the names of people visiting the setting and is usually kept immediately inside the front door. A pen is provided but frequently disappears! Visitors to the setting are asked to sign in when they arrive and sign out when they leave. The main purpose for

asking visitors to follow this procedure is for security. The staff need to know who is on the premises at all times in case there is a fire or something goes missing. In some cases, a visitor is provided with a badge and asked to wear the badge while on the premises. By taking this approach, staff can quickly recognise official visitors as anyone who has not signed in will not be wearing a badge.

Theory into practice

Visit a care setting or invite a professional care worker to your centre to find out the type of records kept of visitors and why.

Date	Name	Visiting	Time in	Signature	Time out
30/06/06	L Lewis	J Cox	10.45	L Lewis	12.00 noon

An entry in a visitors log

Recording accidents or dangerous incidents

What is the difference between a serious accident and a minor injury? A minor injury is one that can be safely dealt with by a first aid person and will heal easily, such as a graze, or a regular asthma attack. A serious injury is one that has caused harm to the service user and which will need some form of further treatment following the first aid procedure. All serious accidents that occur in a care setting must be recorded. Fires, and accidents that cause fractures or unconsciousness, are all serious incidents.

There are no national guidelines as to what should be put into accident and serious incident records, so entries vary from setting to setting. The Health and Safety Executive has provided some guidance which can be found on their website (see p282).

The accident report book is a requirement of RIDDOR, the Reporting of Injuries, Diseases and Dangerous Occurrences Regulations 1995, which came into force in April 1996. Its purpose is to report accidents and ill-health to the **enforcing authorities**, to identify where and how risks arise, and to investigate serious accidents. The enforcing authorities can then advise on any preventative action to reduce injury and ill-health. The reporting also provides a formal record, so that if there are any **repercussions** as a result of the actions taken, legal or medical records are available for reference. The Registered Homes Inspectors for residential and nursing homes will also wish to see these records when undertaking inspections.

Most care settings require every accident, however small, to be recorded. This can be kept in an accident or serious injury book. This is often kept in **triplicate** and copies are often placed in:

Date: 24/07/06   **Time:** 14.30 **hrs**   **Location:** *Main Lounge*

Description of accident:

PH got out of her chair and began to walk across the lounge with the aid of her stick. She turned her head to continue the conversation she had been having with GK, and as she turned back again she appeared not to have noticed that MP's handbag had been left on the floor. PH tripped over the handbag and fell heavily, banging her head on a footstool.

P was very shaken and although she said she was not hurt, there was a large bump on her head. She appeared pale and shaky. I asked J to fetch a blanket and to call Mrs J, deputy officer in charge. I covered P with a blanket. Mrs J arrived immediately. Dr was sent for after P was examined by Ms J.

Dr arrived after about 20 mins and said that P was bruised and shaken, but did not seem to have any injuries.

P wanted to go and lie down. She was helped to bed.

Incident was witnessed by six residents who were in the lounge at the time: GK, MP, IL, MC, CR and BQ.

Signed: **Name:**

An example of an accident/incident report

- the service user's records
- the accident and serious incident folder
- the service user's care plan.

The main information that should be recorded on an accident or dangerous incident form is:

- name of person involved
- date
- time/location/area
- description of accident
- injuries
- witnesses
- action taken
- signature
- name of person making the report.

Purpose of records

The table below shows the different purposes of the records discussed so far.

Some records are kept for different purposes. It must be remembered that settings have a variety of **functions** which means that the law may

Purpose of records	Examples of records
To provide personal details	Admission records, progress reports, care plans
To provide medical history	Admission records, daily statements of service user's health, health records
To monitor	Daily statements of service user's health, health records, progress reports
To inform others	All records kept on service users
To aid planning	Assessment plans, daily statements of service user's health records, progress records
For security	Visitors log
For health and safety	Accident reports
For legal reasons	Admissions records, accident reports, visitors log

require some settings to keep slightly different records from others.

The importance of accuracy

Whatever records are kept, accuracy is important. Staff change shifts, go on holiday or leave to take up other jobs. Therefore it is important that the records are:

- accurate
- legible
- clear
- relevant.

Different people can access records for different reasons, as shown in the table below.

It must be remembered that inaccurate records could lead to:

- incorrect medication being given
- missed appointments
- poor advice
- unnecessary pain or discomfort
- death.

Who can access records?	Why?
Care workers	Part of their job is to follow the care plan, provide treatment, find out what treatment has been given, enter and monitor health records
Other professionals (e.g. physiotherapist, radiographer, dietician)	They are involved in the service user's treatment or care
Service users	They may request to see the records to check certain points or to find out what form of treatment was recommended
Significant others	Other parties such as hospitals, clinics, residential homes and nursing home professionals can the access the records if a different form of accommodation or treatment is being considered

Assessment activity 4.1

Accurate record-keeping and awareness of legislation

Hill Tops Nursing Home cares for service users who require nursing care and support. The setting is trying to improve the knowledge and skills of existing and new care workers. To help them to do this, they have planned a series of training days and would like to prepare a resource pack that can be used for these events.

1 Prepare a presentation (including presentation notes) or other materials for the resource pack. Give a comprehensive account of legislation that impacts record keeping at Hill Tops Nursing Home and show how it influences practice. Include information on:
- Data Protection Act 1998
- Care Standards Act 2000
- Access to Personal Files Act 1987.

2 Provide materials for the resource pack and include a range of examples to illustrate how the legislation influences the access and storage of written and computerised records at Hill Tops Nursing Home.

3 Identify **four** different types of records that would be kept by Hill Tops Nursing Home and give a detailed explanation of their purpose. Try to include some examples of the four types of records chosen.

4 You have been asked to explain to a group of new trainees the importance of completing records accurately. Prepare a presentation (including presentation notes) and a handout that could be used for this purpose.

5 You have been asked to show the new trainees how to complete **three** records. Choose **three** records and complete them accurately.

Spread of infection

Micro-organisms can be harmless, but there are also those that cause disease and infection. There are four main types of micro-organism:

- bacteria
- viruses
- fungi
- protozoa.

> ### Key point
> **Pathogens** are bacteria that cause disease.

Bacteria

Most bacteria are harmless and some can even be beneficial to the environment because they break down and recycle waste material. Those that are harmful cause a range of serious illnesses and diseases, some of which can be fatal. Illnesses that can be caused by bacteria include pneumonia, gastroenteritis, dysentery and whooping cough.

Bacteria can be **inhaled** through the respiratory tract, swallowed though the digestive system or introduced through broken skin.

Viruses

Viruses are the smallest living organisms. They are responsible for the most common diseases such as colds, influenza, mumps, chicken pox and hepatitis.

Viruses can enter the body through the respiratory system via the mouth or nose. Droplets of moisture which have been infected by other people are drawn into the respiratory tract. This is why people, particularly care workers and service users, should always cough or sneeze into a handkerchief to help prevent the spread of infection.

Viral infections can also spread through dust and can be carried in the air, particularly if infected bedding or clothing has been shaken.

Fungi

Fungi include mushroom and toadstools, but there are other types that cause disease. Fungi can live outside the body but the body provides the **optimum conditions**: warmth, moisture and food. Fungi can attack the soft skin areas of the feet, particularly between the toes, causing **athlete's foot**. Ringworm is also caused by fungi attack and can produce a circular swelling on the skin and attack the scalp and the soft skin of the groin. Fungal diseases are spread by airborne **spores**, by contact with infected people and by infected floors and mats. Therefore, care workers and service users need to take particular care in these areas and should make sure that service users are wearing their own footwear and not that belonging to other people.

Protozoa

Protozoa are single-celled complex organisms which vary enormously in size and shape. They are **minute** animals. Very few cause disease in humans. An example of a disease caused by protozoa is **amoebic dysentery**, which is rare in the UK.

Spread of infection through food

Food and water can be vehicles of infection. Food for humans is also food for bacteria, particularly if kept in warm temperatures. In optimum conditions, many bacteria can multiply in high numbers very quickly. Pathogens, for which a high dose is required to cause an infection such as salmonella, can reproduce quickly. Service users and care workers who experience gastrointestinal infection due to eating contaminated food may have a great deal of pain and discomfort and may be more prone to the infection at a future date.

> ### Key point
> **Food poisoning** is an illness caused by eating contaminated food.

The main symptoms of food poisoning are:

- vomiting
- diarrhoea
- nausea
- stomach pains.

The most common cause of food poisoning is bacteria. The table below shows the food that is likely to be infected by bacteria.

Bacteria causing food poisoning	Types of food likely to be infected
Salmonella	Eggs, meat, especially pork and poultry, shellfish
Clostridium perfringens	Meat
Staphylococcus aureus	Ham, tongue, poultry (cooked meats), custards, trifles, cream (desserts)
Bacillus cereus	Rice

To help prevent the spread of infection through food in care settings, care workers should store food as described in the table below.

Food	Stored where?
Uncooked meat	Bottom shelf of the refrigerator
Cooked food	Away from uncooked food, near the top of the refrigerator
Dried, tinned and packet food	In a cool, dark place

Other steps you can take to avoid contamination include:

- not using the same preparation boards for cooked and uncooked meats; colour coding chopping boards
- not storing foods at room temperature for long periods of time
- washing hands before preparing foods and before moving on to prepare other foods

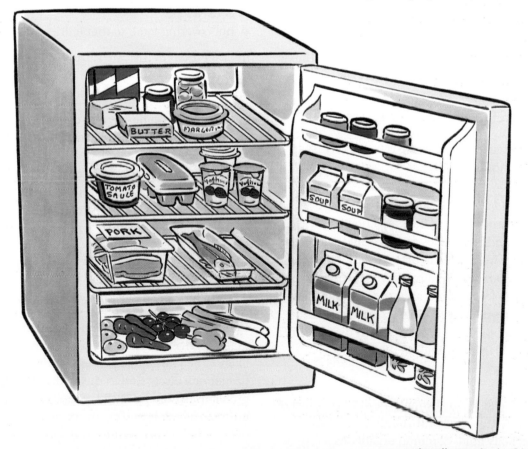

A well-organised refrigerator

- keeping food covered
- using only clean equipment
- cleaning surfaces straight after use
- using colour-coded knives
- handling food indirectly by using plastic gloves
- serving food that is hot, 63°C or above
- making sure the refrigerator is at the correct temperature.

Theory into practice

Try to visit a care setting to find out as much as possible about how they prevent the spread of infection.

Discuss your findings with the whole group.

Did you know

Food handling techniques are ways of making food safe.

Kitchens in care settings should be well planned. For example, vegetables and fruit should be prepared near to their storage area. Raw meat and poultry should be prepared in an area that is set aside for this purpose. The best place for preparation areas are around the sides of the kitchen, leaving the centre islands for cooking equipment. In this way, raw food is kept away from cooked food and waste is kept away from food preparation areas.

Pests

Flies, cockroaches and fleas are known as **vectors** and infection is spread from their feet as they move from place to place to feed. Spread of infection can be from direct contact such as ringworm, from biting (as in the case of rabies) or by **ingestion** of faeces (in the case of toxocariasis). This is how infectious diseases are transferred from animals to man.

Animals

Infection can occur through the direct contact of animals with people or through contact with animal body fluid. Common organisms

transferred from animals to humans in foods include Salmonella enterica, Campylobactor and E. coli. All pets, such as dogs, cats, fish and rodents are capable of spreading disease. In order to prevent the spread of infection from such sources, care workers should ensure that:

- hands are washed after handling pets
- service users do not put their hands to their mouth after handling pets without washing their hands first
- pets are kept out of kitchens.

Cross-infection

Cross-contamination can occur in various ways in care settings. This is because pathogenic organisms and the various forms of illness they produce can easily be spread in such environments. Cross-infection in the cooking area of a care setting could be caused by:

- putting hot food into a refrigerator
- leaving the refrigerator door open
- storing raw meat so it can drip down onto cooked food
- not covering food, so that it dries out.

In other areas of the care setting, cross-infection could be the result of passing an infection from one person to another. This could be caused by:

- the hands of a health and care worker moving from one service user to another without being washed
- the contaminated clothes of a care worker touching another care worker or service user
- lack of sterilisation of instruments or equipment between use with one service user and another
- breathing in droplets of infection or dust from the air
- surfaces and linen not being properly cleaned.

In hospitals and nursing homes, for example, many service users are in poor health and are likely to be vulnerable to infection. There has been much discussion in the media about the problems caused by MRSA (Staphylococcus aureus), which is putting people at risk and costs over £1 billion per year to control.

The four infection **control methods** are:

- surveillance
- isolation
- hand washing
- disinfection.

Control of infection means identifying the cause and spread, and interrupting the cycle of infection.

Promoting a safe working environment when caring for service users with infections

Infections are one of the major causes of human suffering and premature death. The cost of providing care for those who have infections is enormous. For this reason alone, prevention and control of infection are issues of importance for every care manager and care worker.

Service users' rooms

When cleaning a service user's room, using a detergent solution and then drying will usually be adequate for most areas. A regular programme of cleaning should be devised, with service users' rooms being cleaned on a regular basis.

Carpets should be vacuumed daily if these are the floor coverings, but if the floor covering is vinyl or tiled, then it should be cleaned daily with a detergent solution, rinsed and dried. This will help to prevent the spread of any infection that might be present. Disinfectants should not be used for general cleaning.

The table below summarises the process of cleaning a service user's bedroom.

Items to be cleaned	Method to promote safe working practice
Basins and taps	Clean with a detergent solution
Bins	Do not allow to become overfull. Empty daily and clean with a detergent solution
Toilet bowls	Clean daily with a detergent solution
Bed pans	Should be washed in hot detergent solution, dried thoroughly and wiped with hypochlorite solution
Table tops	Should be sanitised before use

Promoting a safe working environment when cleaning service users' bedrooms involves making sure that all cleaning materials are correctly put away. Many cleaning materials are highly **toxic** and can cause injury if drunk.

It may be convenient to have the toilet cleaner next to the toilet, but serious injury could occur or a life could be lost.

Sonia

Sonia lived in a residential home. She was suffering from senile dementia and was very forgetful.

One day she went into the bathroom and found the toilet cleaner left next to the toilet. Sonia picked up the toilet cleaner and drank half a bottle. It was over an hour later that Sonia was found by staff and then taken to hospital.

Sonia died the next day.

Find out from visiting a care setting or through speaking to a care worker how uniforms can help to prevent the spread of infection.

All managers must follow the Management of Health and Safety at Work Regulations 1992 which were amended in 1994 by the Management of Health and Safety at Work (Amendment) Regulations. The regulations require employees to carry out risk assessments to ensure that risks are minimised. Employers must have policies in place and provide adequate training to all staff to prevent accidents in the setting.

Personal safety

If a care worker is suffering from an infectious disease, they should never go into work. Also, any cuts or abrasions to the skin must be covered with a dressing to make sure that the care worker does not risk passing on pathogens to the service user. As a care worker, you must be sure that you are promoting a safe environment by developing an awareness of health and safety risks wherever you are and whatever you are doing.

Contributing to personal safety means being careful about what you wear. Sometimes an employer will insist that their care workers wear uniforms. This is because a uniform protects you from passing on infection to others and also prevents you from becoming infected by others.

Most employers in the health, care and early years sector do not allow their employees to wear jewellery or rings (apart from wedding rings) or to carry anything around in their pockets. This is not only for the sake of personal hygiene and to

reduce the spread of infection, but also to prevent injury to themselves and to others.

Sensible footwear is a must! High heels are not suitable when caring for others and could cause both the care worker and the service user injury.

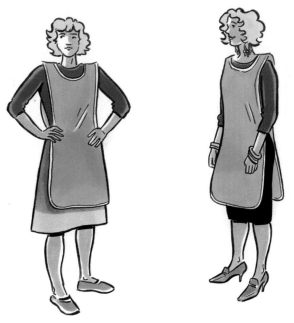

Why is the care worker on the right not suitably dressed for a caring role?

The table opposite shows how service users and carers can be protected from the spread of infection.

Washing hands is an essential contribution to keeping infection under control. Before and after carrying out any procedure, hands should be washed, even if the care worker has worn gloves. It is essential that hands are washed if the care worker has come into contact with:

- blood
- soiled linen
- clinical waste
- any bodily fluids, e.g. sweat, vomit, sputum, or from blowing the nose, using the toilet, etc.

Precaution to protect against spread of infection	Reason	Remember
Wear protective clothing, e.g. plastic apron	Use when carrying out procedure that involves bodily contact to prevent infection getting onto the clothes	Dispose of plastic apron when the job is completed. A new apron should be worn for each individual
Control hair	If hair is not tied back it will come into contact with the individual for whom care is being provided. This means it could spread infection or it could cause the individual harm if it got caught in equipment	Tie hair back and keep it clean by washing regularly
Wear a mask	To prevent breathing in bacteria or breathing them onto other people	Remember to dispose of the mask after each use
Wear gloves	These should be worn when there is any danger of coming into contact with body fluids such as blood, mucus or sweat. Gloves should also be worn when clearing up spillages of blood or soiled dressings. Gloves provides protection against infection	Dispose of gloves after dealing with individual service user. Also, check that the gloves do not have holes or are torn. Always wash your hands after disposing of the gloves
Wear overshoes	Plastic covers or overshoes will help prevent the spread of infection from one place to another and will provide protection from infection	Dispose of overshoes immediately after use

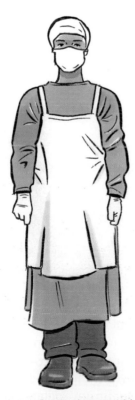

Precautions provide personal safety from the spread of infection

When washing hands:

- use running water in a deep basin – hands can become re-infected if cleaned in still water
- use soap or handwash disinfectants as supplied by the employer
- make sure hands are washed thoroughly, with the surfaces being vigorously massaged with lather
- pay particular attention to fingers, thumbs and underneath wedding rings
- rinse thoroughly and dry with a paper towel
- washing and rinsing should take no less than thirty seconds.

Theory into practice

Practise washing your hands in the correct way.

When ready, ask for an assessment of your demonstration.

Remember to obtain a witness statement which shows the level of competency achieved. This witness statement should be signed and dated by your assessor.

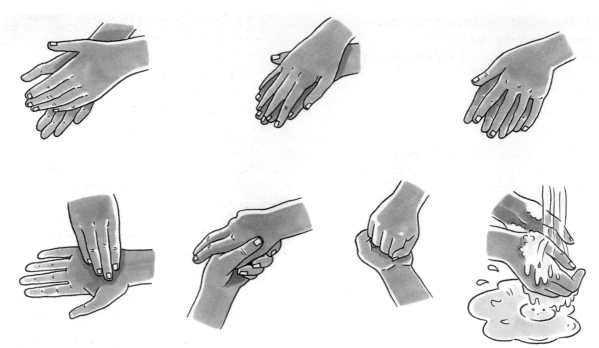

The correct way to wash hands

Dealing with hazardous human waste

Blood-borne viruses are most frequently transmitted in health and social care settings through **percutaneous exposure**, which is when a needle or other sharp instrument which contains the contaminated blood of an infected person penetrates the skin.

> Conditions that run a high risk of being transmitted by percutaneous exposure are:
> - 1 in 3 for hepatitis B
> - 1 in 30 for hepatitis C
> - 1 in 300 for HIV.
>
> (Department of Health figures)

An effective policy must therefore be in place within all care settings to prevent injury through sharp pieces of equipment.

When bodily fluid is splashed into the eye, it is known as **mucocutaneous exposure**. This is not quite as dangerous as when infected blood is transferred from one person to another, but hygiene policies and procedures should be in place in all care settings to prevent and to deal with these situations when they arise.

How to contribute to infection control

Universal precautions

These are basic rules designed to reduce the risk of blood-borne viruses being passed from one person to another in caring. Universal precautions should be followed when there is a risk of anyone being exposed to infected blood-borne viruses and bodily fluids. All blood, tissue and bodily fluids should be thought of as potentially infectious.

Universal precautions are general measures and include the following:

- Change gloves before dealing with new service users. Also wear gloves when cleaning equipment.
- Cover wounds with waterproof dressings and wear protective eye-wear if there is any likelihood of spillage.
- Wear gloves if you think you may come into contact with blood or bodily fluids.
- Handle the disposal of sharp objects carefully.
- Wear footwear that encloses feet so they cannot be covered with blood or bodily fluids.
- Promptly clear up any spillage of blood or bodily fluids.

- Follow safe procedures for the disposal of contaminated waste.
- Wash hands before and after contact with each service user and before and after putting on gloves.

Theory into practice

Try to visit a care setting in your area to find out how, when and which universal precautions are used. Record your findings.

Special precautions

Special precautions are taken when an individual service user has a condition requiring the carer to wear double gloves and/or to wear a gown or mask. The procedures set out must be clearly followed.

Case study

Zoe

Zoe knew that she had responsibility on her next shift to care for a service user who had a severe case of food poisoning. She arrived for work in good time, took off her coat and went straight in to say 'hello' to the service user.

During the conversation the service user vomited. Zoe tried to clean her up and move her into a comfortable position. Her long hair touched the face of the service user, but Zoe told the service user not to worry as she would wash it after her shift.

After attending to the service user, Zoe went straight in to see the service user in the next room and then went to put on her apron and gloves.

The next day Zoe felt very unwell and as the day passed she became very much worse.

1 What did Zoe do wrong?

2 What procedures should Zoe have followed?

3 What would have provided guidance for Zoe on what she should do in these circumstances? How would this have helped?

Assessment activity 4.2

Caring for service users with infections

Case study A: Hill Tops Nursing Home

Fatou, who is responsible for training staff at Hill Tops Nursing Home, is holding a series of training days throughout the year on the subject of 'caring for service users with infections'. You have been asked to prepare materials that can be used on the training days.

Case study B: Brittany Farm Children's Residential Home

Wayne is responsible for training staff At Brittany Farm Children's Residential Home. He is holding a three-day seminar for all staff to try to raise awareness on the subject of caring for children who have infections. You have been asked to prepare materials that can be used on the training days.

Activity

Choose case study A or case study B. For both case studies, remember when responding to meet the required depth of the grading criteria.

1 Prepare materials (including tutor notes) that could be used to show the staff which micro-organisms spread infection, and the routes of infection. Use examples to show a high level of understanding.

   Remember to include the spread of infection through:

- poor personal habits
- contaminated food
- pests
- animals
- cross-infection.

2 Produce materials that could be used as a guide to explain to the staff how they can promote a safe working environment and how to contribute to the control of infection when caring for service users with infections. Try to make informed and reasoned judgements when considering ways of promoting a safe working environment and infection control:

- in service users' rooms
- when considering personal safety/hygiene
- when dealing with hazardous human waste
- by applying universal precautions
- by applying special methods.

3 Demonstrate to a group of staff how to wash their hands correctly.

Note:

Remember to ask your tutor to assess you and to record the level of competency achieved.

You may wish to ask your peers to assess your hand washing to help you when you evaluate the effectiveness of the practical tasks.

Changing a service user's position can involve:

- moving them to a different position in bed
- moving them from a bed to a chair, and vice versa
- changing their position in the chair
- moving them from a chair to the bathroom, and vice versa.

Legal issues associated with moving and handling

The level of assistance a service user needs varies from service user to service user, but all moving and handling is controlled by law. Laws are continually being updated in order to protect both the service user and care workers from harm. Many of the accidents reported each year are associated with the moving and handling of people. These can include back injuries and sprains which are **cumulative** rather than being directly attributable to any single incident.

Health and Safety at Work Act 1974

This is an **enabling** Act that allows the Home Secretary and the Health and Safety Commission to formulate regulations based upon this Act. The table below is a summary of the Act where it is particularly applicable to health, social care and early years settings.

It is obvious from the Health and Safety at Work Act 1974 that everyone has a **duty of care** for others. This responsibility is linked to various **codes of conduct**. A code of conduct sets a framework within which day-to-day work must be carried out. It sets the standard and the quality of care provided. For example, a nurse passing an accident on the road who fails to stop to offer assistance is not providing a duty of care. They could be struck off the nursing council's list for failing to offer others protection.

There are five basic steps within a duty of care:

- organisations involved in caring must have a health and safety policy in place

Area of Health and Safety at Work Act applicable to health, social care and early years settings	What does the Act say?
Employer's responsibility	Ensure the health, safety and welfare of all employees (2.2, Section 7). Protect the health and safety of others, e.g. service users who may need lifting. Prepare a statement of safety policy and the arrangements for carrying it out. Monitor the practical aspects of safety.
Employee's responsibility	Take care of own safety and the safety of others who may be affected by their actions/omissions. Comply with safety instructions given by their employers. Co-operate with any training provided. Report any changes that have an affect on their ability to carry out their work safely.
Employer's and employee's responsibility	Section 37: Where an employer is found to be negligent the line manager or equivalent may also be liable and may be punished accordingly.
	Section 40: If a person is accused of negligence for failure to comply with Health and Safety legislation, they must prove that it was not reasonably practicable to do so.

- staff must be available to implement this policy
- risk assessment and risk avoidance procedures must be in place
- the person responsible must be able to measure the performance of the risk assessment
- there must be regular reviews of the risk assessment and updates when change takes place.

Training of staff in moving and handling is an essential part of the process of managing care. Once training is complete, it should not be forgotten. Failure is often the result of not implementing the training. Regular meetings between teams and the moving and handling co-ordinator is also important.

Duty of care not only involves the delivery of training, but also includes helping people to use that training. Through learning, care workers are enabled to change their practice in a safe and appropriate manner.

Manual Handling Operations Regulations 1992

The Manual Handling Operations Regulations 1992, amended in 2002, require employers to avoid all **manual** handling whenever possible, where there is a risk of injury. There is almost no situation where manual handling should be considered acceptable.

On the rare occasion where manual lifting is absolutely necessary, a risk assessment must be completed first. Care workers must not be put at risk. This means that sufficient staff must be available to move and handle service users safely.

Each time a care worker intends to move or handle a service user, they must undertake a risk assessment. No matter how often a care worker has moved an individual over a period of time, every time that person is moved a risk assessment must be completed.

Risk assessment forms may vary from one care setting to another, but the basic facts included will be the same (see opposite).

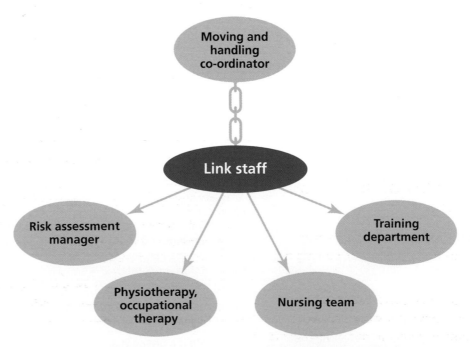

Regular meetings between teams is important

Checklist

1. Is the individual weight bearing?
   - Yes ☐
   - No ☐

2. Is the individual unsteady?
   - Yes ☐
   - No ☐

3. What is the general level of mobility?
   - Good ☐
   - Poor ☐

4. a What is the individual's weight? _____
   b What is the individual's height? _____
   c How many people does this lift require? _____
   (Work this out on the scale devised by your workplace)

5. What lifting equipment is required?
   - Hoist ☐
   - Sling ☐
   - Trapeze ☐
   - Transfer board ☐

6. Is equipment available?
   - Yes ☐
   - No ☐

7. If not, is there a safe alternative?
   - Yes ☐
   - No ☐

8. Is the required number of people available?
   - Yes ☐
   - No ☐

9. What is the purpose of the move? _____
   _____

10. Can this be achieved?
    - Yes ☐
    - No ☐

A checklist for risk assessment before moving a service user

The principles of safe moving and handling

The table at the top of the following page summarises the principles of safe moving and handling.

The individual who is to be moved must be consulted about how they would like to be moved. Discussion is very important to ensure they are moved comfortably and that any pain and discomfort are reduced to a minimum.

Theory into practice

Visit a nursing home or a hospital to find out about the different forms of moving and handling that occur.

Observe care workers using moving and handling techniques. Record your findings.

Principle of safe moving and handling practice	Reason
Assess the situation before moving a service user	Reduces the risks to both care worker and service user
Use equipment to move and handle	Reduces the number of injuries and complies with the law
Check that you are wearing appropriate clothing	Wearing flat shoes prevents twisted ankles and reduces the likelihood of accidents
Always have another care worker present to help with the movement	Reduces the risk of accidents occurring and makes the task easier to manage
Always consult the service user	So that the agreement of the service user is obtained and that the service user knows exactly what is going to happen
Check the immediate environment, e.g. floors. Is the floor even? Is the floor wet/slippery?	Prevents unnecessary accidents
Is the area where the individual is to be placed ready?	Minimises inconvenience to the service user
Check that the equipment is fit for purpose	Prevents danger of using faulty equipment
Always face the person who is being moved	So that the care worker can see the service user's reaction to every situation
Always bend your legs not your back	To prevent injury and to correctly balance the load
Make sure that the brakes on the trolley beds and chairs are on	So that the equipment does not move uncontrollably during the moving process

Case study

Assifa

Assifa is a care worker at Batchfoot Nursing Home. She is asked to prepare handouts to give to new trainees on the legislation and regulations that affect moving and handling at the nursing home.

Assifa has also been asked to explain to her supervisor the principles of safe practice.

1 Role-play this situation with a partner. One person should be the supervisor while the other should be Assifa.

2 Prepare a handout as a result of the role play that could be given to new staff to explain the principles of good practice.

How to use equipment for moving and handling

Hospitals, residential homes, nursing homes and some day-care centres have a variety of equipment that can be used to help move and handle people. These can include hoists, slide boards, transfer boards, monkey poles and sliding sheets.

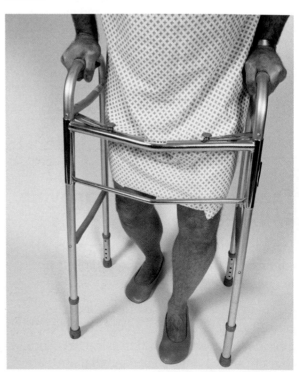

A walking frame in use

Using equipment for moving and handling meets the requirements of legislation as well as helping to prevent injuries. All care settings should have this policy in place, but research has shown that in some care settings manual lifting and handling is still undertaken.

Hoist

Hoists can be:

- manual
- battery-powered.

Mechanical hoists help reduce injury by avoiding unnecessary manual transfers, awkward postures, **forceful exertions** and repetitive motions. Although using these devices may appear to take longer, they can save staff time by reducing the number of employees needed to transfer a service user.

Follow the guidelines in the diagram below when using a hoist.

Theory into practice

Visit a care setting and find out how a hoist is used. Ask if you can be given a demonstration and then try it without a service user being involved.

Slide boards

Slide boards are large plastic boards which reduce friction. Some slide boards have hand-holds. The service user is slid or rolled onto the board and the board is then pushed or pulled to accomplish the transfer. In another common practice, the board goes under the service user who is pulled over the board by use of a draw sheet or incontinence pad.

Slide boards are often designed to be used where the service user is quite active as they can be encouraged to be involved in the moving and handling.

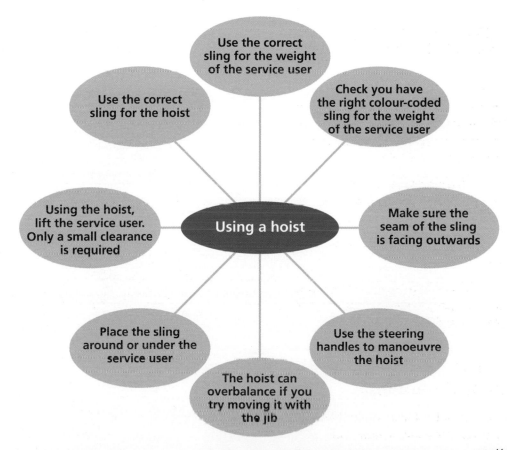

Using a hoist

Central node: **Using a hoist**

- Use the correct sling for the weight of the service user
- Check you have the right colour-coded sling for the weight of the service user
- Use the correct sling for the hoist
- Make sure the seam of the sling is facing outwards
- Using the hoist, lift the service user. Only a small clearance is required
- Use the steering handles to manoeuvre the hoist
- Place the sling around or under the service user
- The hoist can overbalance if you try moving it with the jib

To use a slide board

1 Place the board between a bed and a chair of similar height.

2 Slide the service user onto the board.

3 Help the service user to slide to the required position.

Transfer boards

When using a transfer board, two people are required to stand either side of a bed or trolley. The service user can be moved from a trolley onto a bed or from a bed to a trolley. Transfer boards can be used whether a service user is conscious or not.

To use a transfer board

1 Place the board half under the service user and half under the sheet they are lying on.

2 One care worker pulls while the other pushes.

3 The sheet with the service user then slides easily from one place to another.

Different methods of moving and handling

The method used for moving and handling service users depends on:

- the situation
- the agreement made by the service user
- whether it is an emergency situation.

Other equipment used in care settings for moving and handling is given in the table below.

Other equipment used for moving and handling	Purpose and how used
Monkey pole	Allows service users to assist themselves. A handle is fixed above a bed and swings from a frame. The service user pulls on the bar to help lift their body off the bed.
Standing hoist	Helps a service user to stand. A seat, which is fixed to a frame with arms, is placed under the service user. The seat is gradually raised until it is in an upright position, enabling the service user to stand.
Wheelchair	Moves a service user from one location to another. Can be self-propelled or electrically operated.

Moving and handling

The manager at Hill Tops Nursing Home is concerned that care workers are not sufficiently up-to-date with moving and handling theory and practice. She has asked you to produce materials for several training events on the subject.

1 Give a presentation (including speaker's notes) about the legislation and regulations that affect moving and handling. Remember to include:
   ● the Health and Safety at Work Act
   ● Manual Handling Regulations.

Try to give a comprehensive account that makes significant connections between theory and practice.

2 Prepare a short guide which shows care workers the principles of safe handling. Try to make significant connections between theory and practice.

3 Identify three pieces of moving and handling equipment. Give a talk and demonstration about how to use each piece. Prepare handouts to give the trainees at the end of the session.

Choose equipment to include:
   ● hoist
   ● slideboard
   ● transfer board.

Note: Remember to ask your tutor to assess you on giving the talk and the demonstration.

4 Produce a leaflet to show different methods that could be used when moving and handling and the context for their use.

Support for service users who are receiving health care

When looking after service users, professional staff must consider them as a whole person and not just concentrate on physical problems. The care given should always be adapted to meet the physical needs, but the service user's intellectual, emotional and social needs must also be of concern. Providing support for a service user means:

- matching the care provided to the service user's needs
- determining the level of support required
- identifying the equipment needed to provide health care.

A service user will require support while care is being provided. The purpose of this support is to make the individual as independent as possible and to give them a sense of achievement.

How can this be achieved by care workers? To illustrate the four ways of providing support, let us consider how this could be applied to Mrs F, who is recovering from a fractured hip and hip replacement (see the table below).

If staff do not consider Mrs F holistically, her emotional needs will not be met. She is likely to become depressed, mentally inactive and **socially isolated**. Mrs F must receive support that maintains her dignity and be made aware of the options so that her personal identity and beliefs are maintained and she can make her own choices. To do this, effective communication is a must.

Activity

1 Write a short case study for a service user which shows what their individual needs are.

2 Exchange the case study with another person in the group. Ask them to:
- identify the service user's needs
- determine the level of support required
- identify the equipment needed.

You will do the same for the case study of the other person.

3 Compare answers and draw conclusions about the support provided.

Needs of Mrs F	Determining the level of support for Mrs F	Identifying equipment to support Mrs F
Mobility needs	Unable to turn over in bed unaided.	Monkey pole to help her move in the bed independently. Hoist to move her out of bed. Wheelchair for moving around.
Hygiene needs	Needs help with bathing (washing in bed). Moving from bed to basin for washing (when her condition improves). Toilet needs.	Hoist to move from bed to chair. Wheelchair to take her from bedroom to bathroom. Hoist to move into bath/shower. Seat or seat-lowering device. Commode.
Eating needs	Move to upright position. Move to chair to eat. Support while in upright position in bed.	Monkey pole to get into upright position or hoist to move from bed to chair. Back support – back rest.
Intellectual needs	Meeting with others. Support for activities (e.g. reading) in bed. Support while sitting in chair.	Hoist to move from bed to wheelchair. Monkey pole to achieve upright position. Back rest. Table-top support.

Monitor and record a service user's pulse

A pulse can be felt at different points within the body, for example:

- at the artery in the neck
- at the artery at the wrist.

When taking a pulse, a health care professional such as a health care assistant, nurse or GP is pressing a blood vessel (artery) against something solid such as a muscle or bone. The force of the heart pumping blood around the arteries causes a pulsing sensation that can be felt. This is measured in 'beats per minute'. The only equipment required is a watch with a second hand. When taking the measurement, the health care professional does not usually measure the beat for a full minute, unless the service user has an irregular heart beat. Instead, they measure for thirty seconds and multiply the number by two. For example:

> Pulse rate is 36 beats in 30 seconds
>
> Multiply × 2
>
> 36 × 2 = 72 beats per minute

However, if in doubt, it is a good idea to measure for sixty seconds. The average adult pulse rate is 70–80 beats per minute, but if the adult is very fit their pulse rate could be as low as 60 beats per minute. However, a new born baby's pulse rate can be anything from 120–180 beats per minute, which is considerably higher.

Exercise increases the pulse rate, but as a person rests the beat returns to normal. Pulse rate can be affected by heart disease, lung dysfunction and other illnesses. An increase in pulse rate can be caused by the body not getting enough oxygen, which causes the heart to pump the **oxygenated blood** around the body at a much faster rate.

Theory into practice

Measure another person's pulse rate for fifteen seconds at the point on the wrist. Work out their pulse rate.

The time taken for the pulse to return to normal after exercise is known as the 'recovery rate'. The fitter a person is, the quicker the pulse will return to its normal resting rate after exercise.

Recording the pulse rate accurately is important. Health and social care settings will have different ways of recording the pulse rates.

Measure and record a person's temperature

Normal or average body temperature is a constant 37°C. Measuring a temperature can show whether the service user is suffering from an illness or condition such as influenza. If the body temperature rises too much, then organs such as the brain and the liver begin to fail. Alternatively, if the body temperature falls too low this can also be extremely dangerous. **Hypothermia** could set in, particularly in older people in a very cold winter, causing various organs to fail.

Temperature is measured using a clinical thermometer. A clinical thermometer is very accurate and should always be **sterilised** to prevent infection being transferred from one person to another. Some modern thermometers are disposable and some can take temperature just by being placed briefly in the ear. Sometimes temperature is taken rectally. This involves putting the bulb of a specially designed 'rectal' thermometer into the service user's bottom to take the temperature. This method is often used when the service user has a mouth infection or

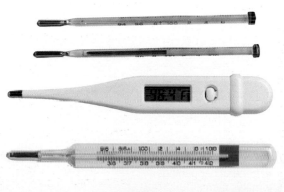

Different types of thermometer

damage, or if they are likely to bite the thermometer.

If temperature is taken by mouth, a standard glass clinical thermometer is placed under the service user's tongue. When the thermometer is removed from the service user's mouth, the thermometer is held horizontally at eye level and rotated until the column of mercury can be seen. After the reading is taken, the thermometer is shaken until the measurement is no longer recorded, sterilised and then replaced in its holder. The frequency of temperature measurements will depend on the service user's condition.

Theory into practice

Either: Take a person's temperature by mouth or by ear.

Or: Visit a care setting and observe a temperature being taken.

How was it recorded?

Recording the temperature and pulse rate accurately is very important. Both give an indication of the service user's condition. The accuracy of the reading from the thermometer will be influenced by the time it is left in position.

It is recommended that the thermometer should be left in for four minutes if taking the temperature by the mouth. If the temperature rises, it is an indication that the service user's condition is worsening and therefore they may need additional medication.

Providing support for service users while taking the pulse and temperature

The amount of support required by a service user depends on:

- their physical condition
- their emotional and intellectual state
- the amount of time being spent on taking and recording their condition
- the equipment being used.

Support for a service user can be given in the ways listed in the table below.

Taking a pulse and temperature are routine measurements that are not regarded as threatening to the service user and are therefore unlikely to cause them distress. However, it is still very important that the service user knows what the care professional is going to do as they are more likely to co-operate.

Support for service user while taking the pulse and temperature	Reason
Explain: • what is going to happen • how it is to be done • why it is being done	This will take away fears and worries about what is going to happen to them
Give information: • about the results • about the effect of the results on the service user	Factual information showing how the service user's measurements relate to the norm reduces stress and aids understanding
Emotional support: • enquire how the service user feels • ask what they would like to see happening as a result of the monitoring	Valuing the service user as an individual improves their self-worth. Asking for their opinions/likes/dislikes provides choice and helps them feel they are in control of their lives
Talking to the service user: • general chat about the weather • general happenings • news items	Helps to relax the service user and takes their mind off the procedures taking place as they have something else to think about. Talking about other things can provide intellectual challenge

Emergency treatment

Emergency first aid treatments and ways of supporting the service user are given in the table on the next page.

Try practising some of the first aid techniques described in this section. Provide support for the casualty. Include:

- changing a dressing
- giving first aid for a minor cut
- dealing with a burn/scald
- giving first aid for a fracture of the lower leg
- dealing with a head injury
- choking.

Emergency treatment for a fall

If it is possible to see that a person is going to fall, then do not try to hold them up. Try to control the fall to reduce the impact to a minimum so that the risks are not so great. Someone could be falling because they are faint, because they have severe pain or because they are about to have an epileptic fit.

If a care worker suddenly finds a person on the floor, they must follow this procedure:

1 Assess the situation
2 Make the area safe
3 Carry out ABC checks (Airway, Breathing, Circulation)
4 Give emergency first aid
5 Call for help.

An individual plan should include the following checks:

- Is the casualty conscious?
- Is the airway open?
- Is the casualty breathing?
- Are there signs of circulation?

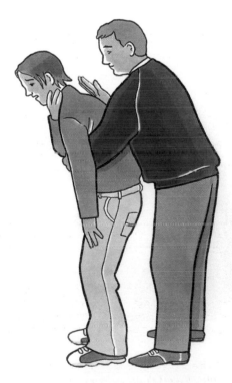

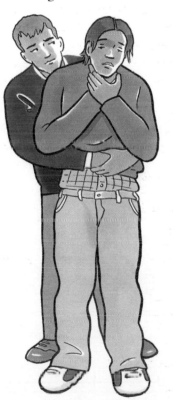

How to help someone who is choking

Emergency	Treatment	Support
Change a simple dressing	**1** Cleanse the wound – remove dirt and gravel **2** Cleanse skin around the wound – to remove dirt and oils and prevent them from entering the wound **3** Protect the wound from further contamination – cover with a sterile dressing in order to keep infection out **NB** Some wounds may need professional care	Service user should be informed about what is being done
Minor cuts	**1** Wash hands thoroughly and put on disposable gloves **2** Clean wound by rinsing carefully under running water **3** Pat the wound dry using a gauze swab **4** Cover with a sterile gauze dressing **5** Elevate the injured part above the level of the heart **6** Support the affected part **7** Clean the surrounding area with soap and water using clean swabs for each stroke	Support service user by talking with them and explaining the first aid treatment that is being given. Also answer any questions they may have
Minor burns and scalds	**1** Place the burn/scald under running cold water for at least 10 minutes **2** Put on disposable gloves **3** Remove any jewellery, watches, belts before the injury begins to swell **4** Cover with a sterile dressing or a clean non-fluffy pad **5** Apply temporary covering, e.g. kitchen film	Never break blisters or skin Do not apply adhesive dressings Do not apply ointments or fats as they may damage tissues and increase the risk of infection Talk to casualty to explain actions being taken Advise referral to hospital if in distress or pain
Fractures There are two types of fracture: ● closed ● open (when the bone protrudes through the skin).	**Closed fracture** **1** Advise the casualty to keep still **2** If possible, bandage the injured part to an unaffected part of the body to give support **3** Arrange to transport the casualty to hospital **4** Check circulation beyond bandage every 10 minutes **Open fracture** **1** Put on gloves **2** Loosely cover wound with a large, clean, non-fluffy dressing **3** Apply pressure to stop bleeding as long as no glass or object is embedded **4** Carefully place clean padding over and around the dressing **5** Secure the dressing and padding with a bandage **6** Immobilise the injured part **7** Treat for shock	Do not press down on protruding bone Prevent the casualty from eating or drinking and from smoking. Do not move the casualty. Talk to the casualty to keep their mind focused on other things
Head injury There are three main types of head injury: ● concussion – brief period of impaired consciousness, sometimes with memory loss ● cerebral compression – deteriorating level of response which may progress to unconsciousness ● skull fracture – wound or bruise to the head with possible loss of clear watery blood from nose or ear.	In all cases: Dial 999 for an ambulance Assume casualty has neck or spinal injury	Explain to the casualty what is happening Reassure the casualty until ambulance arrives
Choking	**1** Give up to five back slaps **2** Check mouth and remove any obstruction **3** Give up to five abdominal thrusts **4** Check mouth and remove anything that may be restricting the abdomen **5** Call an ambulance – continue until help arrives	If at any time the casualty becomes unconscious, open airway (mouth), check breathing and give rescue breaths

	Action at an emergency
1	Assess the situation
2	Make the area safe
3	Give first aid
4	Get help from others
5	Control bystanders

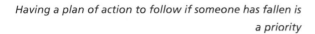

Having a plan of action to follow if someone has fallen is a priority

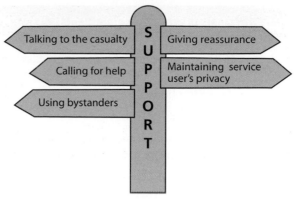

Providing support

Providing support when giving first aid

When a service user is injured, they will need as much support as possible. Support can take various forms such as talking to the casualty, calling for help, making use of bystanders, giving reassurance and maintaining the service user's privacy.

Giving support to a service user allows the service user to feel that they have some control over their life. It also provides encouragement, gives confidence and helps the casualty to remain calm.

It is important for a service user or casualty to know that you, the first aider or carer, is in control of the situation and that you have the ability to cope. They need to know that they can put their trust in you and rely on you at a time when they are finding it difficult to cope with unexpected challenges.

Assessment activity 4.4

First aid procedures

As a health care assistant at Hill Tops Nursing Home, you are required to:
- take the temperature and pulse rate and provide support for a service user (simulated)
- accurately record both monitoring measures.

1 Demonstrate how to do this. Remember to arrange for your tutor to assess you. You may also wish to involve your peers in the assessment. If you do this, provide a document for them to record their opinions.

2 Record the temperature and pulse rate accurately.

3 You have been asked to lead a practical training day to show care workers some first aid procedures. Demonstrate to the group:
- how to change a dressing
- how to treat a minor cut

- how to treat a burn/scald
- what to do if a lower leg is fractured
- how to treat a head injury
- what to do if a service user is choking.

You may wish to prepare posters, handouts or notes to help you when demonstrating the first aid procedures or you could also produce materials for a display.

Remember to arrange for your tutor to assess you carrying out the first aid procedures.

If you follow a first aid course, you must have:
- a list of the procedures demonstrated
- a witness statement showing the level of competency achieved for each first aid procedure.

Try to give support when carrying out each practical task demonstrating confidence, independence and competence.

Making a bed that is comfortable is not an easy task. A large number of hospitals, residential homes and nursing homes do not use duvets on beds. Reasons for this could be:

- the bed may have to be changed several times if a service user has an accident, e.g. if they are incontinent or spill food
- some service users find duvets too heavy
- some service users find sheets and blankets more comfortable
- if sheets and blankets are used, a layer can be removed when the service user becomes too hot.

Correctly making a bed

Care workers make beds on a regular basis as part of their job. If bed-making is not carried out in the correct way, service users could suffer from **musculo-skeletal** problems.

A risk assessment should be carried out before a bed is made to determine the risks to the bed maker and the service user, if the latter is involved. The appropriate control measures must also be considered.

When making a bed, care workers must make sure that they walk around the bed to avoid excessive forward reaching. Often, when bed-making, the arms stretch away from the body, resulting in an awkward shoulder posture. The trunk of the body could be in an awkward posture because of bending forward or sideways to remove dirty linen and to put on clean linen.

Care workers should raise the bed before they start the bed-making process. All care workers should be trained to bend the knees, or to partially kneel on a corner of the bed to avoid bending their back.

Health and care settings are phasing out manual crank beds and are replacing them with beds that can be raised automatically. Beds should always be raised before care workers carry out bed-making tasks.

Using a **mitred** or envelope corner when bed-making will help to make the bed look neater as well as getting the sheets and blankets to stay in place longer. A well-made bed will also help to prevent the service user from getting **bed sores**.

How to make a mitred or envelope corner

1. Take a corner of a sheet between thumb and finger and draw it around the corner of the mattress.

2. At the same time, slide the other hand under the side edge of the sheet and drag it upwards into a diagonal fold.

3. Lay this fold up over the mattress.

4. Turn under the mattress the part of the sheet left hanging.

5. Drop the upper fold and tuck it in under the mattress. This makes a box-like corner.

Procedure for making a bed	Reason
1 Raise the bed	To avoid musculo-skeletal injuries
2 Collect the clean linen and put it near to the bed on the back of a chair	To avoid stretching across the bed to reach the clean linen. Stretching can cause back injury
3 Bed clothes should be pulled back to the bottom of the bed. If possible, place on a chair	To be within easy reach. If they were on the floor, the care worker would need to bend and reach for them. This could cause injury
4 Dirty linen should be removed and placed in an appropriate container	To prevent them being mixed with the clean linen and to prevent the clean linen from becoming soiled
5 The mattress should be turned over	This will help to keep the mattress firm
6 'Mite spray' can be used to spray the mattress	To kill mites
7 Spread the bottom sheet, right side up, wide hem at the top, evenly and straight. Make sure there are no wrinkles	To prevent bed linen from moving to one side or from slipping off
8 Complete envelope corners	To keep bedding firm
9 Place the top sheet evenly and straight, right side down, with wide hem at the top. Envelope the corners	So that when turned back the sheet will have the hem on the inside, not showing outside
10 Spread the blanket, evenly. Envelope the corners	To keep firm
11 Lay the top cover or a throw on the bed smoothly and evenly	To promote a good appearance
12 Put on pillow slip making sure the flaps are folded down correctly. Place opening facing away from the door. Place pillows under or on top of the top cover	So that pillow will not come out of the pillow case. To give a good appearance as open ends cannot be viewed
13 Remove soiled linen	To avoid contamination. To keep the room tidy

What are the reasons for making a bed correctly?

The table above gives the reasons for the correct procedures when making a bed (without the service user present).

Assessment activity 4.5

The staff at Hill Tops Nursing Home are having a training session on the correct way to make a bed.

1 Demonstrate how to make a bed correctly. Remember to ask your tutor to assess you while doing this task. A witness statement will be required for your portfolio.

2 Prepare a handout or a leaflet to give to the care workers giving the reasons for each stage in the bed-making process.

Difficulties with eating

Some service users may be able to eat without experiencing any difficulties. They may be able to enjoy their meals and will be able to select foods from a variety of flavours and textures without experiencing any difficulties. However, other service users may experience difficulties when eating for a variety of reasons, as shown in the diagram below.

- Some service users, particularly older people, may become confused and suffer loss of memory. This could mean that they cannot remember if they have eaten or if they have had the correct amount of food for a particular day. The service user may have forgotten what they have actually eaten and this too can cause a problem as they may not be having a healthy, balanced diet. If the service user is a diabetic, this could be an even more difficult problem as their blood sugar levels could be affected and could result in them collapsing.

- If service users have difficulty swallowing, they are often put off eating because it is too painful. They may only drink liquids, which will meet the needs of some of their dietary intake but would mean that their diet could be lacking roughage. This could cause bowel problems and difficulties when going to the toilet.

- If a service user is unable to see the food properly, they may not want to eat it. Food needs to look good and appeal to the person through smell, texture and flavour. If the service user is unable to see very well, they may not be able to tell whether their meal looks attractive and may wish to give up.

- Foods need to be easy to eat and carefully selected. This is particularly important for the service user who has difficulty in chewing. It is possible that the service user may have false

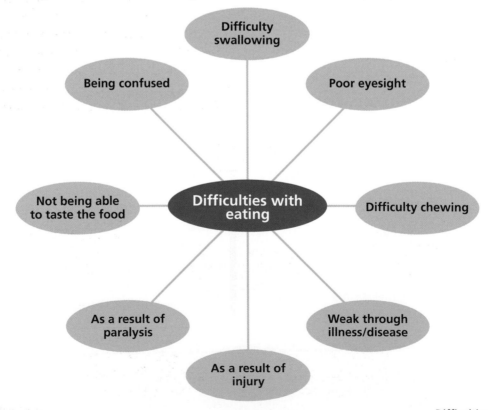

Difficulties with eating

teeth which can make certain foods difficult to chew or the food may get under or between the false teeth. The service user's false teeth may also fit badly or may rub when eating which would put them off the process of eating.

- Having an illness or disease or suffering from body weakness through injury or stroke could also contribute to preventing the service user from eating. In such instances, the service user may require help with eating. The care worker will need to discuss with the service user what they would like to eat and how, and make sure that small amounts are fed to the service user.

The snack

Foods that make interesting snacks will depend on the service user's likes and dislikes. Having sufficient food which gives a well balanced, healthy diet is important whether the service user is experiencing difficulties or not. The function of food within the body is specific and important to health and well-being. Each nutrient has a particular function within the body.

A snack is a light meal which could be served at lunch time, during the day or as an evening meal. Examples of snacks are shown in the diagram below.

Theory into practice

Speak to a child and an older person and find out two snacks that they like to eat.

Nutritional value of foods

A balanced diet is made up of the essential components (nutrients) given in the table below.

Nutrient	Function
Proteins	Body building and repair
Fats	Warmth and energy
Carbohydrates	Energy giving
Vitamins	Maintaining health
Minerals	Maintaining body function
Water	Helps to digest food and dispose of waste
Fibre	Regulating body processes

Proteins

Proteins are the building blocks of the body. They are particularly important for children as they contribute to building the brain, muscle, skin and blood. Proteins also provide the materials needed to repair the cells in the body. Proteins are made up of complex chemicals called **amino acids**. To function properly the body needs twenty-one different amino acids. It can make tweve of these

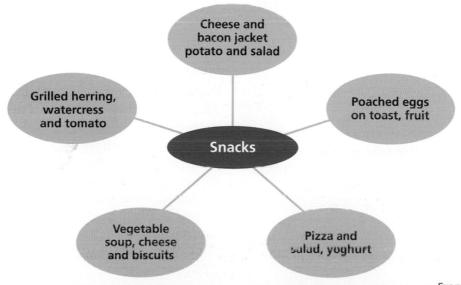

Examples of snacks

itself; the other nine are made from the food that we eat.

There are two types of protein:

- animal protein – obtained from meat, milk, cheese, eggs, fish
- vegetable protein – obtained from nuts, and pulse foods (peas, beans and lentils).

Fats

There are two main types of fat:

- saturated fats – found in both animal and vegetable products, e.g. meat, milk, eggs, cheese and coconut oil. It is important to limit the amount of saturated fat that is eaten because too much can produce high levels of cholesterol. This can increase the risk of heart disease. The increase in cholesterol causes a build-up of fatty deposits in the arteries, which can lead to heart attacks
- unsaturated fats – found in vegetable products such as sunflower oil, olive oil, vegetable oil, herring and cod liver oil. These fats do not turn into cholesterol. They also contain a group known as polyunsaturated fats which are very good at helping the body to repair itself.

Carbohydrates

Carbohydrates provide the body with energy, but the energy value is not as high as fat and the energy is released more quickly. Most carbohydrates come from sugars, starches and fibre. Foods such as biscuits, chocolate, cake, honey and jams are high in carbohydrates as are foods such as pasta, rice and potatoes.

Vitamins

Vitamins are found in most of the food we eat. The main function of vitamins is to regulate the chemical processes that take place in the body. By doing this, they help to promote health. Vitamin A can be found in red vegetables, such as tomatoes and carrots. Vitamin B helps to regulate the nervous system and can be found in Bovril, meat and yeast extracts. Vitamin C can be found in citrus foods and green vegetables.

It is necessary to obtain small amounts of some vitamins from food each day as the body does not store them. If any vitamins are absent from a person's diet, they will suffer from a deficiency disease. A lack of vitamin C, for example, leads to scurvy, whereas a lack of vitamin D (produced by sunlight on the skin) can lead to bone softening and distortion.

Minerals

These are elements such as iron, calcium and potassium. They are found in most of the foods that we eat, though some foods are higher in some minerals than others. Iron is supplied through eating red meat and non-meat sources such as fortified cereals, dried fruit, pulses and green leafy vegetables. Iron is needed by the body to help reduce tiredness and to enable the blood to absorb oxygen. A lack of iron results in anaemia. Minerals such as zinc help to keep the immune system healthy and are needed for healing. Minerals are also essential in maintaining our body functions. Certain minerals, such as calcium, are important for bone growth and repair.

Water

Water is probably the most important part of the diet. Water is the medium in which the body processes take place. It helps us digest food and dispose of waste products. We must not underestimate the value of water. A good rule to follow is to drink half your weight in fluid ounces of water every day.

Fibre

Fibre in our diet adds bulk to the food that we eat. This helps the digestive system to move the food through the intestines. Without these muscular movements, human beings would easily become constipated. Fibre is found in a variety of different foods such as bran, rice, cereals, wholemeal bread, fruit, vegetables (peas, beans, greens). A lack of fibre in a diet results in poor digestion.

1 Karen is living in a nursing home. She is a little confused but eats quite normally. She likes to have a snack for her tea.

Plan a well balanced snack for Karen:
● show the nutritional value of the snack
● explain how the nutrients will meet Karen's needs.

2 Henry is 77 years old and has difficulty swallowing. He is also a resident in the nursing home.

Plan a lunch time snack for Henry. Explain:
● why you have chosen the snack and how it is appropriate for Henry
● the nutritional value of the snack.

Foods suitable for service users' needs

Cultural needs

Some service users will require diets that take into consideration their cultural needs. For example, Muslims and Jews are not allowed to eat pork or pork products, which rules out one source of protein. Many Hindus are vegetarian, which means that their protein will need to be derived from plant products.

Special dietary requirements and allergies

A service user may need a special diet because specific foods, such as wheat, cause a reaction in their system, and so some foods may be restricted. For example, a service user may have coeliac disease or diabetes and may not be able to correctly absorb nutrients or sugar. If the latter is the problem, the body is unable to produce enough insulin to deal with the sugar. The balance between blood sugar levels and the amount of insulin is critical. Too much of either could cause a service user to fall into a coma.

One of the most common allergies to food is nut allergy. Symptoms caused by an allergy can vary from person to person. In some the symptoms will be a rash, while in others the reaction is so severe that they can have an **anaphylactic shock**, which can stop them from breathing.

Care must be taken too when preparing these service users' food to make sure it does not contain anything that they are allergic to.

DRVs

Dietary Reference Values (DRVs) were produced by the Department of Health in 1991 to replace RDA (Recommended Daily Amount). DRVs are the **benchmark** intakes of energy and nutrients which can be used as guidance when planning a meal. As they are only a guide, they should not be seen as exact recommendations. They show the amount of energy that people from different groups need in order to maintain good health. User needs may differ in many ways. Men often need more calories than women. Other factors that can influence the amount of food needed are the type of work that is being done (**sedentary** or manual), a person's age, whether a person is allergic to particular foods, or pregnancy.

DRVs show how many calories a day are needed. On average a person needs 500–700 calories (2,100–2,950 kilojoules) every day to stay alive. While sitting watching the television and resting not much energy is used. At rest, the body burns about twelve calories of energy for every pound that we weigh (approximately 112 kilojoules per kilogram).

The table below shows the DRVs for adults and children over 4, based on 2,000 calories a day.

Food component	DRV
fat	65 g
saturated	fatty acids 20 g
cholesterol	300 milligrams (mg)
total carbohydrate	300 g
fibre	25 g
sodium	2,400 mg
potassium	3,500 mg
protein	50 g

Producing a plan for a snack

A dietary plan will give an outline of:

- the aim and objectives
- the timescales
- what is to be done and how
- the reasons for the actions taken.

When planning snacks for Winsome, you must break down the task into the following smaller parts:

- Find out the recommended DRVs for Winsome.
- Find out Winsome's likes and dislikes.
- Use your research to plan the snack menu.
- Show how the menu meets Winsome's needs.
- Produce one of the snacks.

Work out the timescales, deciding when and how you are going to carry out the objectives and in what order.

The plan could look like the one at the bottom of the page.

From the plan, you can see:

- the timescales involved
- the order in which the tasks are to be carried out
- what is to be done
- any special considerations.

Producing the snack

Before producing the snack, it is important to consider the ingredients to be used, the cost, the time it will take to produce the snack and where the snack is to be made.

A snack is not likely to take very long to make, thirty minutes at the most and usually only about fifteen minutes.

Prepare and serve a snack

Meal times should be pleasant occasions and should provide the service user with the opportunity to enjoy the meal and to chat with others in a relaxed situation. Care workers will

Timescales	Order	What should be done	Notes
Wednesday, 15 Nov	Investigate the DRVs required by Winsome	Use computer to find information on DRVs	Remember he lives a sedentary life
Thursday, 16 Nov	Find out about likes and dislikes Find out what he has for lunch on various days	Talk to Winsome	Make reminder notes
Friday, 17 Nov	Plan three days' snacks Work out nutritional value	Main part of snack: Jacket potato with cheese Vegetable soup with cheese and biscuits Ham and salad sandwich	Do not include cucumber – Winsome does not like it
Monday, etc.	Produce one snack	Etc.	Etc.

need to make an effort to make sure that eating is an enjoyable experience.

Many settings will encourage service users to eat a snack in the dining room so that they can talk to others. Hospitals also encourage those who can walk to sit at a communal table to share their meal. In an early years setting, children meet in the canteen/cafeteria or sit round in a group to eat a packed lunch.

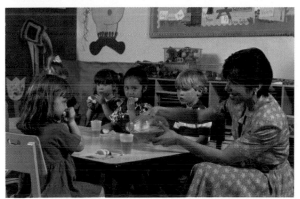

Children enjoying their lunch

Care workers need to make sure that service users have been correctly prepared to make sure that they are comfortable when eating. Preparation can include:

- making sure that the service user has been to the toilet before they eat
- minimising noise and distraction while service users are eating, although playing music quietly in the background can help to create a relaxing atmosphere
- if a service user is in bed and needs help with eating, make sure they are sufficiently supported and are sitting comfortably. The care worker should make sure they are sitting at arms' length from the service user and should ask them what they would like to eat first
- if a service user is able to eat with others but has a special need, like having their food cut up, this should be done before the food is brought to the table, so that the service user is not embarrassed
- a service user may be able to sit at the table but may need to be fed by a care worker. The care worker should sit down next to the service

user to feed them, rather than towering over them. This is more encouraging for the service user and draws less attention to their special need. It also helps the service user to feel more relaxed and less hurried.

Serve a main course to a service user

When preparing and serving food and drink, it should be remembered that 'we eat with our eyes'. Presentation is very important. If the food served looks attractive and appealing to the service user, they are more likely to eat it. When serving a snack to a service user, care workers need to think about:

- colour – include foods with colours that complement one another and are not all the same colour
- appearance – do not serve food that is overcooked
- texture – make sure there is a variety of textures
- flavour.

Care workers will also need to consider the appearance and setting of the table or tray.

Colour is important when serving a meal. If the plate of food looks attractive it is likely to **stimulate** the taste buds of the service user and they will want to eat it. An attractive snack will have different colours.

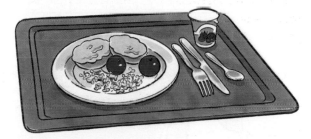

An attractive, colourful snack with a variety of textures

In the snack above, the care worker has given thought to the colour. The jacket potato will be light brown and will contrast with the cheese, green cress and red tomato. When served, this will look attractive. The yoghurt provides a contrast of texture.

Consider this

How are the textures different in the plate of food on the previous page?

Care workers need to be sure that **portion** sizes are not too large, as an overfull plate can put service users off eating. Serving large portions is not a good idea either, as a service user who is not likely to do much exercise and can quickly become overweight which could add to their health problems. Food should be prepared hygienically and hot food should be served at 63°C. A snack that should be served hot and is cold when it arrives is less likely to be eaten.

When setting the table care workers should ensure that the place setting matches the requirements of the meal to be served. Solid coloured plates are less distracting than patterned plates. Any specialist aids, such as special cutlery should be added when laying the table. The table should be laid as follows:

- one non-slip place mat should be used for each service user
- the fork should be placed on the left of the placemat
- the knife should be placed on the right of the place mat
- the spoon and fork for the dessert should be placed above the place mat with the spoon on the outside of the fork. The handle of the spoon should be at right angles with the knife
- a glass for water should be placed above and a short distance from the knife
- a table napkin should be placed to the left of the fork
- salt and pepper should be placed near the middle of the table
- a jug of water should also be placed near the condiments
- flowers, real or artificial, will add an aesthetic finishing touch.

When serving a meal at a table to service users, the plate should be put down for the service user from their left side and the empty plate should be taken from the service user on the right side.

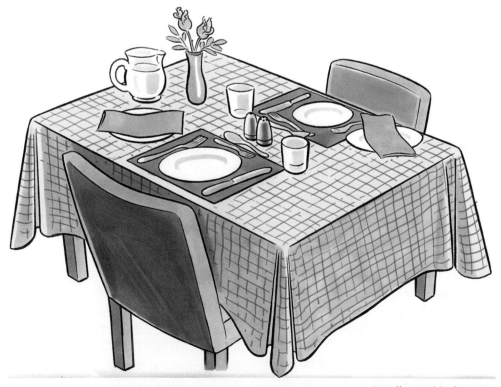

A well-set table for two service users

If a care worker is actually feeding a service user, they should sit next to the service user. The care worker should ask the service user which food they would like to eat first. They should then put small amounts of food on the spoon and place it gently in the mouth. Time should be allowed for the service user to chew and to swallow the food before putting in the next mouthful.

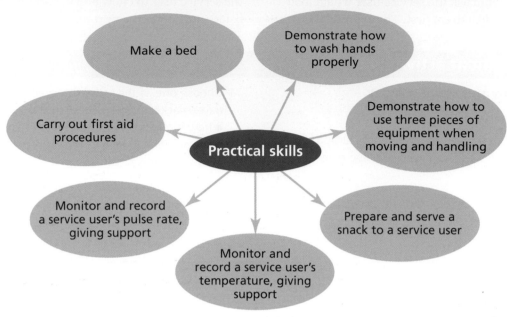

Practical skills

When evaluating practical skills you will need to:

- *reflect* – think about what you have done and how well you did it
- *analyse* – compare what you did with the 'theory' (the correct way of carrying out the task)
- *draw conclusions* – judge your performance, taking account of the opinions of others such as your tutor, the service user or your peers

- *think about improvements* – could you have done anything better or to a higher standard?

You will also need to include information about the different aspects of the task as outlined in the table on the next page.

Max, a care worker, is evaluating the skills he used when taking a service user's pulse, temperature and providing support. He writes:

'My aim was to make sure that the service user knew exactly what I was going to do. For this purpose, I used my communication skills to explain what I would like to do. I went at a pace that the service user could follow and did not use too many technical terms so that the service user was not confused. I asked for the service user's permission to carry out the task, making sure that she still felt in control of the situation. In his book *People Skills*, Neil Thompson states that a carer should "avoid long cumbersome sentences to prevent confusion", so I used short sentences which were clear and easy to follow. My assessors commented on this and confirmed that the sentence construction did provide clarity.

I used mathematical and scientific skills to take the user's pulse rate and temperature. I followed the directions of Nurse X, read the thermometer and then counted the pulse for thirty seconds. I then doubled the score to get a minute's count. I felt quite confident in carrying out these procedures as I had observed them many times before and had practised them by simulating the procedures with my peers.

I achieved my aim as the health monitoring was correctly recorded as confirmed by the nurse on duty. I think I could have been clearer when ...'

Aspect of task	Questions to ask
Aims	What was the aim? How was it met or why was it not met? Was the aim appropriate?
Objectives	What were the objectives? Were they achieved? Were the objectives appropriate?
Skills used	What skills were used? (e.g. Which kinds of practical, scientific or interpersonal skills were used?) How well were they used? Should other skills have been used? Were they effective? Were they used in the same way as suggested by the theory?
Benefits to the service user	What were the benefits? How did they improve the quality of life for the service user? Was the service user empowered?
Timescales	How long did you allow for each task? How long did each task take? Are there any recommended timings that judgements can be made against?
Achieving outcomes	What outcomes were intended? Were these outcomes achieved? What were the benefits to the service user?
Improvements	Where could improvements have been made? Why? What could have been done differently? What do others suggest about improvements that could be made?

This short account shows that Max is considering carefully what he did, how he did it and how effectively he used different skills. When evaluating it is important that:

- judgements are made rather than straight statements

- reference is made to theory (the correct way to carry out a task)
- you give your own and other people's opinions
- your evaluation considers the advantages and disadvantages of different ways of doing things.

Assessment activity 4.7

Evaluating practical skills

You have been asked to demonstrate to the staff at Hill Tops Nursing Home how to write an evaluation of all the practical tasks that you have carried out during training sessions, to help the care workers understand how to undertake the tasks.

Evaluate, in writing, all the practical tasks that need to be carried out. Remember to include:

- aims
- objectives
- skills
- timescales
- achieving outcomes
- improvements.

Try to include a detailed analysis and to make reasoned, informed judgements.

Glossary

Amino acids: the building blocks of proteins

Amoebic dysentery: a disease caused by ingesting substances contaminated with the amoeba Entamoeba histolytica which causes severe diarrhoea, nausea and inflammation of the intestines

Anaphylactic shock: a sudden, severe allergic reaction caused by exposure to a foreign substance brought on by a previous exposure to it

Athlete's foot: a contagious fungal skin infection

Bed sores: ulcers brought about by a long confinement in bed, especially over bony prominences

Benchmark: a point of reference

Care management process: a plan of care for an individual

Codes of conduct: guidelines that are standard and followed by all who are doing a particular job or running a particular type of establishment

Consistent: regular; the ability to do the same thing in the same way

Control methods: ways of controlling (being in charge of) the way something happens

Cumulative: increasing by additions

Deteriorating: getting worse

Domiciliary: dealing with people in their own homes

Duty of care: a responsibility to carry out duties effectively

Enabling: empowering someone to be able to do something

Enforcing authorities: those responsible for seeing that rules and regulations are followed

Food handling techniques: ways of handling food

Food poisoning: causing illness through eating food that is contaminated

Forceful exertions: the bringing about or bearing of power or pressure

Function: a performance or action

Hypothermia: a condition that develops when the body temperature falls too low

Implemented: carried out; put into place

Incontinence: inability to restrain natural discharges

Individualised: personalised; particular to the person concerned

Ingestion: taking into the body

Inhaled: breathed in

Legislation: law

Manual: operated by hand

Micro-organism: organism of microscopic size

Minimum: the least amount; the smallest

Minute: tiny

Mitred: a joint in which a piece is put at 45° to its side giving a right angle

Monitoring: tracking

Mucocutaneous exposure: skin coming into contact with mucus

Musculo-skeletal: muscles and bones

Nominated controller: usually a supervisor or a manager

Optimum condition: the point at which any condition is most favourable

Oxygenated blood: blood carrying oxygen

Pathogen: organism that causes disease

Percutaneous exposure: infection through the skin

Portion: an allotted amount of food

Repercussions: consequences

Sedentary: not active, mainly involves sitting

Socially isolated: not mixing with others

Spore: a unicellular asexual reproductive body

Standardise: to keep to a uniform way; to keep all to the same way

Sterilise: to destroy germs

Stimulate: to make something interesting

Subsume: to include in something else

Toxic: poisonous

Triplicate: three copies

Vector: an organism that carries disease-causing micro-organisms from one host to another

Vulnerable: to be easily affected because of a weakness

Unit 16 Anatomy and physiology for health and care

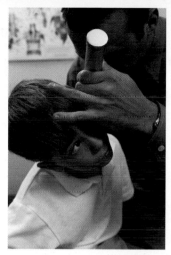

A doctor carrying out an examination of a young patient's ear

Introduction

Everyone can benefit from a better understanding of how our bodies work and what may go wrong. Sometimes, however, body systems **malfunction**, and care workers also need to understand the causes of disease and the treatments available.

This unit introduces the fundamentals of anatomy and physiology and explores different types of dysfunction that may occur.

Dysfunctions may cause an individual extreme pain, worry and fear. With a better understanding of the symptoms, causes and effects, it is possible to adapt our lifestyles to maintain and improve our health.

In this unit you will learn

Learning outcomes

You will learn to:

- investigate the functions and dysfunctions of the digestive system
- investigate the respiratory system and associated dysfunctions
- investigate the cardio-vascular system, explaining the causes of disease
- investigate the functions and dysfunctions of the renal system
- investigate the functions of the musculo-skeletal system and the effects of the ageing process
- review the common dysfunctions of the nervous system
- explain the diagnostic tests, medical care and treatment received by two service users with different needs.

The structure of the digestive system

The digestive system is also known as the **alimentary tract** or **alimentary canal**. It extends from the mouth to the anus. Associated accessory organs, which are part of the digestive system, are located outside it and **secrete** fluids into it.

The digestive system consists of:

- the mouth or oral cavity, with the salivary glands and the tonsils as accessory organs
- the throat or pharynx
- the oesophagus
- the stomach
- the small intestine, with the liver, gall bladder and pancreas as accessory organs
- the large intestine.

The mouth

The mouth, or oral cavity, is bounded by the lips in front (**anterior**), the throat opening into the pharynx at the back (**posterior**), the cheeks on the side (**laterally**) and the palate above. The lower part is formed mainly by the tongue and muscles. The tongue contains specialised cells that are sensitive to taste and known as taste buds.

The teeth surround the palate and the tongue and are set in the tissue of the gums. The ring of muscle formed by the lips, cheeks and tongue helps to keep food in the mouth. The mouth is lined with a **mucous membrane**, which is lubricated with **saliva** produced by three pairs of salivary glands.

The tongue is a large muscular organ, attached at the posterior with the anterior part relatively

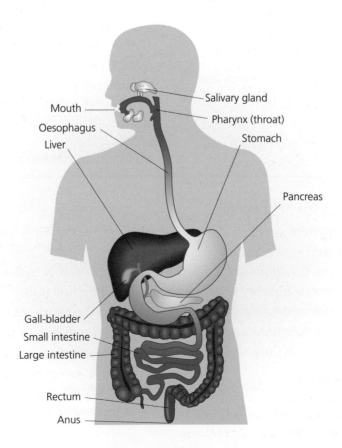

Mouth

Oesophagus

Liver

Salivary gland

Pharynx (throat)

Stomach

Pancreas

Gall-bladder

Small intestine

Large intestine

Rectum

Anus

The digestive system

Swallowing starts with the **tongue** pushing a food bolus to the back of the mouth

The **soft palate** prevents food entering the nose

The **epiglottis** prevents food entering the trachea

Once the food gets to the **oesophagus**, peristalsis takes over

The swallowing process

free. It is attached to the floor of the mouth by a thin fold of tissue called the **frenulum**.

An adult normally has thirty-two permanent or secondary teeth, which replace the first or milk teeth that develop in early childhood.

Functions of the mouth

The functions of the mouth are as follows.

- *Ingestion* *and taste*: fluid and foods are taken into the body through the mouth to commence **digestion**. The taste buds in the tongue are stimulated by salivary action.
- *Mastication* (chewing) is the muscular action and movement of the jaw causing the teeth to break food down into small pieces. The tongue and cheeks help to keep food in the mouth.
- *Digestion* begins with the digestion of carbohydrates (starch) by amylase, an enzyme that is present in saliva.
- *Swallowing*: the muscular action of the tongue moulds the food into a ball (or bolus) and pushes the bolus into the pharynx for swallowing.
- *Protection*: mucin and water in saliva provide lubrication, and an enzyme called lysozyme kills micro-organisms.

The pharynx

The pharynx connects the back of the mouth and nose to the oesophagus. It is lined with mucous membrane and forms part of both the respiratory and digestive systems. A fold of tissue called the epiglottis covers the opening to the larynx (airway) to prevent food and drink entering into the larynx during the swallowing action.

The functions of the pharynx

The main functions of the pharynx are involved in:

- *swallowing*: the bolus (food ball) moves from the mouth to the oesophagus along the pharynx. Particles are prevented from going into the naso-pharynx by the soft palate and from going into the larynx by the epiglottis
- *breathing*: air passes from the nose or the mouth through the pharynx to the respiratory tract
- *protection*: this is provided by the production of mucus.

The oesophagus

The oesophagus (gullet) is about twenty-three centimetres long and extends from the pharynx to the stomach. At each end of the oesophagus there is a **sphincter**, or ring of muscles, that act as a regulating valve to control the passage of food. One is situated at the **distal** (lower) end of the oesophagus, which helps to prevent the reflux of food from the stomach; the other is located in the **proximal** (upper) part and helps to regulate food into the digestive tract and not into the respiratory system.

The functions of the oesophagus

The main function of the oesophagus is the propulsion of food and fluids from the pharynx into the stomach by **peristaltic** (involuntary wave-like) contractions. In the sub-mucosal layer of the oesophageal wall, glands produce mucus, which provides lubrication and also helps to protect the lining from any acid secretions that may escape from the lower end of the stomach.

The stomach

The stomach lies in the left upper section of the abdomen, just beneath the **diaphragm**. It is a bag-like structure capable of holding approximately 1.5 litres.

The stomach has two openings:

- The upper opening from the oesophagus is called the gastro-oesophageal (also referred to as the cardiac opening, being nearer to the heart), and is surrounded by a sphincter.
- The lower opening, where the stomach becomes narrower to form the pyloric canal, before connecting into the first part of the small intestine, is called the pyloric orifice or pylorus (the Latin name for gatekeeper). This orifice is also surrounded by a sphincter.

When empty, the lining of the stomach has large folds known as rugae (wrinkles). These folds lessen as the stomach fills with food.

The functions of the stomach

The stomach has five main functions:

- storage
- digestion
- protection
- absorption
- propulsion.

The stomach can store food by stretching until the food is broken down and ready for digestion. Hydrochloric acid and an enzyme called pepsin prepare proteins for digestion. A secretion known as the **intrinsic factor** is produced by cells in the pyloric end of the stomach. It binds with vitamin B12, to make it more easily absorbed in the small intestine and prevent it from being broken down by stomach acid.

A few substances such as aspirin, water and alcohol are absorbed into the blood stream directly from the stomach; otherwise, very little absorption takes place here.

The stomach is designed to churn food through the action of muscular waves throughout its walls, thus mixing food and fluids with various secretions into a texture called **chyme**. This is propelled into the small intestine through the pyloric orifice by peristaltic contractions. The production of mucus in the stomach helps to prevent the stomach wall itself becoming digested and also helps to kill most micro-organisms.

The small intestine

The greatest amount of digestion and absorption occurs in the small intestine, which consists of three parts:

- the duodenum, approximately twenty-five centimetres long. The duodenum receives secretions from the liver and the pancreas, through ducts or papilla
- the jejunum, approximately 2.5 metres long
- the ileum, approximately 3.5 metres long.

Functions of the small intestine

The functions of the small intestine are summarised in the table on the next page.

Function of the small intestine	What happens
Neutralisation	Bile from the liver and bicarbonate ions from the pancreas neutralise the stomach acid to form a medium that is suitable for the action of the pancreatic and intestinal enzymes.
Digestion	The breakdown of food is completed by the action of the enzymes from the pancreas and the lining of the small intestine. Fats are **emulsified** by bile salts from the liver.
Absorption	The inner lining of the small intestine is increased over 600 times through folds and villi (finger-shaped protrusions). Most nutrients and water are absorbed here.
Mixing and propulsion	Contractions and peristaltic action move the chyme into the large intestine, which takes 3–5 hours.
Excretion	Bile from the liver contains **bilirubin**, cholesterol, fats and fat-soluble hormones.
Protection	The production of mucus protects the intestinal walls against being digested and provides lubrication.

The large intestine

This extends from the ileum to the anus. It is about 1.5 metres long and consists of the caecum, colon, rectum and the anal canal. The walls are quite thick compared with the rest of the digestive tract.

The functions of the large intestine

The main functions of the large intestine are:

- absorption
- storage of faeces
- propulsion of faeces towards the anus
- **defaecation**.

It takes 18–24 hours for material to pass through the large intestine. The movements in the large intestinal walls are slower than the small intestine. Chyme is converted into **faeces** while passing through the colon. Water and salts are absorbed from the contents through the walls of the intestine. Mucus secretion and the extensive action of micro-organisms help in the formation of faeces, which remain in the colon until defaecation.

Mucus also provides lubrication and protection against acid and bacteria.

The function of the rectum is to collect faeces that have been formed in the alimentary tract. Nerve impulses then pass to the brain to trigger the urge to defaecate, although voluntary control may delay this action.

Some dysfunctions of the digestive system

The functioning of the digestive system can be affected by disease, diet, the environment and chemical influences. Some common dysfunctions are illustrated in the spider diagram below.

Crohn's disease

This is a chronic inflammatory disease affecting any part of the gastro-intestinal tract from the mouth to the anus. Once the disease begins, it tends to fluctuate between periods of inactivity (remission) and activity (relapse). Men and

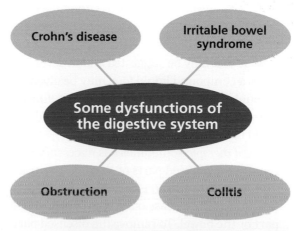

Common dysfunctions of the digestive system

women are equally affected and it may begin at any stage, from childhood to later life.

Cause

The cause is unknown, but some scientists believe that it may be triggered by an extreme response to infection, such as a bacterium or virus. There is also a slight **genetic** link in developing the disease.

Effects

The most common site for inflammation to occur is the distal end of the ileum and symptoms can vary depending on the degree of inflammation and the location. Bloody diarrhoea and abdominal pain are common symptoms. Obstruction of the small intestine may also occur.

The disease is unpredictable, uncomfortable, tiring, embarrassing and disruptive to normal activities. Sufferers are often fearful of leaving the house in the morning because of the frequency of diarrhoea and the inability to control the urge to defaecate. They may avoid eating at times, if this makes their symptoms worse.

Treatment

There is no cure for Crohn's disease, but medication is often prescribed to reduce pain, infection and inflammation.

- *Drug therapy*: the most commonly used drugs are prednisone (a synthetic form of cortisone) and anti-inflammatory drugs. Antibiotics and immuno-suppressive drugs, pain killers, vitamins and minerals may also be used.
- *Nutritional therapy*: some foods can make the symptoms worse. A doctor may recommend changes in the diet to rest the bowel. A low-residue diet may be suggested and in severe cases a compound liquid food may be given through a naso-gastric tube. Intake of fluids, especially water, is strongly recommended to avoid the risk of dehydration.
- *Surgical therapy*: sometimes it is necessary to remove the affected parts of the digestive tract. This usually results in a period of improved health, but the disease often recurs in another part of the bowel. To remove the diseased part

may mean the patient has an ileostomy – the body's fluid-like waste then has to empty into a bag (worn on the outside of the body), through a surgically-prepared opening. The contents of the bag are disposed of by the patient whenever necessary. The psychological and physical effects of the surgery are often distressing, affecting the patient's self-image and confidence, and leading to bouts of depression and anxiety.

Irritable bowel syndrome

Irritable bowel syndrome (IBS) is the most common bowel dysfunction, affecting about 10–20 per cent of adults. The condition is twice as common in women as in men, usually beginning in early or middle adulthood.

Cause

Some doctors consider the main causes of IBS to be psychological, particularly anxiety and emotional stress. People with IBS seem neither to lose nor gain weight because of the condition. The structure of the digestive tract usually shows no abnormalities.

The diagnosis is based on the patient's symptoms, a physical examination, and examination of the faeces, a barium meal, an x-ray examination and a **sigmoidoscopy**.

Effects

There are many symptoms of IBS, as shown in the table below.

Direct symptoms	Indirect symptoms
Abdominal pain	Tiredness
Excessive wind	Agitation
Abdominal distension	Faintness
Constipation	Reduced appetite
Diarrhoea	Backache
	Heartburn

Treatment

Treatment usually includes a high-fibre diet, plus medication to ease the symptoms of diarrhoea and muscular spasms. These treatments do not cure the problem. Patients often find that although the symptoms ease from time to time, the condition recurs throughout life.

Intestinal obstruction

This refers to a partial or complete blockage of any part of the small or large intestine. It is critical the patient receives immediate treatment, otherwise it could prove fatal.

Causes

There are several possible causes of intestinal obstruction, including the following:

- **Paralytic ileus** is the most common cause of obstruction. The rhythmic muscular contractions malfunction causing the intestine to dilate, so that food no longer moves along the digestive tract. This may follow surgery or an abdominal injury. It is vital to prevent dehydration, and treatment involves removal of the content of the bowel by a tube.
- A **hernia** may become strangulated, meaning that the affected part of the bowel becomes twisted, cutting off the blood supply. Emergency surgical treatment is vital.
- A **volvulous**, or twisting of the bowel, causes severe **colic** and vomiting.
- Adhesions are normally unconnected parts of the body binding together with scar tissue. Mostly, they develop as a result of scarring following inflammation. A complication could result in obstruction of the bowel. Urgent surgical intervention to separate the adhesions is paramount.
- Faeces and food may become impacted as in a complication of Crohn's disease, eventually causing obstruction of the bowel.
- **Atresia** refers to a **congenital** absence of an opening or a canal due to failure of development while in the uterus. For example, **oesophageal atresia** would result in the baby not being able to feed due to the oesophagus not opening into the stomach.
- Certain inappropriate objects, if swallowed, could lead to obstruction.

Consider this

What problems may occur in the digestive tract? If obstruction of the intestine is suspected, what precautions should be considered to ensure the care and well-being of the patient?

Colitis

Colitis is inflammation of the colon.

Effects

Patients have diarrhoea, often with blood and mucus in the stools (faeces) and may also complain of abdominal pain and fever.

Causes

Colitis may be caused by organisms such as **campylobacter**, **shigella**, bacteria, viruses or **amoebae**. The prolonged use of antibiotics may upset the balance of the natural bacteria present in the gut, allowing harmful organisms to multiply and spread.

A doctor may diagnose colitis if severe diarrhoea persists, with or without food, for more than five days. He or she would then arrange a pathological test of the faeces and, if no infection is found, a sigmoidoscopy may be performed. A barium meal may also be given to check for areas of inflammation or narrowing of the intestine.

Treatment

If the cause is infection, this usually clears up without treatment, although some infections are treated with antibiotics. Sometimes an area may be damaged and will need to be removed surgically.

Assessment activity 16.1

Functions and dysfunctions of the digestive system

Produce training materials about the digestive system for a resource pack or guide that can be used for trainee nurses.

1 Review the structure and function of the digestive system. Provide clear and accurate diagrams as well as written explanations. Try to give a detailed account of the structure and function of the digestive system.

2 Produce materials to show **one** dysfunction of the digestive system. Include information about its symptoms, causes and effects.

3 Produce a case study to illustrate how a service user who is experiencing this condition could cope with the situation.

Use a wide range of sources when completing these activities, keeping a bibliography or source list to support your evidence.

The respiratory system carries oxygen and air to the bloodstream and expels the waste product of carbon dioxide. Breathing is vital to life because all the living cells of the body need a constant supply of oxygen. The action of breathing involves air passing from the nose through various passages to millions of sacs or balloon-shaped objects called the **alveoli**.

The structure of the respiratory system

The respiratory system consists of:

- the pharynx
- the larynx
- the lungs
- the bronchi and alveoli
- the trachea
- the nose and nasal cavities.

Air may also pass through the mouth, but this is considered to be part of the digestive system and not the respiratory system.

The nose and nasal cavities and their function

This is the first part of the respiratory system and is also the organ of smell. It is divided into two chambers by the **nasal septum**, which is made up of cartilage at the front and bone at the rear. The nasal cavity extends from the nostrils to the openings into the pharynx.

The nose has the following functions.

- The nasal cavity is designed to clean and filter the air. Each vestibule is lined with hairs that trap some of the large particles of dust present in the air.
- The nasal cavity also humidifies and warms the air we breathe in. Moisture from the mucus lining and from the excess of tears that drain from the eyes is added to the air as it passes through the nasal cavities. Warm blood flowing through the mucus membrane lining warms the air before it passes on towards the pharynx. This helps to prevent damage that cold air may cause to the rest of the respiratory tract.
- The sensory organ of smell is located in the uppermost part of the nasal cavity.

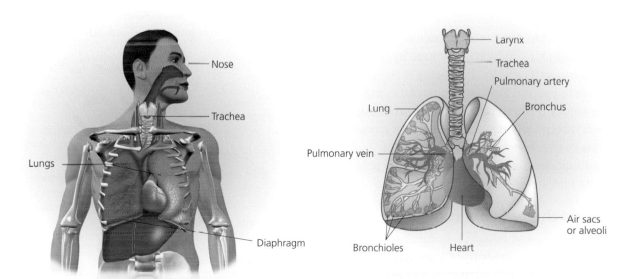

The structure of the respiratory system

Consider this

Which functions of the nose are related to breathing?

The pharynx and its function

The pharynx connects the back of the mouth and nose to the oesophagus. The uppermost part is known as the naso-pharynx and connects the nasal cavity to the area behind the soft palate of the mouth. This is an air passage. The middle section of the pharynx is called the oro-pharynx and is a passage for both air and food. The lowest part of the pharynx, called the laryngo-pharynx, is only concerned with the passage of food and merges with the oesophagus.

A flap of cartilage called the epiglottis lies behind the tongue – during swallowing, it covers the opening to the larynx to prevent food or drink being inhaled.

The larynx and its function

The larynx is in the anterior part of the throat. It is made up of cartilage, muscles and **ligaments**. The thyroid cartilage projects at the front to form the Adam's apple. Two sheets of fibrous tissue stretch to form the vocal cords, which are responsible for voice production.

The larynx has two main functions: one is to prevent choking, which is achieved by the action of the epiglottis and by the closing of the vocal chords to prevent food and liquids entering the respiratory tract; the other is voice production, which occurs when air from the lungs passes through the stretched vocal chords. The resultant vibrations are modified by the tongue, palate and lips to produce speech.

The trachea and its function

The trachea, or windpipe, is immediately below the larynx and is made up of connective tissue, smooth muscle and C-shaped pieces of cartilage. The cartilage supports the trachea, offering protection and maintaining an open passage for air. The back of the trachea is composed of bundles of smooth muscle which are also very elastic. When this muscle contracts, it narrows the diameter of the trachea and causes air to move rapidly through the trachea. The lining produces mucus and the cilia (hairs) that are present sweep any foreign particles that may become trapped into the pharynx, where they are swallowed.

The bronchi and alveoli and their function

Starting with the trachea, all the passages of the respiratory tract are called the tracheobronchial tree. At the distal end, the trachea divides to form two smaller tubes, known as the bronchi, each of which extends to a lung. Each bronchus in turn divides and subdivides to form smaller and smaller bronchioles, until eventually microscopically small tubes and sacs are formed.

As with the trachea, the main bronchi are supported by cartilage. As the bronchioles become smaller, the amount of cartilage becomes less, whilst smooth muscle becomes more abundant. Relaxation and contraction of these muscles can change the diameter of the passages and hence the volume of air moving through them.

Alveoli are microscopic sacs that are found in groups (resembling bunches of grapes) at the ends of the bronchioles. A single sac is called an alveolus and each lung has about 300 million

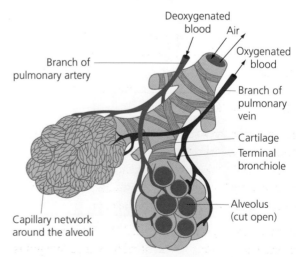

A bunch of alveoli showing the blood supply

alveoli. Each alveolus is surrounded by a capillary network and it is here that the exchange of gases (oxygen and carbon dioxide) takes place. They pass through the alveolar membrane into the blood vessels, and vice versa.

The lungs and their function

These are the main organs of respiration. Each lung is roughly cone-shaped, with the base of the cones resting on the diaphragm (the large muscle separating the chest from the abdomen), while the apex of the cones extends above the clavicles (collar bones) by approximately 2.5 centimetres. The right lung is larger than the left, weighing 620 grams on average. The left lung weighs about 560 grams.

The hilum is a region on the surface of the lung (also referred to as the root of the lung), where the main bronchus, blood vessels, nerves and lymphatic vessels enter or leave the lung.

Each lung is enclosed in a double membrane called the **pleura**, which allows each lung to slide freely as they expand and contract during breathing.

> **Consider this**
>
> *Why do we breathe?*

The respiratory process is the main function of the respiratory system and is explained in the diagram below.

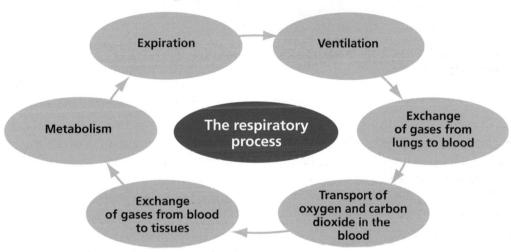

The respiratory process

The process by which oxygen reaches the body cells and how it is utilised is known as **metabolism**, which also includes the production of carbon dioxide before its subsequent elimination from the body.

Respiration provides the energy that is needed by the body and a constant supply of oxygen is required. At the same time, the waste products (mainly carbon dioxide) produced by the body, must be carried away from the cells.

Air rich in oxygen is breathed in and carried along the airways to the alveoli, where oxygen is transferred to the blood. The oxygen-saturated blood is then carried through the circulatory system to reach all parts of the body, where it gives up oxygen and picks up carbon dioxide. When oxygen diffuses from the respiratory system into the blood, most of it combines with **haemoglobin**, while a smaller amount dissolves into the **plasma**. Haemoglobin transports oxygen through the blood vessels to where it is needed in the body.

During exercise, breathing increases automatically, ensuring more oxygen is provided for the increased energy demands.

Metabolism within the cells may be expressed simply as:

glucose + oxygen = energy + carbon dioxide + water

The waste products of carbon dioxide and water are transported through the circulatory system to the lungs to be expelled from the body.

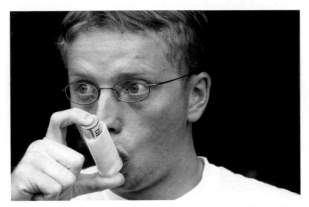

A patient using oxygen to aid breathing

Some dysfunctions of the respiratory system

When the respiratory system is not functioning properly, symptoms can often be frightening.

Asthma

Asthma is a chronic disease of the lungs, characterised by difficulty in breathing when the airways become narrow or constricted. People with asthma have extra-sensitive airways, which react by becoming narrower when they are irritated. The air passages become inflamed and sensitive to certain provoking factors, or triggers. The linings of the airways become swollen and narrow, thus reducing the air flow in and out of the lungs.

Cause

The exact causes of asthma are unknown, but asthma and allergies are more prevalent in some families.

Bronchial asthma is classified into two main types:

- extrinsic, in which an allergy (usually to something inhaled) triggers an attack
- intrinsic, where there is no apparent external cause for the attack.

Extrinsic factors
Pollen
House dust
House dust mites
Animal fur
Feathers
Viral infection
Bacterial infection
Exercise
Tobacco smoke
Food allergy
Drug allergy

Symptoms

Characteristic symptoms of asthma are wheezing, coughing, shortness of breath and tightness in the chest, and they vary in severity. The first symptoms often start in childhood, but more than half of children with asthma grow out of it by the age of twenty-one. The condition can develop at any age, however, and childhood asthmatics are prone to have a recurrence of the condition in later life.

During a severe attack, breathing may become increasingly difficult, causing sweating, rapid heart beat and extreme distress and anxiety. The person may find it difficult to lie down, to speak or to sleep. **Cyanosis** (blue discoloration) of the face and lips may occur in severe attacks.

Treatment

There is no cure for asthma, although much can be done to protect suffers from extrinsic factors. Tests can identify any common causes and precautions can be taken to avoid contact with them. **Prophylactic** treatment, using an inhaler to dispense drugs, is very effective if taken as instructed by a medical practitioner.

Most asthma attacks can be controlled by using an inhaler, but occasionally an attack may be so severe that hospitalisation is necessary, where treatment would include oxygen and a ventilator.

All patients should have a treatment plan agreed with their doctor. This usually involves attending periodic clinics, where the patient's symptoms and records are monitored. Patients usually need to measure and record the air flow in and out of the lungs once or twice daily, to identify whether their condition is under control or getting worse.

Occupational effects

Asthma UK has produced a charter which sets out ten steps for reducing asthma at work.

There are hundreds of known asthmagens relating to people's occupations, including those shown below.

Unlike pre-existing asthma, occupational asthma can be cured if it is identified early.

Key points

Occupational asthma – asthma that is caused by exposure to substances at work

Pre-existing asthma – a previous history of asthma (maybe since childhood)

Asthmagens – substances that can cause asthma in people who did not have it before

Desensitisation – when people develop an allergy after being exposed to even a small amount of an asthmagen

Triggers – things that can set off an asthma attack.

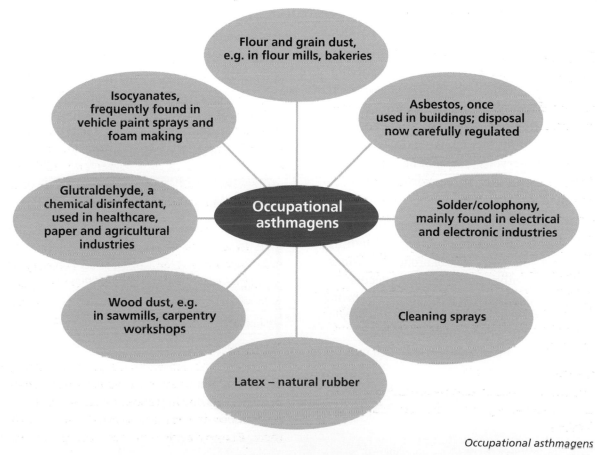

Occupational asthmagens

Case study

Roy

Roy had just retired and was beginning to get used to his new lifestyle. One day he came down with a cold. After a few days, he developed a cough and the **expectoration** was yellow and obviously infected. His GP prescribed an antibiotic, but this produced no improvement. In fact Roy's breathing was becoming noisy, with obvious wheezing and distress. He was not sleeping well, and found it difficult to lie down. A further course of antibiotics was prescribed, still with no lasting improvement. The cough and congestion continued for two to three months and Roy was then referred to the asthma clinic.

1 What do you think should be measured to evaluate the seriousness of Roy's breathing problems?

2 What type of treatment may be prescribed?

3 What other procedures are important in the overall care and prevention of complications?

Broncho-spasm

Broncho-spasm is a term that applies to the narrowing of the bronchi and is caused when the muscles of the walls contract and/or when inflammation is present. The contraction and relaxation of the airways is controlled by the autonomic nervous system. It may also be triggered as an allergic reaction to certain substances.

The result of the narrowing means that air flow out of the lungs causes wheezing or coughing. The most common cause of broncho-spasm is asthma, but other causes include infection, chronic lung disease (e.g. emphysema, chronic bronchitis), anaphylactic shock or an allergic reaction to chemicals. Broncho-spasm is therefore a symptom, or reaction, to a number of underlying conditions.

Pneumothorax

A **pneumothorax** is the condition when air is introduced into the **pleural cavity** through an opening in the thoracic wall or lung.

Cause

Air may enter from the lung, or from outside the body, due to trauma by a knife, bullet, broken rib, etc. Spontaneous pneumothorax usually happens for no apparent reason, but is more common in thin young men. It may also be a complication of lung disease, especially asthma or emphysema.

Symptoms

The most common symptoms are chest pain and shortness of breath. A small pneumothorax may resolve itself, but frequently it is necessary to insert a chest tube into the pleural cavity. This restores the negative pressure necessary for the lung to expand again. Surgery may be necessary to close the opening into the pleural cavity.

Other infections

Infections can affect any part of the respiratory tract (see below). Causes may be bacteria or viruses, but infections may be aggravated by inhaled fumes such as tobacco smoke.

Infections of the upper respiratory tract are very common, especially in childhood. An adult probably develops a natural immunity over the years. The table below gives the most common infections of the respiratory tract.

Upper respiratory tract	Lower respiratory tract
Cold	Bronchitis
Croup	Tracheitis
Laryngitis	Pneumonia
Tonsillitis	Bronchiolitis
Sinusitis	
Pharyngitis	

Haemoptysis is the action of coughing up blood. It may occur due to trauma from swallowed objects, causing injury and bleeding that seeps into or damages the airways. If haemoptysis is associated with lung disease, it is treated as a serious symptom that requires urgent investigation.

Assessment activity 16.2

The respiratory system and associated dysfunctions

Produce training materials about the respiratory system for a resource pack or guide that can be used for trainee nurses.

1 Review the structure and function of the respiratory system. Provide clear and accurate diagrams as well as written explanations. Try to give a detailed account of the structure and function of the respiratory system.

2 Produce materials to show **one** dysfunction of the respiratory system. Include information about its symptoms, causes and effects.

3 Produce a case study to illustrate how a service user who is experiencing this condition could cope with the situation.

Use a wide range of sources when completing these activities, keeping a bibliography or source list to support your evidence.

The heart

The heart is situated in the centre of the chest, with its right side directly beneath the right edge of the **sternum** (breast bone). The rest of the heart extends leftwards, with the apex (tip) of the heart located under the left nipple.

The heart is a muscular pump, consisting mainly of a muscle called the **myocardium**. The myocardium needs oxygen and nutrients and beats rhythmically and automatically with its own nerve supply.

The heart is divided into two by a thick central muscular wall called the septum. It has four chambers, two on the right side and two on the left side. The upper chambers on each side are called the atria (singular: **atrium**) and the larger lower chambers on each side are called the **ventricles**. The lining of the heart is a smooth membrane called the **endocardium** and the complete heart is enclosed in a tough bag, called the **pericardium**.

The heart is continuously pumping blood, but does not receive its own needs from the flow. This is provided by two **coronary** arteries that arise from the **aorta**, leaving the left ventricle and supplying blood to the entire heart muscle.

> ### Consider this
> *Identify the position of the heart in the body and describe the basic structure.*

The heart's pumping action is essential in maintaining a continuous circulation of blood throughout the body. It beats continuously and rhythmically to send blood to the lungs and the rest of the body. It can be thought of as two pumps in one:

- The right side receives **deoxygenated** blood from the body through two large veins called the superior vena cava and the inferior vena

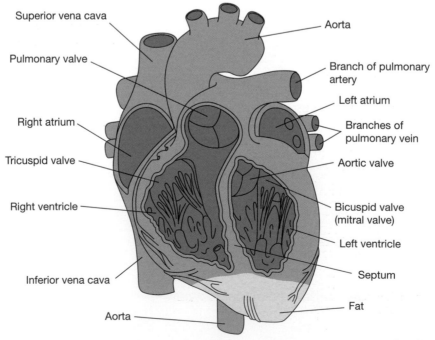

The structure of the heart

cava. This blood is received into the right atrium and transfers through the **tricuspid valve** into the right ventricle. From here it is pumped to the lungs through the pulmonary artery to be oxygenated and to exchange carbon dioxide. This is also known as the pulmonary circulation.

- The left side of the heart receives oxygenated blood from the lungs, through the pulmonary veins which empty into the left atrium. From here, the oxygenated blood transfers through the **mitral valve** in the left ventricle, from where it is pumped to all the tissues of the body via the main artery of the body, known as the aorta, which rises from the left ventricle. The exit to the aorta from the left ventricle is guarded by the aortic valve. This is the **systemic** circulation.

Functions of the heart

The main functions of the heart may be classified as:

- routing of blood
- regulating blood supply
- ensuring one-way blood flow
- generating blood pressure.

Blood pressure is generated by the contractions of the heart, which promote the flow of blood though the blood vessels. The pulmonary and systemic circulations have separate routes. The valves of the heart ensure a one-way system through the heart and blood vessels. The rate and force of the contracting heart muscles match the required delivery of blood to the tissues according to the body's metabolic needs (at rest, exercise, changes in body position, etc.).

Arteries

The ventricles pump blood from the heart into large elastic arteries, which gradually become smaller in size with distance from the heart. The arteries are known collectively as the arterial system.

Arteries are the blood vessels that carry blood *away* from the heart. The largest artery, the aorta, emerges from the left ventricle. The other main arteries of the systemic system (to all parts of the body except the lungs) arise from the aorta. The pulmonary arteries (to the lungs) carry blood from the right ventricle to the lungs. These arteries are shorter, with thinner walls and are under a lower pressure than arteries in the systemic circulation.

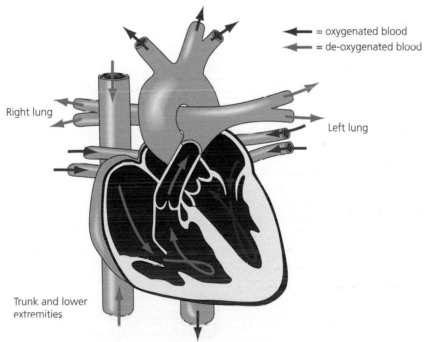

← = oxygenated blood
← = de-oxygenated blood

Right lung

Left lung

Trunk and lower extremities

The flow of blood through the heart

The structure of an artery wall allows it to sustain the high blood pressure which occurs on each heart beat. Arteries are also designed to even out the peaks and troughs of blood pressure caused by the heart beat, enabling the blood to flow at a relatively constant pressure.

Blood flows through the arterial system to the arterioles and then into the capillaries, where the exchanges of oxygen and nutrients occur across the capillary walls. There are more capillaries than any other type of blood vessel.

Capillaries form a fine network throughout the body's organs and tissues and are the vessels that carry the blood between the **arterioles** and the **venules**. Capillaries have a diameter of approximately 0.008 millimetres and the walls are permeable to oxygen, glucose, water and carbon dioxide. They are not open to blood flow all of the time, being in use according to the needs of different organs, depending on activity levels. Capillaries also play an important part in controlling the temperature of the skin.

Veins

Blood returns *from* the arterioles into the **venous system**. The walls of veins are thinner and less elastic than arteries. As the veins return to the heart, they gradually increase in diameter and decrease in number, while their walls become thicker.

Veins return blood *towards* the heart, from the various organs and tissues of the body. The majority of veins carry deoxygenated blood that is collected from the venules, through gradually bigger veins, until they finally converge in the two largest veins in the body, the superior vena cava and the inferior vena cava. The vena cava carries the deoxygenated blood to the right side of the heart to be pumped to the lungs.

A general rule of thumb is that arteries carry blood *away* from the heart, whilst veins carry blood *to* the heart. The two exceptions to this rule are:

- the pulmonary vein in the chest, which carries oxygenated blood from the lungs to the left side of the heart
- the portal vein, which carries nutrient-rich blood from the intestines to the liver.

The inner linings of many veins contain valves to ensure that the flow of blood is controlled towards the heart. The pressure of blood is also lower in veins than in arteries. This explains the fact that if a vein is cut, the blood escapes relatively slowly, whereas blood from a cut artery is pumped out by the action of the heart beat.

Changes in blood and blood pressure

Blood tests

Blood tests are used to diagnose or to eliminate suspected abnormalities, as shown in the diagram at the top of the next page.

- *Haematological tests* look at the components of the blood itself, examining the number, size, shape and appearance of the blood cells and checking the function of clotting. The most important of these tests are blood count, blood clotting time and blood groups.
- *Biochemical tests* measure the chemicals in the blood, such as glucose, sodium, potassium, uric acid, urea, enzymes, gases, digested foods and drugs.
- *Microbiological tests* check for micro-organisms, such as bacteria, viruses, fungi and parasites.

Changes or abnormalities in the blood, or in any of its components, may affect body function and well-being. Some of these are listed in the table opposite.

Blood pressure

Blood pressure refers to the pressure that occurs due to the flow of blood through the main arteries. It rises and falls as the heart reacts to the various demands that are made on the body, such as exercise, sleep or dealing with stressful situations. Two levels of pressure are measured:

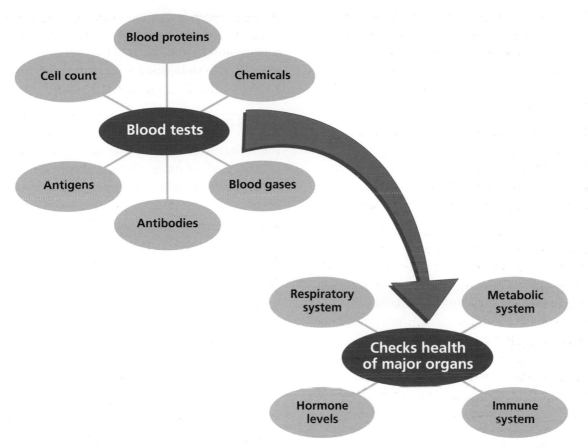

The purposes of blood tests

Condition	Change or abnormality in the blood
Anaemia	A deficiency in the cell pigment haemoglobin
Polycythaemia	Too many red blood cells
Leukaemia	Excessive numbers of white blood cells, crowding out the normal blood cells in the bone marrow
Defects in platelets	Associated with various bleeding disorders
Genetic disorders	These include: sickle cell anaemia, thalassaemia, haemophilia
Nutritional disorders	Iron deficiency anaemia, lack of vitamin B12 or folic acid
Infection	Septicaemia, malaria, amoebic dysentery
Poisons	Lead poisoning, carbon monoxide, toxaemia
Drugs	Alcohol, pharmaceutical drugs at abnormal levels with possible liver or other organ damage

- *systolic pressure* (the top reading), created by the contraction of the heart muscle
- *diastolic pressure* (the lower reading), recorded during the relaxation of the heart between beats.

A healthy young adult has a blood pressure of about 110/75. This often rises with age to about 130/90 at the age of sixty. Abnormally high blood pressure is known as **hypertension** and abnormally low blood pressure is called **hypotension**. The ill effects of hypertension, which puts a considerable strain on the heart and other organs, include:

- giddiness
- shortness of breath
- stroke
- heart disease
- heart failure
- kidney damage
- coronary heart disease
- retinopathy
- confusion
- seizures
- headaches.

Case study

Phyllis

Phyllis was 65 when she had a heart attack. She worked as an ancillary nurse in the community and had retired at the age of 60. Her work had been very demanding and involved being 'on call' for one weekend in three. Over the years her weight had escalated, resulting in her being two and a half stone overweight. Exercise had not been something she had ever enjoyed; she felt she did 'enough running around' with her job. Phyllis enjoyed drinking alcohol at weekends, feeling that it helped her to relax more easily. She used to smoke, but had to give it up four years before she retired, following a severe chest infection.

Her family life had been very stressful, with her son's marriage breaking up and two grandchildren needing extra care during this difficult time. Her husband was in poor health, with pain from arthritis affecting his mobility.

1 What were the risk factors that contributed to Phyllis's heart attack?

2 Bearing in mind her lifestyle, what needs to be considered to prevent a second heart attack?

Postural hypotension may occur if a person stands up quickly, with symptoms of dizziness or even fainting. Other types of hypotension are associated with injuries or burns as a result of shock.

Causes of heart disease

Heart disease is the most common cause of death in developed countries. There are many different causes of heart disease, including those shown below.

Key point

Heart failure is a term used when the heart becomes less efficient at pumping blood around the body.

The causes of heart disease may be related to the following factors:

- ***Inherited*** *or genetic factors*: these may not cause heart disease, but they may increase the possibility of developing **hyperlipidaemia**, and **atherosclerosis**.
- *Congenital defects of the heart*: these are the most common defects in new-born children, as a result of errors in development within the uterus. Defects of the septum (hole in the heart) and some abnormalities of the valves may occur. Fortunately most of the defects are treatable.
- *Infection*: an infection of the lining of the heart and the valves is called **endocarditis**. This is more likely to occur in people who have had a congenital defect. Drug addicts who inject with non-sterile needles are also at risk of developing endocarditis. Infection may cause further damage, affecting the competency of the valves and the heart muscle.
- *Tumours*: these are rare. A **myoxoma** is a benign tumour that grows inside one of the heart chambers and restricts the flow of blood. **Malignant sarcomas** can occasionally develop, and secondary tumours sometimes invade the tissues of the heart.

- *Muscle disorders*: disorders, such as **cardiomyopathy**, may be inherited, or may be caused by vitamin deficiency, alcohol or a viral infection. **Myocarditis** is inflammation of the heart muscle and may also be caused by a viral infection.
- *Injury*: this may be caused by blunt objects, or by an accident, e.g. a car accident, when the steering wheel can cause bruising or even rupture.
- *Nutritional disorders*: the heart muscle may become thin and flabby through lack of protein and too few calories. Vitamin B1 deficiency (common in alcoholics) causes **beriberi**. Obesity is a major risk factor, because it may lead to hypertension, diabetes and high cholesterol levels. Lack of regular exercise also contributes to heart disease.
- *Impaired blood supply*: this is a major cause of heart disease. The coronary arteries become narrow and atherosclerosis develops, depriving the heart muscle of oxygen and leading to a 'heart attack' (**myocardial infarction**).
- *Poisoning*: the most common poison is alcohol. A large intake for many years may lead to a type of cardiomyopathy in which the heart becomes enlarged and leads to heart failure. If alcohol intake is stopped, the heart may recover.
- *Drugs*: certain drugs may disturb the heart beat and even cause permanent damage. Smoking is a major risk factor in developing heart disease, because it damages the lungs and the nicotine causes an increased heart beat.

Assessment activity 16.3

The cardio-vascular system and the causes of disease

Produce training materials about the cardio-vascular system for a resource pack or guide that can be used for trainee nurses.

1 Review the structure and function of the cardio-vascular system. Provide clear and accurate diagrams as well as written explanations. Try to give a detailed account of the structure and function of the cardio-vascular system.

2 Produce materials to show **one** dysfunction of the cardio-vascular system. Include information about its symptoms, causes and effects.

3 Produce a case study to illustrate how a service user who is experiencing this condition could cope with the situation.

Use a wide range of sources when completing these activities, keeping a bibliography or source list to support your evidence.

The structure of the renal system

The kidneys

The kidneys are bean-shaped organs about the size of a tightly clenched fist. Each kidney is 10–12.5 centimetres long and weighs about 170 grams. They lie on the posterior wall of the abdominal cavity, just above the waist on either side of the spinal column.

They receive their blood supply from arteries, branching directly from the aorta. Inside the kidney, the renal arteries gradually become smaller, ending in small capillaries that are called **glomeruli**. Each kidney has about one million glomeruli, which pass the filtered blood through to long **tubules** and into the central part of the kidney, called the **medulla**. Each kidney is surrounded by a layer of fibrous tissue and then embedded in fat, which acts as a shock absorber and helps to protect against injury. Internally, each kidney consists of an outer cortex, an inner medulla and a urinary collecting system.

The ureters

The **ureters** are the two tubes that transport urine from the kidneys to the bladder. Each ureter is 25–30 centimetres long.

Urine passes along the ureters mainly by gravity, but also due to peristaltic movements in the walls of the ureters, which occur several times a minute. The ureters enter the bladder through a tunnel which is angled to prevent **reflux** (back flow) of urine when the bladder contracts.

The bladder

The urinary bladder is a hollow muscular organ that lies in the pelvic cavity, just behind the **symphysis pubis**. It acts as a reservoir for urine, with an adult bladder holding half a litre or more of urine. The bladder walls are muscular and the lining is called the urinary epithelium. The **urethra** carries urine from the bladder to the outside. The opening into the urethra from the bladder is at the lowest point or 'neck' of the bladder. This opening is normally kept tightly closed by a ring of muscle known as the urethral sphincter.

The urethra

The urethra is the tube through which urine is excreted from the bladder. The tube is short in females (about four centimetres) and opens to the outside just above the vaginal opening, between the folds of the **labia minora**. The urethra in males is much longer (about 18–20 centimetres) and forms a conduit throughout the length of the penis. The flow of urine from the bladder is controlled by the muscles and outlet of the bladder.

The prostate gland

This gland surrounds the first part of the urethra in the male. It is solid, resembling a chestnut in shape. It is situated immediately under the bladder and in front of the rectum. Its function is to provide secretions that are part of the fluid

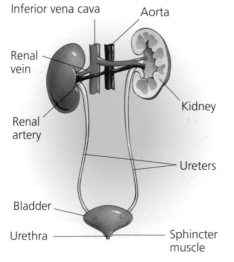

Inferior vena cava

Aorta

Renal vein

Renal artery

Kidney

Ureters

Bladder

Urethra

Sphincter muscle

The renal system

produced during ejaculation. Ejaculatory ducts from the **seminal vesicles** pass through the prostate before entering the urethra. The prostate gland is quite small at birth, weighing only a few grams, becoming larger during puberty. Growth stops at the age of twenty, when it weighs about 20 grams. In later life, usually after the age of fifty, the prostate may enlarge further.

The functions of the renal system

The functions of the renal system include:

- excretion of urine
- vitamin D synthesis
- regulation of:
  - blood pressure and volume
  - concentration of the blood.

Urine production

The kidneys are the major organs responsible for the **excretion** of waste from the body. Although the skin, liver, intestine and lungs eliminate some wastes, if the kidneys fail, the other organs would be unable to compensate adequately.

- The kidneys regulate blood pressure and volume by controlling the extracellular (outside the cells) fluid volume. This is achieved by producing either a large volume of dilute urine, or small amounts of concentrated urine.
- The kidneys regulate the concentrations of nutrients in the blood, as well as regulating the pH (acidity or alkalinity) of the extracellular fluid.
- The manufacture of red blood cells in bone marrow is regulated by a hormone called **erythropoietin**, which is produced in the kidneys.
- The kidneys also play an important role in controlling the levels of calcium by regulating the synthesis of vitamin D.
- Excretion of urine is brought about through the kidneys filtering blood. Large molecules, such as protein and blood cells, are retained in the blood, but smaller molecules pass through. These include metabolic waste and toxic

molecules. Along with other waste products, these result in the formation of urine.

Homeostasis

Homeostasis is the process that maintains a constant internal environment, despite external changes. It is a main function of most organs and includes the regulation of blood pressure, body temperature and blood sugar levels. All the body systems help to control and maintain the internal environment. The digestive, respiratory, circulatory and urinary systems function together to ensure that each cell in the body receives adequate oxygen and nutrients and that waste products do not reach toxic levels.

- Body temperature is a variable that increases in hot weather and decreases in cold weather. Homeostatic mechanisms such as shivering or sweating normally maintain body temperature near an ideal normal value.
- When oxygen levels in the blood are low, breathing is stimulated and when blood pressure falls, the heart rate is increased.

When fluid surrounding cells deviates from homeostasis, the cells do not function normally and can even die. Disease also disrupts homeostasis and sometimes results in death.

> ### Consider this
> *What are the main functions of the renal system?*

Dysfunctions of the renal system

Some of the problems that cause dysfunction in the renal system are:

- infection
- calculi (kidney stones)
- renal failure
- prostrate enlargement
- haematuria (blood present in urine).

Renal infection

Renal infection, or urinary tract infection (UTI), refers to an infection anywhere in the urinary system. Normal urine is sterile, which means it is free of bacteria, viruses and fungi. Infection occurs when micro-organisms, usually bacteria from the digestive tract, enter the opening of the urethra and begin to multiply. Escherichia coli (E. coli), which normally lives in the colon, is the most common cause of urinary tract infections.

The table below lists the types of renal infection.

- **Urethritis** can be caused by a number of micro-organisms, but those that are transmitted during sexual intercourse, such as **gonorrhoea** or non specific urethritis are common.
- **Cystitis** is the most common renal infection, usually caused by a bacterial infection. Urine that is not excreted from the bladder may become stagnant and encourage infection. It is more common in women because the urethra is short and organisms from the exterior have less far to travel. An obstruction, or partial obstruction, may be caused by a **calculus** (stone), a tumour, or a **urethral stricture**, which increase the risk of infection.
- **Ureteritis** can occur as a result of bacteria entering the urinary tract from above, or if reflux of urine from the bladder occurs, also from below. It may also occur due to a stone or calculus becoming lodged in the ureter.
- **Pyelonephritis** may be **acute** (in the form of a sudden attack) or **chronic** (permanent), when previous attacks may have caused damage to the kidneys. Infection spreading from below, from the bladder and ureters, is a common cause. The risks of a urinary tract infection can be reduced by improved personal hygiene, drinking plenty of water and by regular emptying of the bladder.

The main symptoms of renal infections are illustrated in the spider diagram below.

Type of renal infection	Area of inflammation
Urethritis	Inflammation of the urethra. May also be caused by mechanisms other than infection
Cystitis	Inflammation of the bladder
Ureteritis	Inflammation of the ureters
Pyelonephritis	Inflammation of the kidneys

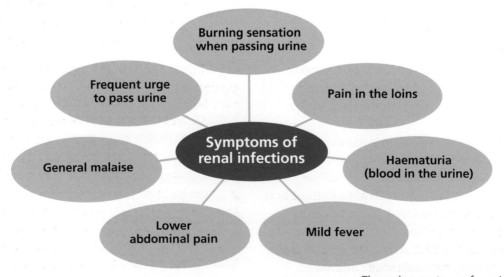

The main symptoms of renal infections

Renal infections can be diagnosed by testing a few drops of urine. Further examinations by x-ray or ultrasound scanning may be necessary.

Most infections are treated with an antibiotic drug. The most appropriate drug will depend on the results of the culture.

Case study

Davina

Davina is 22. She recently had a bout of food poisoning, with frequent abdominal pain and diarrhoea. This took several days to clear, with rest and control of her diet, and some medication from her doctor.

Soon afterwards, Davina found that when passing urine, she experienced a burning sensation at the end of the stream. She also needed to urinate more frequently, although she was unable to pass very much urine. The burning persisted and she tried cutting down on her fluid intake, but this seemed to make matters worse.

1 What do you think may be the cause of Davina's problem?

2 Do you think she should reduce her fluid intake?

3 If left untreated, what complications could develop?

Calculi

A calculus (stone) in the urinary tract is caused by precipitation from solution of the substances in urine, and is more common in the kidneys and ureters than in the bladder. Calculi are three times more common in men than in women, with the incidence being higher in the summer months, possibly because urine is more concentrated in hotter weather, with more fluid being lost due to sweating.

Seventy per cent of the stones consist of calcium oxalate and phosphates. Calcium oxalate is an end product of body metabolism.

The most common symptom of a stone in the kidney or ureter is **renal colic**, whilst the most common symptom of a bladder stone is difficulty in passing urine.

A urine test may reveal red blood cells in the urine. Ninety per cent of urinary tract calculi are visible on an x-ray, which identifies the site of the stone. **Urography** and ultrasound scanning may also be used to assist diagnosis.

Treatment involves bed rest, painkillers and adequate fluid intake to encourage the passing of the stone. The majority of stones are less than five millimetres in diameter. Larger stones may require surgical intervention.

Haematuria

Haematuria is a condition in which blood is present in the urine. It may be visible to the naked eye in some cases. Almost any disorder of the urinary tract can cause bleeding, but the most common cause is renal infection.

Enlarged prostate

Changes in the prostate gland may begin as early as 40 years of age. By 60, as the blood flow to the prostate gland decreases, the epithelial lining thickens and the quantity of smooth muscle decreases. These changes do not affect fertility.

Benign prostatic hypertrophy, or enlargement of the prostate, is common in men over 60, with approximately fifteen per cent of men experiencing difficulties that require medical treatment. This is due to the pressure the enlarged prostate puts on the urethra, resulting in difficulties in urination. Enlargement of the prostate will result in fifty per cent of men experiencing difficulties by the time they are 80. Cancer of the prostate is rare before the age of 50. However, after the age of 55, it is the third leading cause of death from cancer in men. This condition also causes difficulties in urination.

Renal failure

Renal failure (or kidney failure) can result from any condition that interferes with the kidneys' function, i.e. a reduction in their ability to filter the waste products from the blood, to excrete them in the urine, to control the body's water and salt balance or to regulate blood pressure. This causes a build up of urea (**uraemia**) and other waste products that cause dysfunction. The kidneys are susceptible to a number of disorders that may lead to kidney failure; however, only one normal kidney is needed for a person to enjoy good health.

The main causes of kidney failure are outlined in the table below.

Acute	Chronic
Shock	Hypertension
Severe injury	Diabetes mellitus
Illness	Polycystic kidney
Severe bleeding	Urinary obstruction
Myocardial infarction	Calculus
Pancreatitis	Tumours
Calculus	Analgesic drugs
Bladder tumour	
Enlarged prostrate	
Glomerulonephritis	

Renal failure may be acute or chronic. In acute kidney failure, function often returns to normal once the cause has been removed. Chronic failure may progress over months or years to an advanced life-threatening stage, called end stage kidney failure.

The main symptom of kidney failure is reduction in the volume of urine. Less than 400 millilitres per day is called **oliguria**. Complete failure to excrete urine is called **anuria** and will result in a dangerous build up of waste products.

A short time after acute kidney failure starts, more symptoms are obvious, such as drowsiness, nausea, vomiting and breathlessness. A person with suspected kidney failure should undergo kidney function tests to diagnose the problem, before arranging treatment accordingly.

Assessment activity 16.4

Functions and dysfunctions of the renal system

Produce training materials about the renal system for a resource pack or guide that can be used for trainee nurses.

1 Review the structure and function of the renal system. Provide clear and accurate diagrams as well as written explanations. Try to give a detailed account of the structure and function of the renal system.

2 Produce materials to show **one** dysfunction of the renal system. Include information about its symptoms, causes and effects.

3 Produce a case study to illustrate how a service user who is experiencing this condition could cope with the situation.

Use a wide range of sources when completing these activities, keeping a bibliography or source list to support your evidence.

The functions of the musculo-skeletal system

The functions of the skeletal system are:

- support
- protection
- movement
- blood cell production
- storage.

Support

The skeleton of bones is the structural framework that gives the body its shape and provides protection.

The skeletal system has four components:

- bones
- cartilage
- tendons
- ligaments.

Bones

There are approximately 213 bones in the human skeleton. These are joined together with tendons and ligaments to form the protective and supportive framework for muscles and the underlying soft tissues.

The skeleton consists of two main parts:

Axial skeleton		Appendicular skeleton	
Skull	29 bones	Shoulder and upper limbs	64 bones
Spine	33 bones	Pelvis and lower limbs	62 bones
Ribs and sternum	25 bones		

Men's bones tend to be slightly larger and heavier than the corresponding bones in women. Another difference is that the female pelvis is

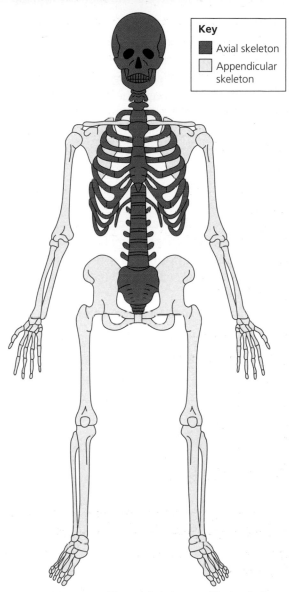

Key
- Axial skeleton
- Appendicular skeleton

The axial and appendicular skeletons

wider than the male, in order to facilitate childbirth.

The bones of the body are connected by three different types of joints, depending on the degree of mobility they permit. These are:

- fixed joints, e.g. the joints between the bones of the skull
- mobile joints, such as a hinge joint of the elbow, or a pivotal joint, e.g. the joint between

the first and second vertebrae, allowing the head to turn from side to side
- ball and socket joints, which allow the widest range of movement, e.g. the shoulder and hip joints.

The skeleton bones contain calcium and phosphorus, which make them hard and rigid. The way that fibres are arranged also makes the bone resilient and strong. The surface of each bone is covered with a thin membrane called the **periosteum**, which contains a network of blood vessels and nerves. The next layer is hard and dense and is referred to as compact, ivory or cortical bone. Inside this layer is a mesh-like structure known as spongy, cancellous, or trabecular bone. The centre cavity in some bones and the spaces in some spongy bones contain fatty tissue, called **bone marrow**, which contains red blood cells, platelets and most of the white blood cells.

Cartilage

This is not as hard as bone, but is an important part of the skeletal system, used mainly as connective tissue and in joints. Most of the skeleton in a foetus is cartilage, which is gradually converted to bone by the process called **ossification**.

Tendons

Tendons are cord-like structures that join muscles together. They are strong and flexible, but inelastic.

Ligaments

Ligaments play an important part in the structure of joints by binding the bone ends together and preventing excessive joint movements. They are also used to support organs such as the uterus, bladder, liver and diaphragm, and help maintain the shape of the breasts.

Movement

There are three main muscle types in the body:

- cardiac or heart muscle
- smooth muscles, found in internal organs
- skeletal muscles, also known as striped or voluntary muscles.

This section will only deal with skeletal muscles.

The skeletal muscles account for 40–45 per cent of the total body weight. They are called skeletal because they are attached to the bones of the skeleton. They are also referred to as voluntary muscles because they can be moved by our conscious control. Each muscle is capable of contraction and relaxation, to bring about movement of the body. There are over 600 skeletal muscles in the body, and they are classified according to the action they perform:

- **extensors** open a joint; **flexors** close it
- **adductors** draw part of the body inwards, **abductors** move it outwards
- **levators** raise a part; **depressors** lower it
- **constrictor** or sphincter muscles surround and close an orifice.

Each muscle is composed of a group of muscle fibres. A small muscle may be made up of only a few bundles, while larger muscles, such as the gluteus maximus, are made up of hundreds of bundles. Movement of these muscles is under voluntary control of the brain, with each muscle fibre supplied with a nerve ending that receives impulses from the brain. These impulses are brought about by the release of **acetylcholine**, which is a type of **neurotransmitter** (a chemical released from nerve endings). This starts a chain of chemical and electrical events. A third of voluntary muscles remains in a state of partial contraction at all times (thus giving muscle tone). **Spasticity** is one form of abnormality, with increased muscle tone.

We use skeletal muscles even when we are not moving. The muscles of posture are contracted to keep us sitting or standing upright. The muscles involved in breathing are constantly working, even when we are asleep. Communication of any kind requires skeletal muscles, whether we are speaking, writing, texting, or using a keyboard. Hand signals and facial expressions all require skeletal muscle function.

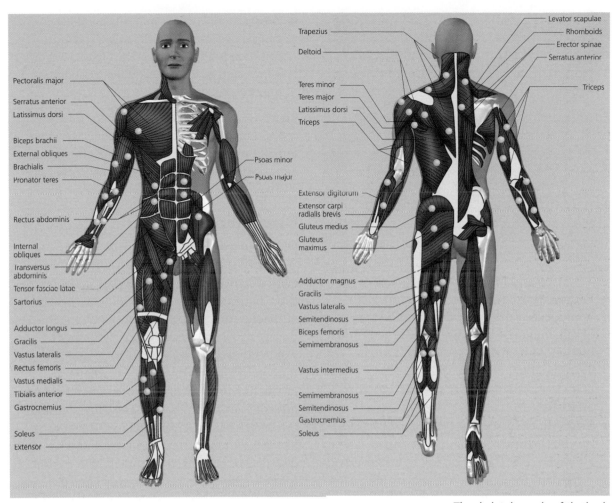

Labels (front view, left side):
Pectoralis major
Serratus anterior
Latissimus dorsi
Biceps brachii
External obliques
Brachialis
Pronator teres
Rectus abdominis
Internal obliques
Transversus abdorninis
Tensor fasciae latae
Sartorius
Adductor longus
Gracilis
Vastus lateralis
Rectus femoris
Vastus medialis
Tibialis anterior
Gastrocnemius
Soleus
Extensor

Labels (front view, right side):
Psoas minor
Psoas major

Labels (back view, left side):
Trapezius
Deltoid
Teres minor
Teres major
Latissimus dorsi
Triceps
Extensor digitorum
Extensor carpi radialis brevis
Gluteus medius
Gluteus maximus
Adductor magnus
Gracilis
Vastus lateralis
Semitendinosus
Biceps femoris
Semimembranosus
Vastus intermedius
Semimembranosus
Semitendinosus
Gastrocnemius
Soleus

Labels (back view, right side):
Levator scapulae
Rhomboids
Erector spinae
Serratus anterior
Triceps

The skeletal muscle of the body

Consider this

What are the three types of muscles in the body? What are the main functions of voluntary muscles?

Degenerative effects on the musculo-skeletal system

Degenerative effects with age can vary considerably. However, a number of changes occur within joints as a person gets older. The changes that take place in the **synovial joints** have the biggest impact, often causing major problems. With age, tissues in the body become less flexible and less elastic. Tissue repair also slows down, the rate of new blood-vessel development decreases, whilst cartilage covering the surfaces of joints wears thin. Some common degenerative conditions are discussed below.

Arthritis

Arthritis is inflammation of a joint. It may affect one joint or several, and symptoms may be mild or severe, from aching and stiffness to extreme pain and deformity.

There are various types of arthritis.

- **Osteoarthritis** is the most common and is also known as degenerative arthritis. It is the result of wear and tear on the joints, and is estimated to affect ten per cent of the world population, but is most common in people over the age of 70.

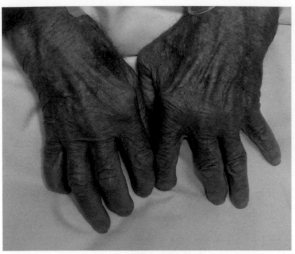

Arthritis in the hands of a patient

- **Rheumatoid arthritis** is due to an auto-immune disorder and is the most severe type of inflammatory joint disease. The body's own immune system damages the joints and surrounding tissues. The joints most commonly affected are the hands, wrists, feet and arms.
- **Still's disease** is a rare condition, also called juvenile arthritis, usually occurring in children under the age of 4. It often starts with a fever and joint pain and clears up after a few years, but could leave the child with permanent deformities.
- **Seronegative arthritis** describes a group of disorders where symptoms of arthritis are present, but blood test results for rheumatoid arthritis are negative. It is often associated with skin disorders and inflammatory bowel disorders such as Crohn's disease.
- **Infective arthritis** is caused by an invasion of bacteria into the joint from a nearby wound, or from the blood stream. It is also referred to as septic or pyogenic arthritis. It may be caused by a complication of chicken pox, rubella, mumps, rheumatic fever, etc.
- **Ankylosing spondylitis** affects the spine and the vertebrae, which become inflamed and gradually fuse together. The cause is unknown, with less than one per cent of the population being affected. It is more common in men than women, often starting between the ages of 20 and 40.

- **Gout** usually occurs in a single joint and is caused by a metabolic disorder. The most common joint affected is the big toe, but other joints such as the knee, ankle, wrist or foot may be affected.

There are specific treatments for the different types of arthritis. These may include the use of antibiotic drugs where there is infection present, or anti-inflammatory drugs to treat conditions such as osteoarthritis or rheumatoid arthritis.

Osteoporosis

Osteoporosis is a condition which makes bones very brittle and susceptible to fractures. It is caused by the loss of protein tissue in the bones. It is a natural process of ageing, with the density of the skeleton diminishing by about one third by the age of 70. It is much more common in women than men, due to the hormonal changes that occur after the menopause, when the production of oestrogen drops and is no longer present to maintain bone mass. Other causes of osteoporosis include removal of the ovaries, a diet deficient in calcium, some hormonal disorders or prolonged treatment with steroids. It is more common in heavy smokers and drinkers.

The first signs of the condition may be fractures following a fall, or spontaneous fractures of one or several of the vertebrae. X-rays and bone density tests confirm the diagnosis.

Rheumatism

Rheumatism refers to any disorder that causes pain and stiffness in muscles and joints.

Paget's disease

Paget's disease occurs most commonly in middle age and in older people. The formation of bone is disrupted, causing the bones to become thicker, weak and deformed. The bones most commonly affected are the pelvis, skull, clavicle, vertebrae and the long bones of the leg. It is thought to be caused by an imbalance between the natural breakdown of cells and the necessary replacement. Infection and possible viral causes are also linked to this condition.

Dysfunctions of the musculo-skeletal system

There are a number of conditions that cause dysfunction of the musculo-skeletal system. The most common are listed in the table below.

Parkinson's disease
General effects
This neurological disorder has certain characteristics:

- a mask-like face
- rigidity and slow movements
- muscle tremor
- stiffness
- muscle weakness
- shuffling and unbalanced movements
- 'pill rolling' movements of fingers.

The first signs are a slight tremor of one hand, which is worse when the hand is at rest and virtually stops when used. The disease is progressive and can eventually cause great difficulties with everyday activities, such as eating, washing and dressing.

Treatment
There is no cure for Parkinson's disease, but help to maintain psychological well-being is important through exercise, whilst supporting independence by introducing aids to improve balance and mobility. Drug therapy may help to minimise symptoms, but cannot halt the **degeneration** of the brain cells.

Bell's palsy
General effects
Bell's palsy is the name given to a paralysis on one side of the face. It is usually temporary and often improves after a few weeks. It usually occurs suddenly with no obvious cause. Most cases occur in people over the age of 40, but it can affect all age groups.

It causes:

- difficulty in speaking
- numbness of the face
- a dry mouth
- loss of taste
- dry, watery eye on affected side
- dribbling when drinking or cleaning teeth
- ear pain
- intolerance to loud noise.

Treatment
Treatment may involve the use of steroids and self-help techniques, such as massage of the face, facial exercises or the application of gentle heat.

Myasthenia gravis
General effects
Myasthenia gravis is a condition which causes the muscles to become weak and tire easily and affects mainly the eyes, face, throat and limb muscles. Drooping eyelids and a blank facial expression are common features. The speech is weak and hesitant. It affects more women than

Dysfunction	Cause	Incidence
Parkinson's disease	Degeneration of nerve cells	1 person in 200. 15,000 new cases each year in the UK
Bell's palsy	Unknown	1 in 60–70 people will be affected at some time in their life
Myasthenia gravis	Auto-immune disorder but reasons are unknown	2–5 new cases per 100,000 people each year
Multiple sclerosis	Unknown but thought to be auto-immune disorder	1 in every 1,000 people

men and, although it can occur at any age, it is usually between the ages of 20 and 30 in women and 50–70 in men.

Treatment

In mild cases, drug therapy is often used to stimulate the transmission of nerve impulses. In severe cases, the removal of the thymus gland often improves the condition considerably. In most cases, the person may lead a comparatively normal life, but sometimes the condition cannot be halted and may progress to respiratory difficulties and death.

Multiple sclerosis

Multiple sclerosis (MS) is a progressive disease of the central nervous system and varies in severity among suffers. The condition is due to the gradual destruction of the protective cover of nerve fibres (myelin), causing symptoms ranging from numbness and tingling to paralysis and incontinence. The pattern of difficulties experienced may change frequently, sufferers sometimes being severely disabled one week and symptom-free the next. There appears to be a genetic factor, with relatives eight times more likely than others to contract the disease.

The first symptoms may appear in early adult life, then regress and subsequently reappear in later life.

General effects

MS may cause symptoms of:

- fatigue
- vertigo
- clumsiness
- muscle weakness

- slurred speech
- unsteady gait
- blurred or double vision
- numbness.

Treatment

Currently, there is no cure. Changes in the diet to include sunflower or evening primrose oils have helped some patients, whilst the drug interferon has also been found to help slow the progress of the disease. Other treatments may include steroids, and physiotherapy to help strengthen weak muscles.

Case study

Ralph

Ralph has a busy life with two young children, a full-time job and a mortgage to pay. He and Joan are happily married, with two children aged 2 and 4. About six months ago, he experienced some difficulty with one of his eyes. His vision was slightly blurred and at times he saw double. He saw his optician, who was unable to detect any problem, although the optician recommended that Ralph consulted his GP. On another occasion he dropped a cup, which just seemed to fall out of his hand. He was definitely clumsier. In general, Ralph felt more tired and did not have much stamina.

1 What do you think Ralph should do to check out the problems he is experiencing?

2 Are some of these symptoms grounds for concern?

Assessment activity 16.5

Functions of the musculo-skeletal system and the effect of the ageing process

Produce training materials about the muculo-skeletal system for a resource pack or guide that can be used for trainee nurses.

1 Review the structure and function of the musculo-skeletal system. Provide clear and accurate diagrams as well as written explanations. Try to give a detailed account of the structure and function of the musculo-skeletal system.

2 Produce materials to show **one** dysfunction of the musculo-skeletal system. Include information about its symptoms, causes and effects.

3 Produce a case study to illustrate how a service user who is experiencing this condition could cope with the situation.

Use a wide range of sources when completing these activities, keeping a bibliography or source list to support your evidence.

The structure and function of the nervous system

The function of the nervous system is to gather information about the external environment and the body's internal state, then analyse this information and initiate responses aimed at satisfying certain drives, the most powerful being survival.

The structure is like a computer system, with the central nervous system (CNS) made up of the brain and spinal column consisting of billions of interconnecting neurons (nerve cells).

Sensory nerves

Nerve endings, called sensory receptors, receive information inside a sense organ, i.e. eye, ear, skin, etc. Sensory nerves send this information to the CNS.

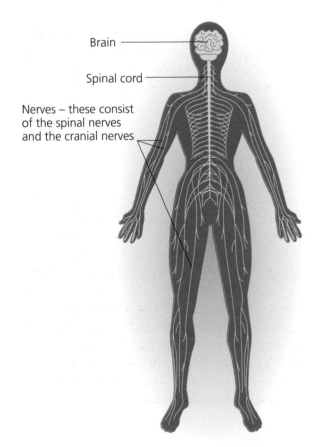

Brain

Spinal cord

Nerves – these consist of the spinal nerves and the cranial nerves

The nervous system

Motor nerves

Motor nerves (or motor transmitters) transmit messages from the CNS to skeletal muscle, muscles controlling speech, internal organs, internal glands and the sweat glands in the skin, to bring about a reaction. This information is transmitted through nerves from the CNS to the entire body.

The motor nerves divide into:

- the somatic nervous system, transmitting messages for potential actions to the skeletal muscles, which are under voluntary control
- the autonomic nervous system (ANS), which transmits messages for potential actions from the CNS to smooth muscle, cardiac muscle and certain glands. Subconscious or involuntary control occurs in this system.

The somatic or voluntary nervous system is under direct control, involving the brain sending messages, via motor nerves, to the muscles to cause the desired reaction. The recognition of the action will be sent back to the brain by the sensory nerves.

The involuntary or autonomic nervous system regulates blood circulation, digestion, breathing, reproductive organs and elimination of waste from the body. It controls important glands and works independently of most of the brain and its cells. It operates entirely by reflexes.

The autonomic nervous system has two parts:

- the sympathetic nervous system, which prepares the body for physical activity
- the parasympathetic nervous system, which is concerned with restoring the body after an emergency.

These two systems work against each other. One system will stimulate an organ and the other stops it from working. First one takes over – then the other. The table opposite shows how this happens. The result is that the organ is kept working at just the right level.

Sympathetic nervous system	Parasympathetic nervous system
Prepares the body for action	Prepares the body for relaxation
Increases heart rate	Slows heart rate
Dilates arteries in skeletal muscles	Dilates arteries in the gut
Slows gut movement	Speeds gut movement
Dilates bronchioles	Constricts bronchioles
Causes sweat glands to secrete	Causes tear and salivary glands to secrete
Causes hair to stand erect	Hair returns to relaxed position
Bladder and anal sphincters contract	Bladder and anal sphincters relax

It is via the sympathetic nervous system that the **hypothalamus** stimulates the production of adrenalin and initiates the alarm reaction.

Common dysfunctions of the nervous system

Common dysfunctions of the nervous system include:

- motor neurone disease
- multiple sclerosis
- Parkinson's disease
- dementia
- hypertension.

Motor neurone disease

Motor neurone disease (MND) is caused by the breakdown of nerve cells in the brain that control muscles. It is a rare condition that usually begins between the ages of 50 and 70. The voluntary muscles enabling movement are affected, but not the nerves that transmit sensation, so there is no numbness, or pins and needles. Intelligence and awareness are not affected. There are three main types of MND, which affect different nerves.

General effects
The first symptoms are weakness in the hands and arms, with muscle wasting. There may also be fasciculations (spontaneous, irregular contractions of areas of muscle), muscle cramps or stiffness. In some cases, symptoms begin in the legs, but usually all four extremities are soon involved.

Diagnosis may be confirmed by a number of tests, including an EMG (measurement of electrical activity in muscle), a muscle biopsy (see page 243), blood tests, myelography (an x-ray examination of the spinal cord) and a CT or MRI scan (see page 242).

There is no cure, but research is on going to find the cause and a possible cure.

Multiple sclerosis

Multiple sclerosis (MS) can affect the brain and the spinal cord. The nerves become damaged and these damaged fibres cannot conduct nerve impulses, so functions such as movements and sensations are lost.

For the general effects of MS, see page 236.

Dementia

Dementia is a general decline in all areas of mental ability. The cause is usually brain disease and it is progressive. The most common feature is decreasing intellectual ability. It is a major problem in modern society, with ten per cent of people over the age of 65, and twenty per cent of people over the age of 75 being affected to some degree. In most cases, dementia is due to cerebro-vascular diseases including strokes and Alzheimer's disease. Cerebro-vascular diseases are often caused by the arteries in the brain becoming narrow or blocked.

General effects

The symptoms of dementia include loss of memory, confusion, emotional outbursts, confabulation (making up stories to fill gaps in memory), loss of care with appearance, irritability and anxiousness. Sufferers may end up needing total nursing care.

Parkinson's disease

This is caused by the degeneration of, or damage to, nerve cells. Degeneration causes a lack of **dopamine** within the brain. As a result muscles are too tense, causing tremor and shaking.

For the general effects of Parkinson's disease, see page 235.

Hypertension

Hypertension is abnormally high blood pressure, even when the person is at rest. Many people have high blood pressure without realising it. If left undiagnosed and untreated, it increases the risks of a stroke or developing heart disease.

The condition is extremely common, affecting 10–20 per cent of the UK adult population.

General effects

Hypertension often causes no symptoms and generally goes undiscovered until diagnosed through routine health checks.

When a person experiences any problem that affects their well-being, they may seek medical advice from their GP. The GP may initially treat the patient to relieve symptoms such as pain or fever. Ultimately, however, the GP will will aim to diagnose the cause of the problem, in order to make a **prognosis** and arrange appropriate treatment.

Case study

Megan

Megan was 75 years of age when she first appeared to be showing signs of confusion. Repeating herself and also forgetting dates and appointments were causing her husband Bryan some concern. She sometimes forgot to wash or change her clothes and needed more and more support and supervision from Bryan. There were times when she would shout and become very irritable and Bryan was very afraid to leave her alone at home to go to the local shops.

1 Does Bryan need to be concerned?

2 What signs and symptoms of ill health is Megan displaying?

3 What needs to be assessed in order to introduce a care plan?

Assessment activity 16.6

Common dysfunctions of the nervous system

Produce training materials about the nervous system for a resource pack or guide that can be used for trainee nurses.

1 Review the structure and function of the nervous system. Provide clear and accurate diagrams as well as written explanations. Try to give a detailed account of the structure and function of the nervous system.

2 Produce materials to show **three** dysfunctions of the nervous system. Include information about their symptoms, causes and effects.

3 Produce case studies to illustrate how service users who are experiencing these conditions could cope with the situation.

Use a wide range of sources when completing these activities, keeping a bibliography or source list to support your evidence.

Making a diagnosis

The two traditional steps to form a diagnosis are to:

- take a careful history of the onset of the illness
- perform a physical examination.

Doctors still attach great importance to these procedures but, in the past twenty years, there have been significant improvements in diagnostic accuracy, due to improvements in equipment and the development of new techniques.

A GP is trained to listen to a patient's account of their symptoms and to observe any signs of ill-health. He or she may also ask questions, e.g. about general lifestyle, eating habits, bowel action, any pain or fever, sleep difficulties, etc.

The GP may then decide to examine the patient physically. The extent of this examination will depend on the nature of the symptoms, but could include any of the techniques listed in the table below.

Depending on the doctor's initial assessment, further tests may be necessary to confirm a diagnosis. This may involve:

- testing urine
- testing blood
- taking a **culture swab**
- referral to hospital.

When a diagnosis has been made, an appropriate course of treatment can be planned.

Diagnostic tests

The main diagnostic tests are listed in the table below. New imaging techniques are being developed all the time to provide detailed pictures of internal organs. **Fibre-optic** scopes enable doctors to look directly into many parts of the body. Biochemical, immunological and microbiological tests are an invaluable part of the technology used today.

X-rays

X-rays are widely used and allow a practitioner to see inside the body. X-rays are absorbed more by the dense parts, such as the ribs or the heart, and less by the finer structures, such as the skin or lungs. A radiographer is able to read the different shadows cast by the x-ray. Dense tissue appears

Body system	Diagnostic techniques that may be used
Musculo-skeletal	Muscle or bone biopsy; x-ray; CT; MRI; arthroscopy; densitometry; blood tests
Reproductive	Men – blood analysis: semen tests; biopsy; culture Women – endoscopy; laparoscopy; colposcopy; mammography; ultrasound; hystosalpingography; cytology; culture; biopsy; blood tests; amniocentesis; chorionic villus sampling
Respiratory	Pulmonary function tests; bronchoscopy; culture; biopsy; blood tests; x-rays; CT; MRI; lung tomography
Endocrine	Thyroid function tests; urinalysis; CT; MRI; arteriography; radionuclide scanning; ECG; sweat tests; blood tests
Digestive	Endoscopy; colonoscopy; gastroscopy; barium meal; CT; MRI; cholecystography; ultrasound; culture; biochemical analysis; liver function tests
Blood and cardio-vascular	Blood tests; clotting time measurements; biopsy; ECG; x-ray; CT; MRI; echocardiography; ultrasound; blood pressure; biopsy
Brain and nervous	EEG; hearing tests; vision tests; intelligence tests; lumbar puncture; myelography; CT; MRI; PET; evoked responses

white and softer tissues a variety of shades of grey.

X-rays cause no sensation when passed through the skin, but frequent or large doses may cause tissue damage to the skin and internal organs and even cancer. Today the risks are very small, because radiation doses are kept to an absolute minimum.

Contrast x-rays involve the use of dyes or fluids that are opaque to x-rays. These are often used to obtain pictures of the urinary tract, using a dye, or the digestive tract, using a barium meal.

CT scanning

This technique may be used to obtain images of virtually any part of the body. It combines the use of x-rays with computer technology to produce a two- or three-dimensional image of an area. These images are more detailed than straight x-rays and can also be manipulated by the computer to give a better view. CT scanning was first used in the 1970s for studying the brain.

Radionuclide scanning

In radionuclide scanning, the images are obtained by x-ray or by CT scanning, but radioactive chemicals are either swallowed by the patient, or injected into the blood stream, before the pictures are taken by a gamma camera. The image shows where metabolic activity is high or low. For example, cancer cells, where the division of cells is rapid, may show as 'hot spots'. The levels of radioactive material are very low, usually considerably lower than conventional x-rays.

MRI scanning

Magnetic resonance imaging (MRI) does not use radiation, but studies the behaviour of the protons or nuclei of hydrogen atoms when they are subjected to a very strong magnetic field and radio waves. The procedure involves the patient lying inside a large hollow cylindrical magnet in which the body is exposed to a magnetic field many thousand times more powerful than that of the Earth. A computer converts the readings into two- or three-dimensional images. As there are

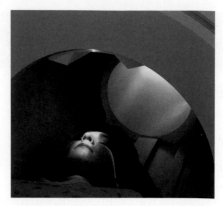

An MRI scanner

more protons in the hydrogen atoms in water molecules, an MRI scan detects the differences in the water content of the tissues.

Ultrasound scanning

This procedure does not cause any discomfort and is thought to be completely safe. A **transducer** is placed on the skin and transmits inaudible high-frequency sound waves into the body. These are reflected by the internal structures of the body and the transducer detects the echoes, converts them into numerical data and then displays them on a screen. Alternatively, they can be analysed by computer to produce an image of the structures. This technique is useful in pregnancy for measuring the size of the foetus, for detecting multiple pregnancies and also various defects that may be present, without risk either to the baby or mother.

Echocardiography

Echocardiography provides information about the heart, including the structure and flexibility of the heart valves, the condition of the heart muscle and the flow of blood within the heart.

PET scanning

As with radionuclide scanning, positron emission tomography (PET) scanning uses radioactive substances to produce an image that shows the level of metabolic activity of cells within the tissues. It is often used to investigate brain tumours, for studying brain function in various mental illnesses, and to investigate the function of the heart and other organs.

Biochemical analysis

Biochemical tests may be carried out on:

- blood
- urine
- spinal fluid
- saliva
- sweat.

Biochemical tests may also be used to assess the function of the liver or the kidneys.

Biopsy

A biopsy involves the removal of a sample of tissue, or cells, from a living patient. The sample is then examined under a microscope. This procedure is useful for investigating:

- tumours
- breast cysts
- ovarian tumours or cysts
- testicular tissue
- thyroid tissue.

Case study

Ruby

Ruby was a very healthy baby born weighing 7lb 12oz. Her parents, Jane and Robert, were delighted to have a little girl.

Around the age of 2½, Ruby complained of tummy pains and had frequent bouts of diarrhoea. She also began to lose her appetite, but craved sweet foods and chocolate. Jane remembered that earlier that year, while she was pegging out the clothes in the garden, Ruby had been standing by the side of the fish pond, holding a small spoon from her play kitchen. She may have been drinking the pond water. Jane stopped her and Ruby had no immediate after-effects.

When the bouts of diarrhoea continued, Jane went to see her GP for advice. During the history-taking by the GP, Jane recalled the incident in the garden. The GP arranged for a stool culture to be done and offered advice on diet and fluid intake, recommending that Jane reduced Ruby's milk intake and increased the amount of water she drank. The result of the stool culture proved to be negative, showing no infection or micro-organisms present. The GP advised Jane that Ruby had 'toddler diarrhoea' and this would eventually clear up.

After several weeks, Ruby's problem with loose stools became worse and the odour was foul. She was potty trained, but the urgency to reach the toilet meant that sometimes she didn't make it in time. On her next visit to the GP, Jane asked for a referral for a second opinion. Ruby was seen by a paediatric gastroenterologist. By this time, Ruby was also looking very pale and lacking in energy. She was unable to keep up with play activities at her nursery or with her friends without becoming very tired.

When Ruby was seen by the consultant gastroenterologist on the first visit to the hospital, a blood test showed that she was severely **anaemic**, with a haemoglobin of 4.5 g/dl (normal is 11 g/dl or above). Tests were done to check her blood cells, bones, liver and endocrine system.

High doses of iron were prescribed, to be taken by mouth to improve her haemoglobin levels immediately.

Jane discussed the history again with the consultant, who arranged for another stool test to test for the presence of Entamoeba Histolytica, the parasite that causes amoebiasis (amoebic dysentery). The stool specimen was sent urgently (within twenty minutes) the micro-biology laboratory. If the specimen had been left too long before testing, the parasite would have been more difficult to locate. This test showed that Ruby was harbouring the parasite. The treatment of amoebiasis is with drugs such as **metronidazole**, which kills the parasite within weeks and leads to full recovery.

Ruby's haemoglobin is now normal and she has made a full recovery, although she still attends the hospital for an annual check-up.

1 What were some of the difficulties in reaching an earlier diagnosis?

2 How did Ruby ingest the parasite?

3 Identify some of the other causes of anaemia that may have been considered?

A biopsy can provide evidence as to whether a tumour, or lump, may be malignant or **benign**. It may also help to determine the cause of disorders affecting the degeneration of the skin, liver, kidneys or muscle.

Endoscopy

Endoscopy is an investigative procedure that allows a doctor to look directly into a patient's body using an endoscope. It is currently used to investigate problems in:

- the digestive tract
- nasal sinuses
- the lungs
- the bladder
- the abdominal cavity
- joints of the musculo- skeletal system.

Some endoscopes are also fitted with a video camera, which projects an image onto a screen in the operating theatre. These developments have led to minimal invasive surgery.

Case study

Pradeep

Pradeep enjoys a busy, active lifestyle and considers himself a bit of a workaholic, often eating lunch at his desk and rushing from one meeting to another. He survives on coffee during the day, but his wife makes sure that he has plenty of leafy vegetables and fruit.

Following an exceptionally busy week at work and a hectic weekend, Pradeep felt a severe pain in the left **loin** area and he felt faint and sick. His wife immediately spoke to the GP, who promised to visit as soon as possible. In the meantime, he recommended that Pradeep should return to bed and try to sip small amounts of water.

The doctor came an hour later. After talking to Pradeep, taking the history of the onset and assessing the nature of the pain, he suggested that it may be due to a kidney stone lodged in the left ureter, resulting in renal colic. The pain is caused by the ureter contracting and trying to move the stone along its channel. The doctor explained that with rest, adequate fluid intake and a narcotic analgesic drug to ease the pain, the stone may be encouraged to pass along the ureter, into the bladder, and be expelled through the urethra.

The doctor left a form and a sterile pot for a urine sample to be sent for analysis and culture. He also arranged to call again the next day. Pradeep had a reasonable amount of sleep and the medication helped to control the pain to some extent. His wife encouraged him to drink as much as possible and to continue to rest.

The next morning, when the GP called, Pradeep continued to complain of pain and tenderness in the left loin area and the doctor thought that the stone had not passed along the ureter. Pradeep was admitted to hospital as an emergency, where an x-ray was immediately carried out to locate the position and size of the stone. A genito-urinary specialist was contacted and Pradeep was prepared for theatre. He was informed that a special x-ray would show whether there was an obstruction caused by the stone. This could also be monitored by ultrasound scanning.

The stone was found to be in the lower part of the ureter, just before the opening into the bladder. Using a **cystoscope** and a very fine tube with a crushing device, the surgeon successfully crushed and removed the stone from Pradeep's ureter. He made a good recovery from the anaesthetic and was very pleased that he did not need to have 'open surgery'.

1 What was the main symptom experienced by Pradeep?

2 If the stone had not been successfully removed via the bladder, what would have been the next step?

3 When caring for someone in extreme pain, what are the main considerations?

4 Following any surgery on the urinary tract, what should the patient be encouraged to do to prevent complications occurring?

Diagnostic tests, medical care and treatment for two service users with different needs

Produce case studies for two service users with different needs for a resource pack or guide that can be used for trainee nurses. Within the case studies:

1 Explain in detail **two** different testing or screening methods, one for each service user. Make sure you make significant connections between the monitoring procedures, tests, and the medical care and treatment.

2 Explain how the monitoring procedures, tests and medical treatment have improved the quality of life for each service user. Show how they contribute to the physiological well-being of each service user.

Remember

- Use a wide range of sources when completing these activities, keeping a bibliography or source list to support your evidence.
- Make reasoned, informed judgements and be critical when drawing conclusions.
- Use different sources of evidence.

Glossary

Abductors: muscles that move the limb away from the body

Acetylcholine: a hormone that transmits messages between nerve cells and muscle cells

Acute: of sudden onset

Adductors: muscles that move the limb towards the body

Adhesions: joining of normally unconnected body parts

Alimentary tract/canal: digestive tract

Alveoli: tiny sacs at the end of a bronchiole where gases are exchanged during respiration

Amoebae: tiny single-celled parasites

Anaemia: a condition where the level of haemoglobin in the blood is below the normal range

Anterior: front

Anuria: complete cessation of urine output

Aorta: the main artery of the body

Arterioles: the small end-branches of arteries, e.g. those that connect with capillaries

Arthritis: inflammation of a joint

Atherosclerosis: disease of the arterial walls

Atresia: congenital absence of a body opening or canal

Atrium: either the right or left upper chamber of the heart

Benign: harmless; used to describe a condition, e.g. a tumour, which is not life-threatening

Beriberi: disorder due to lack of vitamin B

Bilirubin: the main pigment found in bile

Bone marrow: a soft fatty tissue found in bone cavities

Broncho-spasm: a temporary narrowing of the airways to the lungs

Calculus (urinary): a stone in the kidneys, ureter or bladder

Campylobacter: a micro-organism that can cause colitis

Capillaries: the vessels that carry blood between the smallest arteries and the smallest veins

Cardiomyopathy: a disease of the heart muscle causing a decrease in efficiency

Chronic: describes a disorder or symptoms that have persisted for some time

Chyme: ingested fluid and stomach secretions mixed together

Cilia: brush-like filaments found on the surface of linings in the respiratory tract

Colic: a severe spasmodic pain occurring in waves of intensity

Colitis: inflammation of the colon

Congenital: present at birth

Constrictor: see Sphincter

Coronary: to do with the heart

Culture swab: a laboratory test that isolates and identifies organisms that may cause infection

Cyanosis: a bluish coloration of the skin

Cystitis: inflammation of the lining of the bladder

Cystoscope: an instrument for inspecting the inside of the bladder

Defaecation: the expulsion of faeces from the body

Degeneration: changes in cells or tissues that reduce efficiency

Degenerative: progressive impairment of both structure and function

Deoxygenated: where most of the oxygen has been removed

Depressor: a muscle that lowers a part

Diaphragm: dome-shaped muscle that separates the chest from the abdomen

Digestion: the function of breaking down food in the digestive tract

Distal: the end furthest away from the body

Dopamine: a chemical released by nerve endings found in the brain

Emulsified: to have become an emulsion – the product of mixing an oily liquid with another liquid so that it is completely dispersed and the mixture does not separate out into its original components

Endocarditis: inflammation of the lining of the heart

Endocardium: the lining of the heart

Erythropoietin: a protein that helps in the formation of bone marrow

Excretion: a discharge of waste material from the body

Expectoration: the coughing up and spitting out of sputum (phlegm)

Extensor: a muscle which opens a joint

Faeces: waste material from the digestive tract

Fibre-optics: transmission of images along thin flexible glass or plastic threads

Flexors: muscles responsible for bending a limb

Frenulum: fold from the floor of the mouth to the under surface of the tongue

Genetic: inherited

Glomeruli: filtering units in the kidney

Gonorrhoea: a common sexually transmitted disease

Haematuria: red blood cells in the urine

Haemoglobin: the oxygen carrying pigment found in red blood cells

Haemoptysis: coughing-up of blood

Hernia: protrusion of an organ or tissue through a weak area of muscle.

Homeostasis: state of equilibrium in the body to maintain balance

Hyperlipidaemia: metabolic disorder with high levels of lipids (fats) in the blood

Hypertension: high blood pressure

Hypotension: low blood pressure

Hypothalamus: small area of the brain that controls the sympathetic nervous system

Ingestion: taking in of any substance through the mouth

Inherited: traits, characteristics passed to offspring through genes

Intrinsic factor: a substance secreted by gastric cells necessary for vitamin B absorption

Irritable bowel syndrome (IBS): intermittent abdominal pain and irregular bowel habits

Labia minora: the smaller hairless inner folds of the female external genital organs

Lateral: side

Levator: a muscle which raises a part

Ligament: strong material that joins the bones together

Loin: area of the back on each side of the spine below the lowest ribs and above the pelvis

Malfunction: not functioning properly

Malignant: a term used to describe conditions that become progressively worse and result in death

Medulla: innermost part or an organ or body structure

Metabolism: the chemical processes that take place in the body

Metronidazole: an antibiotic drug

Mitral valve: a heart valve found in the left side of the heart between the atrium and the ventricle

Mucous membrane: often lines cavities that open to the outside of the body and secrete mucus

Myocardial infarction: a heart attack

Myocarditis: inflammation of the heart muscle

Myocardium: the heart muscle

Myoxoma: a benign jelly-like tumour

Nasal septum: the central partition inside the nose

Neurotransmitter: a chemical released from nerve endings that transmits impulses from one neuron to another, or to a muscle

Oesophageal atresia: a birth defect where the oesophagus is not fully developed and ends as a 'blind tube'

Oliguria: production of small quantities of urine

Ossification: the process by which bone is formed

Osteoporosis: loss of protein matrix tissue from bone, causing it to become brittle

Paget's disease: disease where the normal process of bone formation is disrupted

Paralytic ileus: a failure of the muscles of the small intestine to contract

Pericardium: the membrane around the heart

Periosteum: the membrane covering bone

Peristaltic: wave-like rhythmic contractions

Plasma: the fluid part of the blood after the cells are removed

Glossary continued

Pleura: a two-layered membrane on the outside of the lungs

Pleural cavity: the space between the two layers of the pleura

Pneumothorax: a condition when air enters the pleural cavity and may cause the lung to collapse

Posterior: back

Prognosis: the probable course and outcome of a disease

Prophylactic: procedure to prevent disease

Proximal: the end nearest to the body

Pulmonary: to do with the lungs

Pyelonephritis: inflammation of the kidney

Reflux: abnormal back-flow of fluid

Renal colic: spasms of severe pain on one side of the back, usually caused by a kidney stone

Rheumatism: any disorder that causes pain and stiffness in muscles and joints

Saliva: a watery secretion produced by the salivary glands that are in the membranes lining the mouth

Sarcoma: a cancer of connective or supportive tissue e.g. bone, cartlilage, fat, muscle, blood vessels

Secrete: release liquid-like mixture

Seminal vesicles: one of two glands that produce liquid to transmit semen during ejaculation

Septum: partition

Shigella: a bacteria that causes dysentery

Sigmoidoscopy: examination of the lower bowel and colon through a viewing instrument passed through the rectum

Spasticity: increased rigidity in a group of muscles

Sphincter: a ring of muscle around a natural opening

Sternum: breast bone

Symphysis pubis: the joint between the two pelvic bones at the lower front of the body

Synovial joints: a joint that contains synovial fluid which protects and lubricates it

Systemic: the whole body

Tendons: the fibrous cords that join muscle to bone

Transducer: a device that converts input energy of one form into output energy of another

Tricuspid valve: the heart valve between the right atrium and right ventricle

Tubules: tiny tubes to be found in the kidney

Uraemia: the presence of excess urea and other waste products in the blood as a result of kidney failure

Ureteritis: inflammation of the ureters

Ureters: the tubes that carry urine from the kidneys to the bladder

Urethra: the tube through which urine is excreted from the bladder

Urethral stricture: a narrowing of the urethra

Urethritis: inflammation of the urethra

Urography: a procedure for obtaining x-ray pictures of the urinary tract; may also be called pyelography

Venous system: the circulatory system through the veins of the body

Venules: small veins, e.g. those joining capillaries to larger veins

Ventricles: the lower two chambers of the heart

Volvulous: a twisted loop of intestine that can cause strangulation of the gut

Unit 17 Health education and promotion

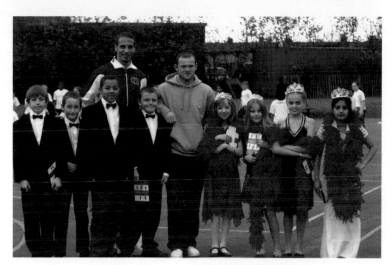

Health education brings many benefits

Health is important to everyone at every life stage, be it infancy or adolescence or later adulthood. Money cannot buy health, but lifestyle choices can affect it. Although health education campaigns can be costly, they can save the NHS billions of pounds in the long term. This is because health campaigns can empower service users by giving them information to help them decide to make life-changing choices which could improve their health and well-being.

Local health promotion teams (from the primary care trusts) base their campaigns around nationally set health events. Local teams choose their own particular targets depending on the health issues within their area. For example, from the NHS Health Events 2006 (see poster on page 251), one local area might have chosen one of the following as their prime health campaign for 2006:

- No Smoking Day in March
- Heart Week in June
- World Mental Health Day in October
- World AIDS Day in December.

Another area of the country might have chosen entirely different events from the calendar, depending upon local needs.

The Health Improvement Programmes (HImP) came about as a result of the 1997 white paper, *The New NHS – Modern and Dependable* which required that primary care trusts (PCTs) take responsibility for health issues within their own local area. These HImPs must show how the local area will help to meet national aims, priorities and targets. Once the local area has identified their health improvement priorities, they can then plan their health education campaign and decide which model or educational approach would be most suited to their target audience.

Communication methods, too, must be analysed by the health promotion team to ensure they choose the most effective method of reaching the target audience. For example, if the campaign is aimed at raising the awareness of adolescents, then the delivery method must appeal to this age group in order to have maximum impact. Boring or inappropriate methods of communication could mean the campaign is ignored from the beginning.

Evaluation methods must be planned into the health promotion campaign so that the team will know whether their health promotion event has been successful and has achieved its expected outcomes. Simple methods of evaluation could be used to see if the objectives were met.

Planning and implementing your own small-scale campaign based on local health improvement priorities will provide a challenging experience. Within the plan it will be necessary to make decisions about:

- target chosen
- reasons for your campaign
- your target group(s)

- your objectives
- the approach (model) you will use
- the communication methods you will use.

The campaign will need to be analysed to find out how successful it has been. This means that the evaluation will need to show judgements. To do this, you will need to reflect, to analyse and to consider improvements that could be made.

In this unit you will learn

Learning outcomes

You will learn to:

- describe local health improvement priorities for a health education campaign and the population group targeted.
- review the health education approaches (models) used
- analyse the main communication methods used in health education campaigns
- describe methods to evaluate health education campaigns
- plan and implement a small-scale health education campaign based on local health improvement priorities, using materials from an existing campaign
- evaluate the small-scale health education campaign.

HEALTH EVENTS 2006

The information included is correct at the time of going to press. For the latest updates, visit the events section at www.dh.gov.uk/NewsHome/EventsDiary/fs/en. Inclusion does not necessarily imply recommendation by the Department of Health

JANUARY

Jan 3 - 8 Arthritis Research Week Arthritis Research Campaign Ph: 01246 558033 Fax: 01246 558007 Email: info@arc.org.uk www.arc.org.uk

Jan 24 - 28 Food Allergy & Food Intolerance Week Allergy UK Ph: 01322 619898 Fax: 01322 663480 Email: info@allergyuk.org www.allergyuk.org

Jan 31 Bug Busting Day - Head Lice Beware! Community Hygiene Concern Ph: 020 7686 4321 Fax: 020 7686 4322 Email: bugbusters2k@yahoo.co.uk www.nits.net/bugbusting

FEBRUARY

Feb 1 - 28 Raynaud's Awareness Month Raynaud's & Scleroderma Association Helpline: 0800 917 2494 Ph: 01270 872 776 Fax: 01270 883 556 Email: info@raynauds.org.uk www.raynauds.org.uk

Feb 14 National Impotence Day Sexual Dysfunction Association Ph: 0870 774 3571 Fax: 0870 774 3572 Email: info@sda.uk.net www.sda.uk.net

Feb 13 - 19 Contraceptive Awareness Week fpa Helpline: 0845 310 1334 Ph: 020 7923 5216 Fax: 020 7837 6785 Email: caw@fpa.org.uk www.fpa.org.uk

MARCH

Mar 1 - 31 Great Daffodil Appeal Marie Curie Cancer Care Ph: 0845 601 3107 Fax: 020 7599 7700 Email: info@mariecurie.org.uk www.mariecurie.org.uk/daffodil

Mar 1 - 31 WellBeing of Women's Ovarian Cancer Awareness Campaign WellBeing of Women Ph: 020 7772 6400 Fax: 020 7724 7725 Email: wellbeingofwomen@rcog.org.uk www.wellbeingofwomen.org.uk

Mar 8 No Smoking Day No Smoking Day Ph: 0870 770 7909 Fax: 0870 770 7910 Email: mail@nosmokingday.org.uk www.nosmokingday.org.uk

Mar 8 UN Day for Women's Rights and International Peace United Nations www.un.org

Mar 13 - 19 Obesity Awareness Week TOAST (The Obesity Awareness & Solutions Trust) Helpline: 0845 045 0225 Ph: 01279 866010 Fax: 01279 866010 Email: enquiries@toast-uk.org.uk www.toast.uk.org.uk

Mar 13 - 19 Brain Injury Awareness Week Headway – The Brain Injury Association Helpline: 0808 800 2244 Ph: 0115 924 0800 Fax: 0115 958 4446 Email: enquiries@headway.org.uk www.headway.org.uk

Mar 18 - 26 CF Week Cystic Fibrosis Trust Ph: 020 8464 7211 Fax: 020 8313 0472 Email: events@cftrust.org.uk www.cftrust.org.uk

Mar 21 International Day for the Elimination of Racial Discrimination United Nations www.un.org

Mar 20 - 26 Prostate Cancer Awareness Week The Prostate Cancer Charity Helpline: 0845 300 8383 Ph: 020 8222 7622 Fax: 020 8222 7639 Email: info@prostate-cancer.org.uk www.prostate-cancer.org.uk

APRIL

Apr 7 World Health Day: Healthy Mothers and Children World Health Organisation www.who.int

Apr 16 - 22 Mental Health Action Week The Mental Health Foundation Ph: 020 7803 1100 Fax: 020 7803 1111 Email: mhf@mhf.org.uk www.mentalhealth.org.uk

Apr 17 - 23 National Depression Week Depression Alliance Infoline: 08451 23 23 20 Fax: 020 7278 6747 Email: information@depressionalliance.org www.depressionalliance.org

Apr 22 - 29 National MS Week Multiple Sclerosis Society Helpline: 0808 800 8000 Ph: 020 8438 0700 Fax: 020 8438 0701 Email: info@mssociety.org.uk www.mssociety.org.uk

Apr 23 - 29 Parkinson's Awareness Week Parkinson's Disease Society Helpline: 0808 800 0303 Ph: 020 7963 9370 Fax 020 7630 8745 Email: pr@parkinsons.org.uk www.parkinsons.org.uk

MAY

May 2 World Asthma Day Asthma UK Helpline: 08457 01 02 03 Ph: 020 7786 4900 Fax: 020 7256 6075 Email: info@asthma.org.uk www.asthma.org.uk

May 7 - 13 Dystonia Awareness Week The Dystonia Society Helpline: 08450 95 65 75 Ph: 020 7490 5671 Fax: 020 7490 5672 Email: info@dystonia.org.uk www.dystonia.org.uk

May 8 - 15 Baby Safety Week Foundation for the Study of Infant Deaths Helpline: 0870 787 0554 Ph: 0870 787 0885 Fax: 0870 787 0725 Email: info@sids.org.uk www.sids.org.uk/fsid/

May 14 - 20 National Breastfeeding Awareness Week Department of Health Ph: 020 7972 1339 Fax: 020 7972 4877 www.breastfeeding.gov.uk

May 14 - 20 National Epilepsy Week National Society for Epilepsy Helpline: 01494 601 400 Ph: 01494 601 300 Fax: 01494 871 927 Email: margaret.thomas@epilepsynse.org.uk www.epilepsynse.org.uk
National Epilepsy Week Epilepsy Action Helpline: 0808 800 5050 Ph: 0113 210 8800 Fax: 0113 391 0300 Email: epilepsy@epilepsy.org.uk www.epilepsy.org.uk

May 14 - 20 National Smile Week British Dental Health Foundation Helpline: 0845 063 1188 Ph: 0870 770 4000 Fax: 0870 770 4010 Email: mail@dentalhealth.org.uk www.dentalhealth.org.uk

May 15 - 19 National Allergy Week Allergy UK Ph: 01322 619898 Fax: 01322 663480 Email: info@allergyuk.org www.allergyuk.org

May 22 - 28 Cancer Prevention Week (incorporating Fruity Friday May 26) World Cancer Research Fund (WCRF UK) Helpline: 020 7343 4205 Ph: 020 7343 4200 Fax: 020 7343 4201 Email: l.brown@wcrf.org www.fruityfriday.org

May 22 - 26 Walk to School Week Living Streets Ph: 020 7820 1010 Fax: 020 7820 8208 Email: jo@livingstreets.org.uk www.walktoschool.org.uk

May 22 - 28 National Hypnotherapy Awareness Week London College of Clinical Hypnosis Helpline: 0800 389 4453 Fax: 020 7486 1123 Email: info@hypnotherapyawareness.co.uk www.hypnotherapyawareness.co.uk

May 31 World No Tobacco Day World Health Organisation www.euro.who.int/tobaccofree

JUNE

Jun 1 - 30 Everyman Male Cancer Awareness Month Institute of Cancer Research Infoline: 0800 731 9468 Fax: 020 7153 5313 Email: everyman@icr.ac.uk www.icr.ac.uk/everyman

Jun 1 - 30 National Osteoporosis Month National Osteoporosis Society Helpline: 0845 450 0230 Ph: 01761 471 771 Fax: 01761 471 104 Email: info@nos.org.uk www.nos.org.uk

Jun 3 - 11 Heart Week British Heart Foundation Infoline: 0845 070 8070 Ph: 020 7487 9485 Fax: 020 7486 3815 Email: heartweek@bhf.org.uk www.bhf.org.uk

Jun 5 World Environment Day United Nations www.un.org

Jun 5 - 10 Tampon Alert Week (incorporating National Tampon Alert Day on June 8) Tampon Alert Ph/Fax: 0161 748 3123 Email: enquiries@tamponalert.org.uk www.tamponalert.org.uk

Jun 5 - 11 Down's Syndrome Awareness Week Down's Syndrome Association Helpline: 0845 230 0372 Fax: 0845 230 0373 Email: info@downs-syndrome.org.uk www.downs-syndrome.org.uk

Jun 5 - 12 Glaucoma Awareness Week International Glaucoma Association Helpline: 0870 609 1870 Ph: 0870 609 1871 Fax: 01233 648179 Email: info@iga.org.uk www.glaucoma-association.com

Jun 11 - 17 Diabetes Week Diabetes UK Helpline: 0845 120 2960 Ph: 020 7424 1000 Fax: 020 7424 1001 Email: info@diabetes.org.uk www.diabetes.org.uk

Jun 12 - 18 National Food Safety Week Food and Drink Federation Ph: 020 7836 2460 Fax: 020 7379 0481 Email: foodlink@fdf.org.uk www.foodlink.org.uk

Jun 12 - 18 National Men's Health Week Men's Health Forum Ph: 020 7388 4449 Fax: 020 7388 4477 Email: mhw@menshealthforum.org.uk www.menshealthforum.org.uk

Jun 14 - 21 Homeopathy Awareness Week The Society of Homeopaths Ph: 0845 450 6611 Fax: 0845 450 6622 Email: info@homeopathy-soh.org www.homeopathy-soh.org

Jun 15 Bug Busting Day – Head Lice Beware Community Hygiene Concern Ph: 020 7686 4321 Fax: 020 7686 4322 Email: bugbusters2k@yahoo.co.uk www.nits.net/bugbusting

Jun 17 - 25 Bike Week (including Bike2Work) Bike Week Helpline: 0845 612 0661 Ph: 01243 527 444 Fax: 0845 612 0662 Email: hq@bikeweek.org.uk www.bikeweek.org.uk

Jun 17 - 25 MND Week Motor Neurone Disease Association Helpline: 0845 762 6262 Ph: 01604 250 505 Fax: 01604 624 726 Email: enquiries@mndassociation.org www.mndassociation.org

Jun 18 - 25 Learning Disability Week Mencap Helpline: 0808 808 1111 Ph: 020 7696 5524 Fax: 020 7454 9193 Email: press.office@mencap.org.uk www.mencap.org.uk

Jun 19 - 25 Child Safety Week Child Accident Prevention Trust Ph: 020 7608 3828 Fax: 020 7608 3674 Email: csw@capt.org.uk www.capt.org.uk

Jun 26 International Day Against Drug Abuse and Illicit Trafficking United Nations www.un.org

Jun 26 - Jul 2 National Deafblind Awareness Week Deafblind UK Helpline: 0800 132 320 Ph: 01733 358 100 Fax: 01733 358 356 Email: info@deafblind.org.uk www.deafblind.org.uk

JULY

Jul 2 - 8 Alzheimer's Awareness Week Alzheimer's Society Helpline: 0845 300 0336 Ph: 020 7306 0606 Fax: 020 7306 0808 Email: info@alzheimers.org.uk www.alzheimers.org.uk

Jul 2 - 8 Metabolic Disease Awareness Week CLIMB The National Information and Advice Centre for Metabolic Disease Helpline: 0800 652 3181 Ph: 0870 77 00 325 Fax: 0870 77 00 327 Email: info@climb.org.uk www.climb.org.uk

Jul 3 - 8 Twins, Triplets & More Week Twins & Multiple Birth Association (TAMBA) Ph: 0870 77 03 305 Fax: 0870 77 03 303 Email: enquiries@tamba.org.uk www.tamba.org.uk

Jul 9 - 15 National Transplant Week Transplants In Mind Ph/Fax: 0117 931 4638 Email: sue@transplantsinmind.fsnet.co.uk www.transplantsinmind.co.uk

AUG

Aug 7 - 13 Sexual Health Week fpa Helpline: 0845 310 1334 Ph: 020 7923 5216 Fax: 020 7837 6785 Email: shw@fpa.org.uk www.fpa.org.uk

SEPTEMBER

Sep 3 - 8 Hughes Syndrome Awareness Week Hughes Syndrome Foundation Ph: 020 7188 8217 Fax: 020 7633 0462 Email: hsf@btconnect.com www.hughes-syndrome.org

Sep 3 - 9 Migraine Awareness Week Migraine Action Association Ph: 01536 461 333 Fax: 01536 461 444 Email: info@migraine.org.uk www.migraine.org.uk

Sep 4 - 10 National Pregnancy Week Tommy's, The Baby Charity Helpline: 08707 77 30 60 Ph: 08707 70 70 70 Fax: 08707 70 70 75 Email: mailbox@tommys.org www.tommys.org

Sep 11 - 17 Continence Awareness Week Continence Foundation Helpline: 0845 345 0165 Ph: 020 7404 6875 Fax: 020 7404 6876 Email: aware@continence-foundation.org.uk www.continence-foundation.org.uk

Sep 16 - 23 Children's Hospice Week Association for Children's Hospices Ph: 0845 203 2233 Fax: 0117 905 5340 Email: info@childhospice.org.uk www.childhospice.org.uk

Sep 16 - 23 National Eczema Week National Eczema Society Helpline: 0870 241 3604 Ph: 020 7281 3553 Fax: 020 7281 6395 Email: helpline@eczema.org www.eczema.org

Sep 21 World Alzheimer's Day Alzheimer's Disease International Ph: 020 7981 0880 Fax: 020 7928 2357 Email: info@alz.co.uk www.alz.co.uk

OCTOBER

Oct 1 International Day of Older Persons United Nations www.un.org

Oct 1 - 31 Breast Cancer Awareness Month Breast Cancer Care Helpline: 0808 800 6000 Ph: 020 7384 2984 Fax: 020 7384 3387 Email: info@breastcancercare.org.uk www.breastcancercare.org.uk
Breast Cancer Awareness Month Breakthrough Breast Cancer Ph: 020 7025 2400 Fax: 020 7025 2401 Email: info@breakthrough.org.uk www.breakthrough.org.uk

Oct 1 - 31 Lupus Awareness Month Lupus UK Ph: 01708 731251 Fax: 01708 731252 Email: headoffice@lupusuk.org.uk www.lupusuk.org.uk

Oct 2 - 6 Walk to School Week Living Streets Ph: 020 7820 1010 Fax: 020 7820 8208 Email: jo@livingstreets.org.uk www.livingstreets.org.uk

Oct 10 World Mental Health Day World Federation for Mental Health www.wmhday.net

Oct 20 World Osteoporosis Day The National Osteoporosis Society Helpline: 0845 450 0230 Ph: 01761 471771 Fax: 01761 471104 Email: info@nos.org.uk www.nos.org.uk

Oct 31 Bug Busting Day – Head Lice Beware Community Hygiene Concern Ph: 020 7686 4321 Fax: 020 7686 4322 Email: bugbusters2k@yahoo.co.uk www.nits.net/bugbusting

NOV

Nov 6 - 12 Scleroderma Awareness Week Raynaud's & Scleroderma Association Helpline: 0800 917 2494 Ph: 01270 872776 Fax: 01270 883556 Email: info@scleroderma.org.uk www.scleroderma.org.uk

Nov 12 - 18 Mouth Cancer Awareness Week British Dental Health Foundation Helpline: 0845 063 1188 Ph: 0870 770 4000 Fax: 0870 770 4010 Email: mail@dentalhealth.org.uk www.dentalhealth.org.uk

Nov 14 - 18 Indoor Allergy Week Allergy UK Ph: 01322 619898 Fax: 01322 663480 Email: info@allergyuk.org www.allergyuk.org

DEC

Dec 1 World AIDS Day National AIDS Trust Ph: 020 7814 6767 Fax: 020 7216 0111 Email: info@nat.org.uk www.worldAIDSday.org

Dec 3 International Day of Disabled Persons United Nations www.un.org

Dec 10 Human Rights Day United Nations www.un.org

Produced by COI for the Department of Health
Available online only at www.dh.gov.uk

© Crown copyright 2005 Last updated October 2005

NHS

Source: Department of Health website: www.dh.gov.uk. Crown copyright material is reproduced with permission of the Controller of HMSO.

NHS Health Events 2006

Origins of the campaign

In 1992 the Conservative government published a white paper *The Health of the Nation*. This document is important as it represented the first attempt by the government to provide a targeted approach to improving the overall health of the population. From 1992 to 1997 *The Health of the Nation* was the basis of health policy in England and was used in the planning of NHS services.

Our Healthier Nation

As a result of this initiative, in 1997 the Labour government published *Saving Lives: Our Healthier Nation*. This white paper was basically an action plan to:

- improve the health of everyone
- improve the health of the worst-off especially.

The government targeted the main killers listed in the diagram at the bottom of this page.

Theory into practice

Look up the main causes of death at the beginning of the twentieth century. Compared with the main causes of death at the beginning of the twenty-first century, what differences do you notice? Give reasons for your answer.

The table opposite indicates the areas that were targeted by the government and what they hoped to achieve.

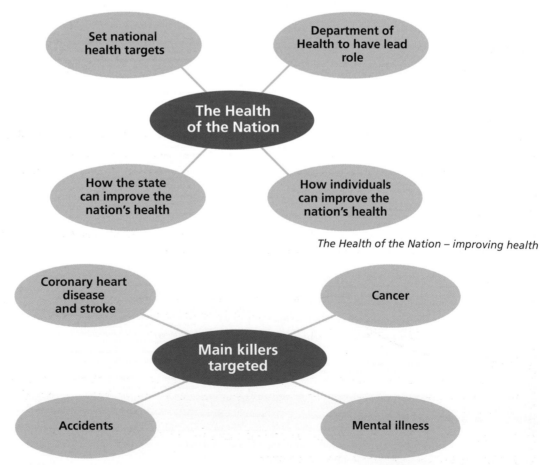

The Health of the Nation – improving health

Government-targeted main killers

| Main killer of under-75s | Government targets to be achieved by 2010 | |
	Reduce death rate by	Number of lives to be saved
Cancer	20%	100,000
Coronary heart disease and stroke	40%	200,000
Accidents	20% (serious surgery at least 10%)	12,000
Mental health	20%	4,000

In order to achieve better health for everyone, and especially for the worst-off, the government decided to:

- give an extra £21 billion to the NHS to help secure a healthier population
- tackle smoking as the biggest preventable cause of ill health
- integrate national and local government, working to improve health
- stress health improvement as a key role for the NHS
- press for high health standards for everyone.

Saving Lives: Our Healthier Nation stated quite clearly that, in order to improve health, a partnership was needed between:

- people
- communities
- government.

People
People could improve their own health through:

- physical activity
- better diet
- giving up smoking.

Activity

Improving health

Alan
Alan is a 20-year-old full-time student. He attends lectures three times a week. For the rest of the week he gets up at midday. He usually eats the leftovers from the previous night's take-away for breakfast. He doesn't bother with any more food until he is on his way back from the pub when he picks up another take-away.

Jacinta
Jacinta is a 35-year-old single woman. She watches her diet very carefully. She allows herself one small meal each day, usually in the evening. She runs five miles every day.

Molly
Molly is overweight and does very little exercise. She feels she eats very little so she cannot understand how her weight keeps going up. She has tried lots of different diets, but soon loses interest as the weight comes off too slowly and she feels hungry all the time.

Makis
Makis does a lot of exercise at the gym. He feels fit and is careful about his diet. He drinks little alcohol. He has a very stressful job where he feels under constant pressure. He spends three nights a week in a smoky gambling club.

1 What advice would you give each individual in the case studies regarding their health?

2 What type of campaign might help each one?

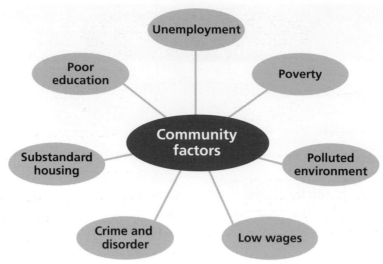

Community factors affecting health

Health promotion would be particularly important as people would need to be properly informed about risks if they were to make decisions.

Communities

It was also decided that communities could tackle poor health. This was to be through community factors that affected the areas in which people lived (see the diagram above).

(see the diagram above)

Theory into practice

Choose one of the community factors affecting health from the diagram above. Research why your chosen factor can contribute to poor health. Discuss your findings with the group.

Government

Health **inequality** is widespread, with the most disadvantaged people likely to be suffering most from poor health. The government decided it could address this inequality with a series of initiatives on education, welfare-to-work, housing, neighbourhoods, transport and environment which would improve health.

Other important health issues which would be tackled include:

- sexual health
- drugs
- alcohol
- food safety
- water fluoridation
- communicable diseases.

Theory into practice

Explore one of the health issues which the government intended to tackle. Produce a colourful, informative poster on your chosen issue which could be displayed to provide information for the rest of your group.

Saving Lives: Our Healthier Nation sought to **integrate** health improvement into local delivery of health care. Local authorities would work in partnership with the NHS to plan improvements.

Health Action Zones

As a result of the white paper, Health Action Zones (HAZ) were created in March 1998 to target areas of disadvantage in the community. This recognised the effect of social deprivation on health and the need to tackle the root causes of ill health.

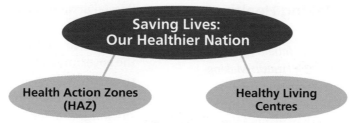

Saving Lives:
Our Healthier Nation

Health Action Zones
(HAZ)

Healthy Living
Centres

Initiatives created as a result of Saving Lives: Our Healthier Nation

As the Health Action Zone website states:

'The purpose of a Health Action Zone (HAZ) is to act as a catalyst to bring together in a working partnership all those contributing to the health of their local population – including health organisations, District Councils, other statutory organisations, the voluntary community and private sectors – to implement locally agreed strategies for improving health.'

Healthy Living Centres

Healthy Living Centres is another initiative resulting from *Saving Lives: Our Healthier Nation*. This programme aims to educate and support people on all aspects of keeping healthy. Healthy Living Centres ensure people have the knowledge and expertise they need. Having the best information available helps people to make informed decisions about their health and their lifestyle. They therefore have a better understanding of risks involved in their lifestyle choices, for example the consequences of drinking too much alcohol. Healthy Living Centres help people struggling with health problems which may not need medical treatment, for instance obesity, which could be helped by giving dietary advice. Health screening facilities are also available.

Healthy Living Centres aim to reach across the different age groups within a community from the very young to the older service user. For example, a parent of a young child would be offered support, advice and courses if required. Courses could include first aid, budgeting or keeping fit. Older service users might benefit from the social and leisure activities as well as being able to attend workshops on topics such as ICT.

Healthy Living Centres involve groups working together from voluntary and statutory organisations. They are **holistic** services offered to the community, as shown in the diagram below.

Healthy Living Centres aim to fulfil the World Health Organisation's (WHO) definition of health: 'The extent to which an individual or group is able, on one hand, to realise **aspirations** and satisfy needs and, on the other hand, to change or cope with the environment. Health is therefore seen as a resource for everyday life, not the objective of living: it is a positive concept emphasising social and personal resources as well as physical capabilities.'

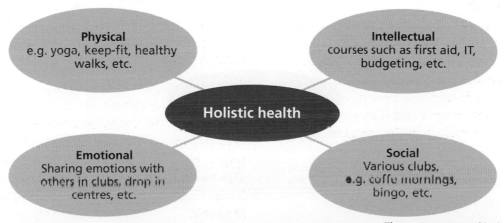

Physical
e.g. yoga, keep-fit, healthy walks, etc.

Intellectual
courses such as first aid, IT, budgeting, etc.

Holistic health

Emotional
Sharing emotions with others in clubs, drop in centres, etc.

Social
Various clubs, e.g. coffee mornings, bingo, etc.

The components of holistic health

Choosing Health: Making Healthy Choices Easier

As a follow-up to *Our Healthier Nation*, the government published *Choosing Health: Making Choices Easier* in November 2004. For the first time, it was the people of Britain who set the agenda and identified when they wanted the government to intervene and when they did not. This paper re-emphasised the benefits of agencies working together to improve public health. It also reiterated the government's role in tackling social inequality. It established three core principles of a new public health approach which would underpin the whole of the new strategy, as shown in the diagram below.

- *Informed choice*: it was stressed that people needed and wanted to make their own decisions, but needed reliable and trustworthy information to enable them to make the right choices. This principle was subject to two qualifications:
  - Special responsibility needs to be exercised for children who are too young to make their own informed choices. For example, parents have to make the decision about whether to have their child immunised against diseases such as polio, tetanus and whooping cough. Considering all the **adverse** publicity against the MMR vaccine, would you still advise parents to have their child immunised using this vaccine?
  - Special arrangements are needed where one person's choice may cause harm or nuisance to another, such as smoking. Does the government ban smoking in restaurants, bars and clubs so that non-smokers are not harmed by passive smoking? If it does, does this go far enough or should smoking be banned in *all* public places?
- *Personalisation*: to be effective in tackling health inequalities, the support has to be tailored to the individual, with services and support provided flexibly and conveniently.
- *Working together*: there must be a partnership across communities which should include local government, the NHS, businesses, advertisers, retailers, the voluntary sector, communities, the media, faith organisations and others.

The main priorities of *Choosing Health: Making Healthy Choices Easier* were to:

- reduce the number of people who smoke
- reduce obesity and improving diet and nutrition
- encourage and supporting sensible drinking
- increase exercise
- improve sexual health
- improve mental health.

A number of areas for action came out of *Choosing Health*, as shown in the diagram opposite.

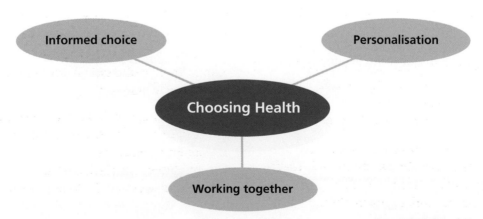

Core principles of Choosing Health

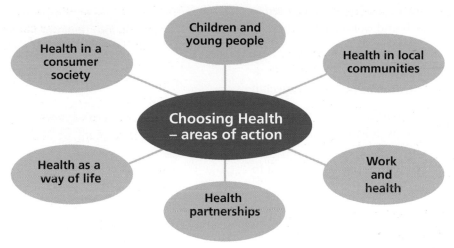

Areas for action as a result of Choosing Health

The Governance Framework for health and social care

The Governance Framework is part of the modernisation process of the NHS as laid down by the Department of Health in the first edition published in 2001. This was updated in April 2005.

The introduction of **clinical governance** in 1998 was designed to introduce a systematic approach to the delivery of high quality health care. Clinical governance is the system through which NHS organisations are accountable for continuously improving the quality of their services and safeguarding high standards of care, by creating an environment in which clinical excellence will flourish.

Clinical excellence comes under the guidance of the National Institute for Clinical Excellence (NICE). NICE is the independent organisation responsible for providing national guidance on the promotion of good health and the prevention and treatment of ill health. On 1 April 2005 NICE joined with the Health Development Agency to become the new National Institute for Health and Clinical Excellence, still to be known as NICE.

Health and social care research and governance in the Department of Health

The Department of Health needed a research and governance framework to ensure that:

- policy for health care and social care is based on reliable evidence of needs and of what works best to meet those needs
- improved interventions are developed to promote health, treat ill health and provide social care
- information is available to those responsible for health and social care services on what works and what does not, and on proven ways of improving quality, access and efficiency.

Health Improvement Programmes (HImP)

Health Improvement Programmes (HImP) consist of a local plan of action which will improve health and modernise services. The first HImP began in 1999–2000 as a result of the 1997 white paper, *The New NHS – Modern Dependable*.

HImPs embody the government's aim of building high-quality public services. They set out to bring together a local team from the NHS with local authorities and others from the voluntary sector. Jointly they would set:

- targets to improve health, tackle inequalities and develop more efficient services
- high-level objectives
- commitments of the local team
- measurable targets for improvement

- guidelines for how resources are to be used to improve the health and well-being of the population
- guidelines to modernise the NHS.

All those interested would be involved, especially:

- primary care groups in the planning process, to ensure the HImP is guided by needs of the local community
- hospital clinicians who could say how best to meet local needs
- the local community and its leaders who would have the opportunity to influence strategy.

HImPs would describe how local actions would help to meet national targets. Action plans were produced which would identify targets and describe what needed to be done to meet them locally. The funding, too, needed to be addressed.

HImPs are now called Health Improvement and Modernisation Plans (HIMPs) to reflect their importance in bringing together planning for health improvement, including health inequalities, with the NHS modernisation agenda.

How a local health promotion campaign is initiated

The diagram top right shows the origins of a local campaign in a simplified way.

The government produces a white paper which highlights areas of concern. The Department of Health (DoH) then produces its Health Events calendar for the year ahead. The events listed here will reflect the current white paper.

For example, the calendar for 2005 showed that people who smoke were addressed specially on:

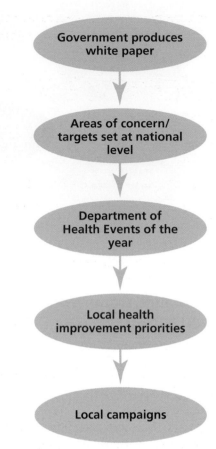

How local health promotion campaigns are initiated

- 9 March – No Smoking Day
- 31 May – World No Tobacco Day.

Similarly, mental health was addressed on:

- 27 Mar–2 April – Mental Health Action Week
- 18–24 April – National Depression Week
- 21 April–8 May – Samaritan Week
- 10 October – World Mental Health Day.

If you remember, reducing the number of people who smoke and improving mental health were two of the main priorities of the white paper, *Choosing Health*.

From the DoH's Health Events, local health promotion groups will choose campaigns which are especially relevant to their own area. Their campaign must impact on the needs of the service users within their area. As stated earlier, if smoking is a problem in the local area then one of the features for that year would be 'No Smoking' and 'No Tobacco Day'. Using the same day as the national event makes sense as then events can be co-ordinated and money can be saved as the national event will generate health promotion materials which will be free of charge to the local health promotion units.

Activity

Health Events calendar

1 Contact your local health promotion unit and find out their calendar of events for the year.

2 Look at the Department of Health's website for the Health Events calendar for this year (see p282).

3 Which local events match the national promotions? Research the reasons for this.

Reasons for health education campaigns

There are many reasons for health campaigns. One key reason is to promote up-to-date information regarding health messages to as wide an audience as possible. Health campaigns also raise the profile of health issues and empower service users by allowing them to bring about a change in their behaviour as a result of informed choice.

The other key reasons for health education campaigns are to:

> ## Consider this
>
> *Think of a recent health campaign. What were the key reasons for this campaign?*

- improve health and well-being
- encourage the use of preventative methods
- increase skills to enable people to take control of their lives

- aid understanding of environmental causes of ill health.

Improving health and well-being

A service user may not know how many units of alcohol they are consuming each week or indeed what the current safe number of units is. Once alerted to the safe level the service user could then moderate their alcohol consumption which could lead to improved health and well-being.

Activity

Alcohol units

For this activity, you will need informaton about the units of alcohol contained in various drinks.

1 Do students in your centre know about units of alcohol? Prepare a questionnaire about the number of units of alcohol in a cross-section of alcoholic drinks.

2 Interview 100 students (from 14 years old upwards) and collate the results. Are there any unexpected results?

3 Repeat the exercise outside a local busy shopping centre (having first contacted the management to seek permission). Collate the information.

4 Compare the results with your earlier survey at your school/college. What conclusions can you draw?

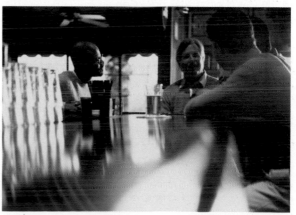

How many units?

Encouraging the use of preventative methods

A condom, while primarily used to prevent pregnancy during sexual intercourse, could also prevent Chlamydia or another sexually-transmitted infection. Some adolescents think that the contraceptive pill will protect them from a sexually-transmitted infection. It will not – it will prevent pregnancy, but will not prevent infection.

> ### Consider this
>
> *Did you know Chlamydia is the commonest sexually-transmitted infection in the UK, with 103,763 diagnoses in clinics in 2004? The highest rate is seen in young men and women under 24 years of age. Why do you think this is so?*
>
> *Use the Health Protection Agency website to find out about Chlamydia (see p282).*

Increasing skills to enable people to take control of their lives

If people understand the risks of smoking it can help them to say 'No' to a cigarette, especially if they are supported by a smoking cessation programme. This will let them have control, rather than the cigarette.

To aid understanding of environmental causes of ill-health

A service user could be helped to understand that the unsuitable housing they are living in is causing the new baby's chest infection. This could empower the service user when they realise that it is not their actions that have affected the baby, but rather, the environment.

Other reasons for health education campaigns are to:

- encourage people to change their behaviour
- prevent the development of disease
- address social issues such as housing, poverty, etc.
- try to change policies so that people are helped to make healthy choices.

Activity

Alex

Alex is a successful stockbroker who takes care of his health. He watches his weight and eats carefully. He has lots of business lunches and dinners but he always eats plain food with plenty of vegetables. He never has desserts. However, his partner is worried about him as she feels he drinks too much without realising it. This is what Alex drinks on an average weekday:

- lunch – 1 gin and tonic, 2 large glasses of wine
- dinner – 1 gin and tonic, 2–3 large glasses of wine, 1 brandy.

At weekends, Alex and his partner drink one bottle of wine between them on Saturday evening and the same again on Sunday evening,

1 Is Alex's partner right to be worried about his alcohol intake?

2 How many units of alcohol does Alex consume over the course of one week? How might this affect his health?

3 Suggest ways for Alex to cut down on his alcohol intake.

Target audiences

Most people can benefit from health promotion materials even if they learn just one new fact. Some people are targeted, such as those who are at risk from:

- *disease*, e.g. women over 50 who should have breast screening. This could be because post-menopause women are more likely to develop breast cancer
- *early death*, e.g. people who have parents who died from coronary heart disease (CHD) before the age of 50. This is because research shows that heart disease can be hereditary. Whether this is because a person inherits the same

genetic make-up or merely adopts a similar lifestyle to the parent is at present not proven

- *their lifestyle*, e.g. smokers. This is because smoking is the biggest cause of premature death. Smoking is a key factor in deaths from coronary heart disease and cancer
- *their environment*, e.g. people living in substandard accommodation. This could be because: too many people are living in a certain amount of space; hygiene facilities are poor and, therefore, people do not care for themselves properly; cooking facilities are broken or limited so that ready-prepared foods are the main dietary sources.

Activity

If the following people were targeted in a campaign, how could they be persuaded to change their way of thinking?

1 Doria is a sexually active 62-year-old who has never been for breast screening despite numerous reminders. She feels it would be far too embarrassing.

2 George, aged 47, is a long-distance lorry driver. He is overweight and does little exercise. His father died from coronary heart disease (CHD) at 53 years of age. George is far too scared to go to his GP in case he has high blood pressure or his cholesterol level is too high.

3 Dan is a 38 year-old heavy smoker who says, 'You have to die from something; it might as well be cigarettes.'

Assessment activity 17.1

A local health education campaign

1 Contact your local Health Promotion Team to find out what their local health improvement priorities are.

2 How does their choice of health promotion campaigns match their health improvement targets?

3 Who is the main target audience and why?

4 In light of the information you have collected from your local team, choose **one** of their health promotion campaigns. Write a comprehensive account of the origins of this chosen campaign and the reasons for it.

5 Write about their main target audience, showing a high level of understanding of why they have targeted this group.

There are three different approaches to health promotion:

- **health education**, which includes formal health education programmes and campaigns as well as health advice and information given to service users by health practitioners, such as health visitors, community nurses, etc.
- **prevention**, which is anything associated with preventing illness and includes preventative medical services, such as immunisation and screening
- **health protection**, which is when the government works with other agencies to make sure public health is looked after and protected. Legislation could be passed to look after physical and social environments. Safe working conditions and public health measures fit into this category.

These approaches to health promotion are summarised in the table below.

Traditional health education aims to change people's behaviour and encourages them to adopt a healthier lifestyle.

Health education programmes can be divided into three different areas:

- *Primary health education* is aimed at healthy people to prevent them suffering from ill health. Targets are children and young people with topics ranging from hygiene to nutrition to contraception. Quality of health is improved by primary health education, which in turn leads to improvement in quality of life.
- *Secondary health education* is aimed at people with health problems to try to stop their ill health becoming worse and advancing to the next stage. They may have to make a change to their lifestyle in order to regain good health, e.g. they may have to eat a healthier diet or stop smoking.
- *Tertiary health education* is about educating service users, who already have a serious health problem, on how to make the most of their remaining potential for healthy living. An example of this could be a person who is suffering from cancer is helped to control pain and is taught to manage their symptoms. It allows people to lead as 'normal' a life as possible.

In the delivery of health education, there are five main approaches or models:

- the preventative model
- the empowerment model
- the educational approach
- the use of fear as an approach
- the medical model.

These are the most common approaches to health promotion but there are more. No one model is the correct way; they are all useful in their own right. The approach used will depend on several different factors, for example, the service users targeted by the health campaign or

1	Preventative measures	e.g. immunisation, breast screening, cervical screening, screening for hypertension
2	Preventative health education	e.g. aims to discourage misuse of alcohol; could be in a school's health education programme
3	Preventative health protection	e.g. fluoridation of water supplies
4	Health education for preventative health protection	e.g. providing education to support (3)
5	Positive health education	e.g. promotion of low-alcohol drinks
6	Positive health protection	e.g. government legislation, for example banning sale of alcohol to under-18s
7	Health education for positive health protection	e.g. lobbying to ensure alcohol is not sold to under-18s

the experience or personal perspectives of the promoter.

The preventative model

This model is also known as the behaviour change, behaviourist or persuasive model. This model aims to change people's attitudes and behaviour so that they will then follow a healthy lifestyle. People will be encouraged to follow a healthy eating plan, give up smoking, take more exercise, drink less alcohol and generally look after themselves following 'healthy' guidelines. Health promoters using this approach will genuinely believe that a healthy lifestyle is in the best interests of the service user and will feel it is part of their duty to encourage people to adopt the healthy lifestyle they are promoting. This is probably the most commonly used method.

The empowerment model

This model is also known as the client-directed approach. The aim of this model is to inform the service user by giving them the information they require. This will then enable them to make their own well-informed decisions independently.

The health practitioners following this model will act as guides, helping service users to identify their concerns and to gain the skills and knowledge they need to bring about change. Self-empowerment is crucial to this aim. Service users are seen as equals who have the right to be in charge of their own lives and therefore their health decisions.

The educational approach

Also known as the informative approach, this model will give service users information and make sure they understand it, and the health issues involved. Service users are encouraged to look at their own decisions.

Health promoters using this method will respect service users' rights to choose their own health behaviour, but will see it is their responsibility to raise any health issues they think will best suit the service users' interests.

Theory into practice

Ossie is a 26-year-old who lives a promiscuous lifestyle. He is unsure if he is heterosexual or homosexual so at present he is bisexual. He does not have a regular partner as he can usually 'get lucky' and pull a new partner when he goes clubbing at least three times each week. He has been treated for a STI but feels this is just bad luck. He thinks that as he is young he deserves to take any opportunity that life gives him.

Discuss which health education approaches or models would be best suited to Ossie. Give reasons for your choices.

The use of fear as an approach

The aim of this approach is to frighten people into choosing a healthier lifestyle. It is possible that a hard-hitting anti-smoking campaign is too frightening for some people and they may, for example, switch off the television to avoid listening to, or acknowledging, a featured interview with a real service user suffering from terminal lung cancer.

Health promoters using this method will explain in graphic detail the unpleasant effects of an unhealthy lifestyle, as in the sort of campaign mentioned above, which was shown at peak viewing time on television. In this campaign, the person was dying from cancer and was genuinely not going to get better.

Consider this

Does fear work? Have you ever been frightened into choosing a healthier lifestyle? Did the posters showing Leah Betts in intensive care with the caption, 'Sorted. Just one Ecstasy tablet killed Leah Betts', affect teenagers? Do you think that this campaign had the desired effect and frightened Ecstasy users? Or did it confuse young people by trying to scare them rather than explain the dangers and how to avoid them?

The medical model

Also known as the interventionist model, this approach aims to ensure the service user is free from medically-defined disease. The approach involves medical staff, such as a nurse or a doctor, persuading a service user to make use of preventative medicine, e.g. encouraging women over 50 to take advantage of breast screening services.

Relevant health promoters would usually be medically trained as this model relies on using medical intervention to prevent ill health.

Activity

1 Which health promotion model would make the biggest impact on you?

2 Why do you think this is?

3 Can you think of the health campaign which has had the most effect on you? Which model did this use?

4 Is this consistent with your first answer?

Case study

Examine the following scenarios and decide which health education model has been used in each one.

1 A tutor shows her group a DVD/video about a teenager who buys an Ecstasy tablet at a rave and dies as a consequence of taking it.

2 When Mrs A goes to the nurse to have her blood pressure measured she is encouraged to lose weight and increase her amount of daily exercise.

3 Julie is advised by her doctor to have regular smear tests.

4 Mr F asks for advice to help him to stop smoking and the practice nurse spends time explaining his options. She gives him some leaflets after discussing the contents with him.

The table below summarises the commonly used health promotion approaches.

Approach	Aim	Example
Preventative or behavioural change, behaviourist or persuasive	To persuade service user to adopt a healthier lifestyle to change their existing attitude to health	Behaviour change by service user from drinking a lot of alcohol to drinking little or none. Trying to discourage non-drinkers from starting. Discourage drinking to excess
Client-directed approach or empowerment or client-centred	Explore health services as defined by service user	Service user is advised to give up smoking to enjoy healthier lifestyle but they decide to cut down on alcohol intake instead. Service user is empowered by making the decision and choosing the issue, whilst being supported by the health promoter
Educational or informative	To provide service user with relevant information, allowing them to make an informed decision	Service user is given information about the effect of alcohol on their health. They have to decide how much alcohol they may safely drink
Use of fear	To scare or frighten people into choosing a healthier lifestyle	Using television as medium to show accidents caused by drinking and driving, e.g. killing a child because of being over the alcohol limit
Medical or interventionalist	To make service user free from medically defined disease, e.g. cirrhosis of the liver	Freedom from, e.g. heart disease, stomach cancer or cirrhosis of the liver, by seeking medical intervention early on

Review the health education approaches

1 Giving a comprehensive account, review the health education model used in the health promotion campaign you chose in Assessment activity 17.1.

2 What other model or approach could have been used?

3 Critically compare the model used with a different model which could have been used for the chosen campaign.

Methods of communication used

Health promotion campaigns need to use communication methods to get the message across. Different campaigns use different methods. The main methods, shown in the diagram below, are:

- mass media techniques
- peer group education.

Effectiveness of the main communication methods used in health education campaigns

Mass media

Reaching target audience

Mass media techniques can reach large numbers of people. For example, television, radio, newspapers and magazines can reach a much larger audience than a whiteboard or poster could.

At first glance you could be forgiven for thinking that the mass media techniques would be the most effective method of transmitting health promotion materials, but this is not always so. Although they do reach a wide audience they are examples of non-personal communication. This means that there is no personal contact and, therefore, no feedback from the service user. However, it is a highly public means of

transmitting a message and it can be persuasive especially if the message is repeated over and over. An example of this is the 'Don't drink and drive' campaign.

Achieving aims and objectives

It is very difficult to judge if the aims and objectives of the campaign have been reached as the mass media campaign is accessible to a wide cross-section of the public and there is little feedback from the audience. It is a good way of transferring simple messages to the public, but any message that is too complicated is likely to be lost. Anything too threatening or uncomfortable could be rejected by the audience. Mass media campaigns need to be very well thought out if they are to succeed.

Suitability for target audience

As the mass media campaign will reach a wide cross-section of the public, it is difficult to target one group. Audiences search for relevant facts relating to them in a health promotion message and if there are any inaccuracies, then the message will be rejected.

Readability

The message must be easy to read and easily recognisable. It should be simple and easy to understand as there is no one to clarify any points. The message must be obvious straight away in order to have the maximum impact.

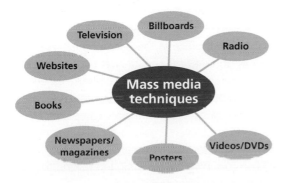

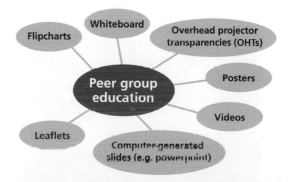

Main communication methods in health promotion

	Advantages	Disadvantages
Mass media (such as radio, television, internet)	Reaches mass audience Raises public awareness of health issues Comes into privacy of your home If famous person fronts campaign, this may generate interest	Not individualised Expensive programme No opportunity to clarify message No immediate feedback One-way communication Service users can 'switch off'

Cost-effectiveness

Campaigns that use the media are very expensive and in order to be value for money they must be very well planned. Although they do reach a wide audience, they are unlikely to be successful on their own. But they can raise general awareness of health promotion issues.

The advantages and disadvantages of mass media campaigns are summarised in the table above.

As you can see, the disadvantages of mass media campaigns outweigh the advantages, and mass media alone will not produce dramatic long-term changes in health behaviour. Due to the lack of two-way communication in mass media, it is best used for conveying simple rather than complex messages.

Activity

Mass media campaigns

1 Think of an example of a mass media campaign which made an impact on you. Why do you think it was successful?

2 Think of a mass media campaign which was less than successful as far as you were concerned. Why was this?

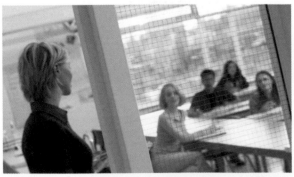

Peer group education can be very effective

Peer group education
Reaching the target audience

The personal touch of peer group education must not be underestimated. Generally speaking, messages in peer group education are individualised to a particular age group and there is plenty of opportunity for interaction between information presenter and information recipient. This is an interpersonal approach. The information presenters must have good interpersonal skills and their presentation should be well rehearsed and pitched at the right level for their audience.

Case study

An example of peer group education

A group of Year 12 Health, Social Care and Early Years students decided to promote 'Say yes to safer sex' to a Year 10 class during a PSE session.

A month before the session the selected Year 10 class was given questionnaires to fill in. The year 12 group was then able to analyse the completed questionnaires so that gaps in Year 10's knowledge could be identified.

On the day of the talk, the Year 12s were very nervous but well prepared. They had planned an interactive session with Year 10 showing how to put a condom onto a cucumber. Year 10 then had their turn. The form tutor, who had remained in the office at the back of the classroom, thought the session went very well indeed. After initial giggling and embarrassment, the Year 10 group settled down and asked some sensible questions. Questionnaires completed by Year 10 after the event showed their knowledge had increased. Year 10 commented that they felt more comfortable and less inhibited talking to students of their own age group.

Peer group education has been successful, for example, ex-alcoholics have been effective when working with alcoholics to get the anti-alcohol message across and to get them to give up alcohol. Peers in schools, too, have been very successful when talking to other groups in their school or in other schools. This could be because they can relate to their target group because they are a similar age.

Achieving aims and objectives

If the aims and objectives are well thought out and chosen especially for the target audience, then there is every chance that the audience will relate to them. The audience will feel the programme has been designed around them and their needs. Therefore they are more likely to listen to and follow the health promotion advice given.

Suitability for the target audience

Just as the aims and objectives are designed around the target audience, so too should the appearance of the health promotion materials. For example, if the campaign is targeting junior school children, then the presentation of the materials should reflect the type of language they will use and understand, and leaflets, posters, etc. can use popular cartoon figures that this age group relates to. 'Text speak' could be used for older children. Messages can be explained and clarified where necessary.

Readability

If using materials specifically for a certain age group, then the language should reflect this. Leaflets and fact sheets should not contain too many words, which might be off-putting to some people. Eye-catching presentation encourages people to use material, as does local information.

Cost-effectiveness

Usually peer group campaigns are cheap to run and offer value for money. Although materials may not be professionally produced, they can still be effective. This could be more so if the audience realises that the materials have been especially prepared for them

The advantages and disadvantages of peer group education are summarised in the table below.

	Advantages	Disadvantages
Peer group education	Individual to targeted group Cheap to run Presenters often of similar age/experience, so on same 'wavelength' Immediate feedback Can clarify/repeat message Two-way communication	Narrow target audience Materials not as professionally produced Limited knowledge base

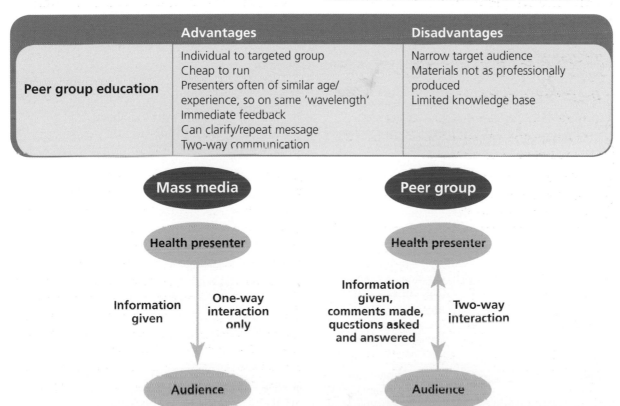

Comparison of mass media and peer group communication

Theory into practice

Compare mass media with peer group education. What conclusion can you draw? Which method would you prefer?

Peer group education materials

There is a wide variety of materials available to you and it is up to you to decide which would be the most appropriate communication method. You have to plan and implement a small-scale health promotion campaign using an existing campaign. You may be able to use all the existing materials or you may feel you would like to supplement the campaign with some of your own additional resources. Either way, it is useful to know the advantages and limitations of the range of presentation methods, which are summarised in the table below.

Guidelines for choosing health promotion materials

Ask yourself:

● *Is it appropriate for achieving your aims and objectives?* Think about the context. For

Method	Advantages	Disadvantages
Flipcharts	Good for 'thought showers' Pages can be prepared in advance Easily portable Cheap Nothing to break down	Easy to get 'dog-eared' or torn Useful for groups of around 20
Whiteboard/blackboard	Good for highlighting points Cheap and readily available Can be re-used Nothing to break down	Whiteboards can be damaged by use of incorrect pens and/or incorrect cleaning Too small for groups of more than 20
Overhead projector transparencies	Can be prepared in advance Can be used with any size audience Cheap to buy and produce by hand Equipment widely available Presenter faces audience, so maintains rapport	Requires electricity supply Can break down
Videos	Suitable for small to medium audiences Can convey reality Educational programmes for TV can be recorded for later use Easily stopped and started to allow discussion	Small screen can limit audience Requires electricity supply Can break down
Computer-generated slides	Can be prepared in advance Can be projected onto large screen Can be animated with sound effects	Requires electricity supply Can break down Equipment is costly
Leaflets, handouts and other written materials	Service users can go over health materials at their own pace Information can be shared afterwards with others Reduce need for note-taking Cheap to produce (non-commercially) Can give references for further information, e.g. websites	Mass-produced materials may not be suitable for targeted group Can end up in bin as unread waste if service user does not use material Not durable, easily lost Literacy skills required for service user to read and understand information
Posters	Cheap, easily made Can raise awareness of health issues Can direct people to other help, e.g. give telephone numbers	Quickly become 'dog-eared' or damaged Must be changed regularly or will be ignored

example, if you are talking to a group of teenagers about the dangers of excessive alcohol consumption, a leaflet called 'Stop Drinking' will be of little value if they are planning to go to a party that evening. You might be better off bringing someone of their own age group to talk about their experiences, leading to a group discussion.

- *Is it the most appropriate material?* Could you use photographs which would be cheaper and work just as effectively as a video? Could real fruits and vegetables be brought to a class of 6–7-year-olds rather than pictures? They could then taste them.
- *Is it suitable for the target audience you are working with?* If you are working with a group of 6–7-year-olds, you must ensure that the language is appropriate. Can they understand it? If the service user group is older, is the language patronising? You also need to ensure you reflect the values and cultures of the group. You must be careful that your material is not racist or sexist.

- *Is the material up-to-date?* The material must be current and totally unbiased.
- *Is the material readable?* You should ensure that the material is in plain English and service users will be able to understand it. It should be neatly laid out and easy to follow.
- *Is it cost-effective?* A low-budget campaign can be just as effective as a high-budget one. For example, as already stated mass-media campaigns which cost lots of money are not effective on their own but do complement interpersonal approaches.

Assessment activity 17.3

Communication methods

1 Demonstrating a high level of understanding, write a description of the communication methods used in your chosen local health campaign.

2 Give detailed reasons for the choices of communication methods used.

Whatever the question, your research will involve you finding out information. This information is called data.

Quantitative data

Numerical data, which can be analysed using statistical methods is known as **quantitative** data. An example of this could be to find out *how many* service users like the new appointment system at their local GP surgery. Quantitative data tells the researcher information such as how much, how often or how long. This data is measurable and quantifiable.

Working with quantitative data

Quantitative data is numerical pieces of information. Analysing a set of numerical data relies on the use of arithmetic and statistical methods, i.e. counting and grouping together the answers given to the questions.

For example, answers may be coded. Coding means giving a number to a response so that similar responses may be grouped together under the same number, as in this question:

What is your gender?	
	Code
Male	(1)
Female	(2)

In the question above, all the female responses would be coded 2.

The first part of data analysis involves preparing the data into a form which may be analysed. There are two things you must do:

- code the responses
- collate them into a table of responses.

You will find your main method of collecting quantitative data will be questionnaires. You will have a mixture of open and closed questions.

Quantitative data is generally produced by closed questions and is easy to code. You need to code all your closed questions before collecting any data. When you have collected all your data, you should be able to feed your information into a computer programme which will calculate simple statistics for you.

Qualitative data

If you were to ask service users what they *felt* about the new appointments, you would be asking for their views and feelings. This information you collect would be called **qualitative** data. This data cannot be statistically analysed as it involves words rather than numbers. It is non-numerical data.

Most well balanced examples of good research contain both quantitative and qualitative data. For both types of data, you could use:

- **primary research** – research that you have done yourself, i.e. your own original research
- *secondary research* – information gathered from sources such as books, newspapers, magazines, the internet, etc., i.e. other people's findings.

Once you have collected all your information you can then begin to analyse it. Quantitative data is much easier to analyse than qualitative data.

Working with qualitative data

Responses to open questions are hard to predict and this can cause problems when you are trying to make sense of the data.

As with quantitative data, the first stage is the preparation of the data. Generally, qualitative data is part of a much larger body of information. Analysing qualitative data is a time-consuming and very involved process. This is because you need to organise the data into a manageable form. You could draw up a framing code for each possible focus so you can read through and assess each answer. You could also look for similarities or themes in the data. This will take time and practice. When themes and patterns have been identified, you could use direct quotes in the discussion of your findings. You may also want to try to convert some of your qualitative data into a quantitative format. This can be done by counting the similar answers. They can then be presented in a graph or chart format.

Presenting data

Generally, quantitative data is presented in statistical and graphical formats. As it is numerical, it is easy to present. Qualitative data is more complicated and is usually presented as a written discussion. Quotes from interviewees are included to clarify and add depth to issues. Diagrams and flow charts could also be used for presenting qualitative data.

Pre-set criteria

Pre-set criteria are decided upon before beginning the campaign. They are targets often set alongside objectives. These state how the targets/objectives will be achieved in terms of quantity, quality and a set time by which they will be achieved. Pre-set criteria should be as measurable as possible. For example, in a smoking cessation programme, the pre-set criteria might be to find out what percentage of service users who enrolled on the programme are still not smoking after three months, six months and one year.

Theory into practice

Arrange an interview with a member of your local health promotion team or ask them to come into your centre. Prepare a list of questions to ask them about the pre-set criteria for some of this year's health promotion topics. This will help you to decide on your pre-set criteria for your small-scale campaign.

Presenting information

There are many different ways of presenting data. These include:

- charts
- graphs
- statistics.

Charts

The two most popular charts used for presenting information are:

- bar charts
- pie charts.

Bar charts

A popular choice for presenting simple data, bar charts are easy to draw and to understand. Bar charts can be used as an alternative to pie charts, for displaying percentages or whole numbers, where there are too many groups for a pie chart. They are especially useful when you have a lot of categories to display.

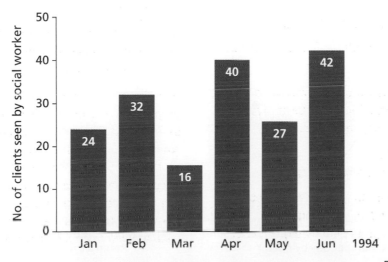

Example of a bar chart

When presenting information on a bar chart, ensure that:

- the chart has an appropriate title
- the vertical axes are clearly labelled
- the bars are same width
- the units of measurement are identified.

Pie charts

A pie chart is a circular chart which resembles a pie which has been cut into slices. Each slice represents a proportion/percentage of the whole.

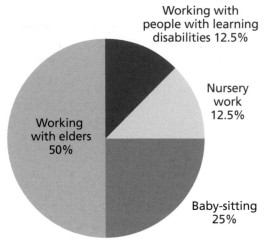

Example of a pie chart

When producing a pie chart, ensure that:

- it has a clear appropriate title
- each slice is labelled
- each slice is shaded/coloured to differentiate it.

Pie charts are best avoided when there are fewer than three, or more than nine, categories of data to display.

Graphs

Line graphs are a good way of showing trends, especially trends over a period of time. They are the most popular type of chart when the researcher has a lot of data to display. Although more than one line may be displayed, it is important to avoid having too many different lines on the graph as it can become messy and difficult to read.

When producing a line graph, ensure that:

- it has a clear appropriate title
- the vertical and horizontal axes are clearly labelled
- the units of measurement are clearly indicated.

Statistics

Statistics are a valuable way of presenting and interpreting researched information. However, statistics are open to abuse and are sometimes misleading. They can be manipulated to show what the researcher wants to show, while the collected data actually shows an entirely different story.

As well as problems with the presentation and interpretation of statistics, problems can also happen due to the research process. To ensure your statistics are accurate you must:

- be focused on your topic – what is it you wish to find out?
- use the correct method of research related to your study. Ensure your results are valid and reliable

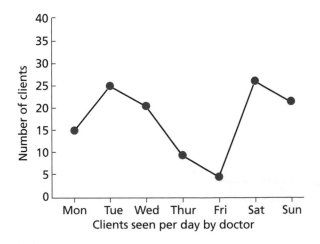

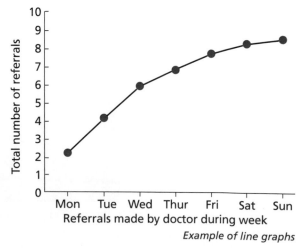

Example of line graphs

- ensure your sample represents the area of the population you are interested in. For example, if your research is looking at the number of women over 50 who take advantage of the breast screening programme, it would be inappropriate to ask women under 50 for their opinions
- be honest – make sure your graphs, etc. match your data and make sure they are accurate
- look at your results carefully and do not misinterpret your data
- draw conclusions which are real and accurate.

Assessment activity 17.4

Methods of evaluating health education campaigns

Describe the methods used to evaluate the local health education campaign that you chose in Assessment activity 17.1.

Showing a high level of understanding, write up:

1 the pre-set criteria which would be used to measure your chosen health promotion campaign

2 the methods of presenting information for your chosen health promotion campaign.

Planning a small-scale health education campaign

Planning a health promotion campaign will help you to decide:

- what you want to achieve
- how you are going to do it
- whether you have been successful.

Remember that this is a small-scale health education campaign and you must be realistic about what you set out to achieve. You can use health promotion materials already produced by national or local health promoters. You must check your facts are correct and up-to-date. For example, current thinking of maximum units of alcohol per week for males is now 28 units rather than 21 units as previously recommended. You must also beware that you do not exceed your knowledge base.

If you ask someone to fill in a questionnaire, make sure that you do not ask for names for confidentiality reasons. You must also ensure that you do not reveal any information discussed during your discussion.

Ewles and Simnet (1992) produced the seven-stage flow chart below for planning and evaluating a health campaign.

Identify priorities

First, you need to identify your needs and priorities. You can use your local health improvement priorities to help you to choose your campaign theme. Just as the local health education campaigns fall into the national targets, so you can feed into your local targets. Ensure you have a clear focus to your campaign.

Reasons for the campaign

You need to give reasons for your campaign and decide which age group you are going to target. Again this could be linked to your local improvement priorities. For example, you may decide to target 13–14-year-olds in your area because there has been an increase in alcohol consumption in that age group.

Aims and objectives

Aims and objectives are very important. These words are often mixed up as they can both be defined as a 'purpose'. An aim however, is the overall purpose or goal, whereas objectives are the specific ways you are going to achieve your aim.

1 Identify needs and priorities

2 Set aims and objectives

3 Decide the best way of achieving the aims

4 Identify resources

5 Plan evaluation methods

6 Set up an action plan

7 ACTION! Implement your plan, including your evaluation

A seven-step flow chart for planning a health campaign (Ewles and Simnet, 1992)

Objectives need to be SMART:

- **S**pecific – must be clear and not vague
- **M**easurable – has the objective been achieved or not?
- **A**chievable – must have a realistic target
- **R**elevant – focused on an issue within broad aims
- **T**imed – must have agreed timescale for delivering objectives.

Approach

The approach needs to be considered. Look back to Unit 17.2. Which method do you think will best meet the needs of your service user group? Remember, you can choose from:

- the preventative model
- the empowerment model
- the educational model
- the use of fear as an approach
- the medical model.

Communication methods

Since you have chosen a local health improvement priority, you will be able to use materials produced nationally as well as those produced by your local team. These could include:

- posters
- handouts
- information guides
- leaflets
- videos/DVDs.

You will need to contact your local health promotion unit to check which materials are available for your chosen subject.

Check through the health promotion material carefully to make sure it is suitable for your chosen target group. For example, if you are educating young children, some of the material may be too difficult for them to understand and you may need to simplify it. Check the resources available to reinforce the health message you wish to give.

Remember that the evaluation needs to be integral to the campaign and must take place from the beginning of the campaign planning. It might be a good idea to keep a diary of everything you do throughout the planning and implementation process of your campaign.

Assessment activity 17.5

A small-scale health education campaign

Plan and implement a small-scale health education campaign based on your local health improvement priorities, showing both confidence and competence.

Evaluating your health promotion campaign means you have to make a judgement about the value of your work. You need to look critically at your campaign and decide what was good about it, what was poor about it and how it could be improved.

Evaluation consists of four main components:

- *reflection* – look back over all areas of your work from the planning stage to the end of the campaign
- *analysis* – examine in minute detail all aspects of your performance. Are you aware of your strengths and areas that need improvement?
- *make informed decisions* – use your knowledge and understanding to help you make a decision or judgement. For example, you may have chosen to carry out an anti-bullying campaign for younger children. Although this is not listed as a target in *Our Healthier Nation* or *Choosing Health*, you recognise that it could come under the mental health banner
- *plan for improvement* – list all the areas that you feel need to be improved, explaining the actions you need to take to achieve your improvements.

You should consider the following when assessing the success of your health campaign:

- pre-set criteria used to measure outcomes
- intended and unintended outcomes
- costs
- time spent
- presenting and interpreting data
- impact of campaign on target audience.

Pre-set criteria used to measure outcomes

Were your pre-set criteria appropriate? If not, why not? If yes, explain why.

You can judge what has been achieved (the outcome) and whether you achieved the aim and objectives you set. If you based your campaign around teenage drinking, did your group understand the use of units to measure alcohol consumption? How do you know? Did you produce a questionnaire so you have some evidence?

Case study

Marsha and Rabina

Marsha and Rabina decided to look at breast cancer. They collected most of their health promotion materials through the charity Breakthrough Breast Cancer. Their aim was to raise awareness regarding breast cancer.

Some objectives were to encourage members of the teaching staff at their school to carry out breast examinations at least once each month and to persuade teachers over 50 to go for screening.

With their class teacher, they drew up a questionnaire (before the talk) to find out what was already known about breast awareness. After their talk, another questionnaire was given out so that Marsha and Rabina could see if the staff's knowledge had increased. Like a lot of professional women, the female staff were aware of breast examinations but very few took the time to check their breasts for any abnormalities on a regular basis.

Although ten members of staff were originally targeted for the promotion, other members did ask the girls for their breast examination leaflet.

Other unintended outcomes were that some of the male staff asked for leaflets for their partners. Marsha and Rabina sold some Breakthrough Breast Cancer 'diamond' ribbons. A coffee morning was also arranged for the charity.

Examples of pre-set criteria you could have used are:

- How many people came or were involved in the health promotion campaign?
- How many people came to seek further information by questioning the presenter? If there is a website, how many people accessed it?
- How many people took away prepared health promotion materials?
- How many people went to seek medical help or advice as a result of the health promotion campaign?

Resources	Cost	Supplier
Breast cancer video	Nil	Health Promotion Unit
Coloured card	Nil	School resource
White card	Nil	School resource
Leaflets	Nil	Health Promotion Unit
Leaflets (made at school)	£1.48 for photocopying	School
Posters	Nil	Health Promotion Unit
Information	Nil	School internet
Ludo	75p	School

Intended and unintended outcomes

Did you meet your intended outcomes? Were there any unintended outcomes? For example, in your alcohol awareness campaign for Year 9, a student may have approached you after the session seeking your help and advice because they were worried about a parent who is drinking heavily.

Costs and time spent

Was your campaign value for money? In order to judge this you need to record everything that went into your health promotion activity, in terms of time, money, effort and materials. Then you can make an informed judgement about whether the outcome was worth the cost.

An example of recording costs for a health promotion campaign is given in the table at the top of the next column.

Presenting information and data

If you were to repeat the campaign, would you use the same materials? Why? Would you have any advice for your local health promotion team/ graphics unit? Did you produce any materials yourself? Were they successful? How do you know? Were your posters bold and eye-catching? Was your data correct, unbiased and presented in an interesting way? Did service users take your leaflets away with them?

An example of an evaluation of materials is shown in the table at the bottom of the page.

Impact of campaign on target audience

Was feedback from a supervisor given? Did the target audience look interested? If you observe the audience, you can soon see if they are bored

Material used	Successful	Why?
Ludo-type game	Yes	Students enjoyed playing interactive game
Video	Partially	Too long – students started to lose interest after 10 minutes
Posters	Yes	Students liked the 'cool' image presented
Leaflets	No	Could have been more eye-catching – use of colour would have helped but would have more than doubled cost of photocopying. Students did not take them away with them at the end of talk

or alert. Did the audience ask for further information? If you had interactive activities, did they take part? Were questions answered or asked? Did the audience pay attention? Did you ask the audience to fill in an evaluation sheet? Were they asked to answer a questionnaire on the health promotion area before and after the presentation so you could see an improvement, or not, in their knowledge? Did you work with other agencies to help you get the message across? Did you choose appropriate communication methods?

Your evaluation could start in a similar way to the example given below:

The aim of our health promotion campaign was to encourage female teachers on the staff to go for breast screening (if they were in the over-50 age bracket) or for younger members to carry out breast examination on a regular basis. I think we achieved our aim as our questionnaire (given out at the beginning of the talk) showed that most of the staff did not know much about breast cancer before our talk. (Only thirty per cent were aware of the information we gave out.)

Our objectives were to:
- raise awareness of breast screening and cancer
- raise awareness of the success of treatment of breast cancer if detected early
- find out how much staff knew compared with national figures.

I think we raised awareness of breast screening as the staff were keen to question us when we had finished our presentation. I think we could have been better prepared as some of the questions were too difficult for us to answer and we had to refer staff to our prepared leaflet (from the health promotion unit). Surprisingly, not many staff were aware of breast cancer campaigns with the exception of the 'Pink Ribbon' campaign. The main place that staff saw information on breast cancer was in leaflets in surgeries and clinics, but everyone thought that campaigns are worthwhile and that awareness should be raised.

Our pre-set criteria were to see how many staff came to the presentation and how many were really interested and asked questions. We also asked staff if they were going to follow through our advice on breast examination and breast screening. Fifteen female members of staff attended our presentation. This is out of a possible fifty-eight people so we felt this was a good turnout. All the staff said they would follow the guidelines we gave them on either breast examination or screening.

One unexpected outcome of the presentation was that one of the male members of staff asked if he could have the leaflets to take home for his wife. Apparently, some of the female members of staff who had attended the presentation and talked to other staff members about how interesting the presentation had been.

If we had to do the presentation again we would use the same presentation methods but we would try to be sure of our facts so we could answer questions more competently.

We would also rehearse the presentation a few more times before the real one. This would improve our delivery as we would be more 'polished'. We would also ensure that we faced the audience throughout our presentation. We would also have noticed the two spelling mistakes on the computer presentation.

Evaluation

Evaluate your health education campaign, reflecting your ability to interpret information accurately.

You must cover all the following criteria:
- pre-set criteria used to measure outcomes
- intended and unintended outcomes
- costs
- time spent
- presenting and interpreting data
- impact of campaign on target audience.

Demonstrate evidence of synthesis and the ability to critically analyse and make judgements.

Demonstrate a high level of understanding of the pre-set criteria ensuring you use primary sources of evidence within your evaluation.

Glossary

Adverse: unfavourable to anyone's interests

Aspiration: a strong desire to achieve something such as success

Catalyst: a person or thing that causes a change

Clinical governance: the system through which NHS organisations are accountable for continuously improving the quality of their services and safeguarding high standards of care, by creating an environment in which clinical excellence will flourish

Holistic: referring to the body as 'a whole', i.e. the physical, emotional, etc., aspects which combine to form good health

Inequality: the state of being unequal

Integrate: to mix with

Primary research: one's own, original research

Qualitative: data which is not measurable in numerical form as it involves views and opinions

Quantitative: data that is measurable in numerical form

Statistics: the collection, classification and interpretation of quantitative data

Bibliography

Unit 1

Hucker, K., *Research Methods in Health, Care and Early Years*, Heinemann, Oxford, 2001

Payne, M., *Modern Social Work Theory*, Palgrave Macmillan, London, 1997

Units 2 and 3

Argyle, M., *The Psychology of Interpersonal Behaviour*, Penguin, London, 1994

Cooley, C.H., *Human Nature and the Social Order*, Scribner, New York, 2002

Egan, G., *The Skilled Helper (7th edition)*, Thomson Learning, 2004

Houston, G., *The Red Book of Groups*, Rochester foundation, Rochester, MA, USA, 1990

Houston, G., *Brief Gestalt Therapy*, Sage Publications Ltd, 2003

Noonan, E., *Counselling Young People*, Methuen, London, 1983

Rogers, C.R., *On Becoming a Person*, Houghton Mifflin, Boston, 1961

Rogers, C.R., *A Way of Being*, Houghton Mifflin, Boston, 1980

Thompson, N., *Communication and Language: A Handbook of Theory and Practice,* Palgrave Macmillan, London 2003

Unit 16

Connor, J., Godfrey, S., Milsom, G., *Beauty Therapy Sciences,* Heinemann, Oxford, 2004

Mills, R. and Parker-Bennett, S., *Sports Massage*, Heinemann, Oxford, 2004

Moonie, N. (ed.), *Health and Social Care*, Heinemann, Oxford, 2005

Seeley, R.R., Stephens, T.R., Tate, P., Anatomy and Physiology, 7th edition, McGraw Hill, New York, 2005

Smith, T. (ed.), *The British Medical Association Complete Family Health Encyclopaedia*, Dorling Kindersley, London (1997)

Unit 17

Ewles, L. and Simnett, I., *Promoting Health: A Practical Guide*, Scutari Press, London, 1992

Miller, J. (ed.), *Care in Practice for Higher Still*, Hodder & Stoughton, London, 2005

Moonie, N. (ed.), *AS Level for OCR Health and Social Care*, Heinemann, Oxford, 2005

Naidoo, J. and Wills, J., *Health Promotion – Foundation for Practice*, Baillière Tindall, London, 2000

Nazarko, L., *Nursing in Care Homes* (2nd edition), Heinemann, Oxford, 2002

Nolan, Y., *Care S/NVQ Level 3*, Heinemann, Oxford, 2001

Stretch, B., *BTEC Nationals Health Studies*, Heinemann, Oxford, 2002

Walsh, M., Stephens, P. and Moore, S., *Social Policy and Welfare*, Stanley Thornes, Cheltenham, 2000

Walsh, M., Stretch, B., Moonie, N., Herne D., Miller, E. and Webb, D., *BTEC National Care*, Heinemann, Oxford, 2003

Useful websites

Unit 3

www.drugfree.org
(information and guidance on substance abuse)

www.mentalhealth.org.uk
(for a leaflet on substance abuse and mental health, and information on personality disorders)

www.bild.org.uk
(British Institute of Learning Disabilities)

Unit 17

www.investingforhealth.gov.uk
(information on Health Action Zones and
related topics)

www.hpa.org.uk
(Health Protection Agency)

www.timesonline.co.uk
(*The Times* newspaper)

www.parliament.uk
(trends in UK statistics since 1900)

www.hda.nhs.uk
(information on health inequalities)

www.nimhe.org.uk
(*Celebrating our Cultures: Guidelines for
Mental Health Promotion with the South East
Asian community*)

www.archive.official-documents.co.uk
(Independent Inquiry into Inequalities in Health
– Black Report)

www.immunisation.nhs.uk
(information on immunisation)

www.nhsia.nhs.uk
www.dh.gov.uk
(both have information on proposals for NHS
Plan, 2000)

www.wiredforhealth.gov.uk
(information on the Healthy Schools Award)

www.babycentre.co.uk
(information on antenatal tests)

www.cancerresearch.uk.org
www.cancerbacup.org.uk
(information on self-examination for testicular
and breast cancer)

Index

codes of conduct 40, 179
codes of practice 37–8
cognitive approach to counselling
132
cognitive development 108–9
colitis 211
Commission for Racial Equality 42
communication 70–80
  barriers to 81–6
  computerised 75
  contributing factors 77–80
  cycle 70–1
  effective 55, 87–9, 139
  emotional, social and physical
    factors 80
  ending conversations 92–3
  environmental factors 78, 81,
    87–8
  positive positioning 88
  providing clear channels 139–40
  purpose of 76–7
  skills 77–8, 79, 91, 140
  SOLER 77
  special needs 75–6, 88
  transference 81
  verbal 70–2
  written 72–3
  see also interaction with service
    user
communication with service users
  55, 61–2
complaints procedures 12, 24, 28–9,
  39, 41–3, 75, 161
  support for service users 42–3
  workers' responsibilities 42
confidentiality
  care workers' responsibilities 30–1
  maintaining 60–1
  organisational requirements 28–
    30
  policies and procedures 28–9, 30
  rights to 6–7, 8, 26–31
  support available 31
  see also information
Cooley, C.H. 103
counselling 125–7
  for depression 114
  person-centred approach 107
  skilled helper model 106, 129
  theories 128–32
Crohn's disease 209–10
CT scanning 242
culture 120–1
  as barrier to communication 84

and food 197
and self-identity 66
values 20
cystitis 228

Data Protection Acts 12, 26–7, 29,
  61, 75, 143, 158–9, 163
  principles 26
decision-making, participation in 5, 6
dementia 239–40
democracy 17–18
depression 113–14
diagnostic tests 241–4
dietary requirements 195–7
digestive system 206–11, 241
  dysfunctions 209–11
  structure 206–9
disability discrimination 18, 19, 33–4
Disability Discrimination Acts 12,
  33–4
Disability Rights Commission 42–3
disclosure of information 6, 7, 31
discrimination
  basis of 19–20
  beliefs and actions 20–1
  challenging 20–1
  development of 18–19
  direct 21, 22, 33
  disability 12, 18, 19, 33–4
  effects of 22–3
  historical oppression 17
  indirect 21–2, 33
  and language 32
  links with prejudice 20
  naming service users 32, 60
  origins of 17–19
  types of 21–2
diversity 45
Down's syndrome 113
dressings, changing 190
drug abuse 118–19
DRVs (Dietary Reference Values) 197
duty of care 179–80

e-mail 75
early years care 44
  values 46
eating see food
echocardiography 242
education, and self-identity 66
Egan, Gerard 77, 82, 106, 126,
  128–9
emergency treatment 189–91
  fall 189

empathy 72, 79, 140
employment discrimination 32
empowerment 15
empty nest syndrome 121
endocrine system 241
endoscopy 244
environment
  appropriate 145, 146
  and behaviour 122
  effect of 119, 121
  and ill-health 260–1
  and self-identity 66
environment, positive 139–40,
  143–52
  checklist 148–9
  evaluation 150–2
  managing and coping skills 148–9
  physical and psychological 145–8
  planning for 143–9
  recording meetings 147–8
  skills 144–5
environmental abuse 69
equal opportunities
  codes of practice 37–8, 40
  legislation 32–7, 39–40
  organisational policies 38–40
Equal Opportunities Commission 33,
  38, 42
equal pay 34–5
Equal Pay Acts 34–5, 42
equality and diversity, promoting
  23–5, 45, 60
  care workers' practice 23
  formal and informal structures
    25
  organisational practice 23–5
  policies and procedures 24–5
Erikson, Erik 107–8, 119, 122
evaluating 95–8, 150–2
  analysis 278
  contribution of others 98
  drawing conclusions 97–8, 151,
    202
  health promotion campaign
    272–80
  making informed decisions 278
  planning for improvement 98,
    151–2, 202, 203, 278
  practical care 202–3
  referring to theory 203
  reflection 95, 97, 202, 278
  skills 95
Ewles, L. 276
eye contact 74–5, 78, 84

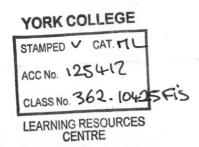